Download the Gunner Goggles App Now!

Go to the App Store from your iPhone or iPad and search for **Gunner Goggles**

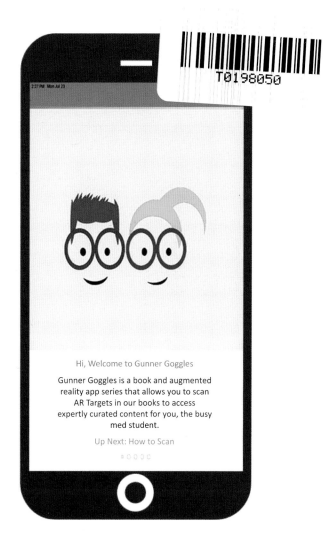

Each Gunner Goggles specialty has its own app;
you can purchase other titles at:
ElsevierHealth.com/GunnerGoggles

Surgery

HONORS SHELF REVIEW

EDITORS:

Hao-Hua Wu, MD
Resident, Department of Orthopaedic Surgery
University of California–San Francisco
San Francisco, California

Leo Wang, MS, PhD
Perelman School of Medicine
University of Pennsylvania
Philadelphia, Pennsylvania

Rebecca Gao, MS
Stanford University School of Medicine
Stanford, California

FACULTY EDITORS:

Sean Harbison, MD
Clinical Professor of Surgery
Chief, Division of General Surgery at
Penn Presbyterian Medical Center
Perelman School of Medicine
University of Pennsylvania
Philadelphia, Pennsylvania

DaCarla Albright, MD
Associate Professor of Clinical
Obstetrics and Gynecology
Perelman School of Medicine
University of Pennsylvania
Philadelphia, Pennsylvania

Temitayo Ogunleye, MD
Assistant Professor of Clinical
Dermatology
Perelman School of Medicine
University of Pennsylvania
Philadelphia, Pennsylvania

Wanda Ronner, MD
Professor of Clinical Obstetrics and
Gynecology
Perelman School of Medicine
University of Pennsylvania
Philadelphia, Pennsylvania

Neil Sheth, MD
Assistant Professor of Orthopaedic
Surgery
Perelman School of Medicine
University of Pennsylvania
Philadelphia, Pennsylvania

Chuang-Kuo Wu, MD, PhD
Professor of Medicine
University of California–Irvine
School of Medicine
Irvine, California

ELSEVIER

ELSEVIER

1600 John F. Kennedy Blvd.
Ste 1800
Philadelphia, PA 19103-2899

GUNNER GOGGLES SURGERY, HONORS SHELF REVIEW   ISBN: 978-0-323-51040-0

Notices

Library of Congress Cataloging-in-Publication Data
Names: Wu, Hao-Hua, editor.
Title: Gunner goggles surgery : honors shelf review / editors, Hao-Hua Wu,
   Leo Wang ; faculty editors, DaCarla Albright, Sean Harbison, Temitayo
   Ogunleye, Wanda Ronner, Neil Sheth, Chuang-Kuo Wu.
Description: Philadelphia : Elsevier, 2018. | Includes bibliographical
   references.
Identifiers: LCCN 2017051683 | ISBN 9780323510400 (pbk. : alk. paper)
Subjects: | MESH: Surgical Procedures, Operative | Test Taking Skills |
   User-Computer Interface | Study Guide
Classification: LCC RD37 | NLM WO 18.2 | DDC 617.9--dc23 LC record available at
https://lccn.loc.gov/2017051683

Executive Content Strategist: Jim Merritt
Content Development Manager: Lucia Gunzel
Publishing Services Manager: Patricia Tannian
Senior Project Manager: Cindy Thoms
Senior Book Designer: Maggie Reid

Printed in China

Last digit is the print number: 9 8 7 6 5 4 3 2 1

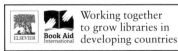

Gunner Goggles Honors Shelf Review Series

Gunner Goggles Family Medicine	978-0-323-51034-9
Gunner Goggles Medicine	978-0-323-51035-6
Gunner Goggles Neurology	978-0-323-51036-3
Gunner Goggles Obstetrics and Gynecology	978-0-323-51037-0
Gunner Goggles Pediatrics	978-0-323-51038-7
Gunner Goggles Psychiatry	978-0-323-51039-4
Gunner Goggles Surgery	978-0-323-51040-0

Contributors

QUESTIONS EDITOR

Kaitlyn Barkley, MD
Resident Physician
Department of Neurosurgery
University of Florida
Gainesville, Florida

Drake Lebrun, MD, MPH
Resident Physician
Department of Orthopaedic Surgery
Hospital for Special Surgery
New York, New York

CONTRIBUTING AUTHORS

Rachel Dillinger, MD
Resident Physician
Department of Psychiatry
University of Maryland
Sheppard Pratt Psychiatry
Training Program
Baltimore, Maryland

Jonathan Hunt, MD, MBA
Resident Physician
Department of Obstetrics and Gynecology
Cleveland Clinic
Cleveland, Ohio

Diana Kim, MD
Resident Physician
Department of Ophthalmology
University of Pennsylvania
Philadelphia, Pennsylvania
Diseases of the Blood and Blood-Forming Organs

Rafael Madero-Marroquin, MD
Johns Hopkins School of Medicine
Baltimore, Maryland
Diseases of the Musculoskeletal System and Connective Tissue

Kumar Nadhan
Temple University School of Medicine
Philadelphia, Pennsylvania
Renal, Urinary, and Male Reproductive System

William Plum, MD
Resident Physician
Department of Ophthalmology
Columbia University
New York, New York
Diseases of the Respiratory System
Nutritional and Digestive Disorders

Alejandro Suárez-Pierre, MD
Johns Hopkins School of Medicine
Baltimore, Maryland
Nutritional and Digestive Disorders

Junqian Zhang, MD
Resident Physician
Department of Dermatology
University of Pennsylvania
Philadelphia, Pennsylvania
Cardiovascular Disorders

Acknowledgments

"If I have seen further than others, it is by standing upon the shoulders of giants."
– Isaac Newton

We would like to thank the many exceptional innovators who helped transform our vision of *Gunner Goggles Surgery* into reality.

To our editorial team at Elsevier, thank you for your unrelenting support throughout the publication process. Jim Merritt believed in *Gunner Goggles* from day one and used his experience as an executive content strategist to point us in the right direction with respect to book proposal, product pitch, and manuscript development. Lucia Gunzel expertly guided us through manuscript submission and revision, no easy feat with two first-time authors. Maggie Reid collaborated with us closely to create the layout design and color schemes. Cindy Thoms and the copy editing team made sure our written content adhered to a high professional standard.

To the editors, authors, and student reviewers of *Gunner Goggles Surgery*, thank you for your scholarship and unwavering enthusiasm. Our outstanding faculty editors—Dr. Sean Harbison, Dr. Wanda Ronner, Dr. DaCarla Albright, Dr. Temitayo Ogunle, Dr. Neil Sheth, Dr. Chuang-Kuo Wu—took time out of their busy schedules to meticulously edit each chapter and provide numerous invaluable insights on how to improve quality and accuracy. A number of outstanding residents and medical students contributed to the content of this textbook and provided us feedback on high-yield topics for the NBME Surgery Subject Exam, notably Dr. Kaitlyn Barkley, Dr. Rachel Dillinger, Dr. Jonathan Hunt, Dr. Diana Kim, Dr. Drake Lebrun, Dr. Rafael Madero-Marroquin, Kumar Nadhan, Dr. William Plum, Dr. Alejandro Suarez-Pierre, and Dr. Junqian Zhang.

To our augmented reality (AR) team, thank you for your creativity and dedication during the development of the *Gunner Goggles* AR application. Nadir Bilici, Brian Mayo, Vlad Obsekov, Clare Teng, and Yinka Orafidiya helped us develop and test the initial *Gunner Goggles* AR prototype. Tammy Bui designed the *Gunner Goggles* logo and AR app icon.

We would also like to thank the Wharton Innovation Fund for awarding us seed money to help pursue development of *Gunner Goggles* AR.

You all continue to inspire us, and we are incredibly grateful and deeply appreciative for your support.

– Hao-Hua, Leo, and Rebecca

Contents

Introduction

Hao-Hua Wu and Leo Wang

I. Gunner's Guide to a Better Test Score

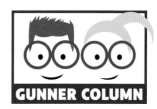

GUNNER COLUMN

Curious why certain classmates perform well on every exam? Frustrated by how few of these "gunner" peers share study secrets?

At *Gunner Goggle*s, our goal is to reveal and demystify. By integrating *augmented reality* into this review book, we **reveal** how the best students approach topics, conceptualize complex disease, and allocate study time efficiently. By organizing each topic according to the National Board of Medical Examiners (NBME) format, we **demystify** exam content and the types of questions one can expect on test day.

Of the tests medical students strive to conquer, shelf exams boast the highest ratio of importance to study resource quality. For instance, performance on shelf exams typically informs final clerkship grades, which are the most important criteria on the medical school transcript for residency application. Yet, there is no single authoritative study resource for the shelf across all disciplines. Most importantly, no current book specifically targets shelf exam prep. So students must rely on miscellaneous resources and anecdotal advice to get the job done.

In light of this void in authoritative test prep, we have created the *Gunner Goggles* series to provide you with the most effective shelf exam testing resource. *GG* stands out for three important reasons:

First, readers have the opportunity to enhance understanding of important shelf topics by utilizing the **augmented reality (AR)** features on each page. With an iPhone or iPad, users can download the *Gunner Goggles* AR iOS app and use it to turn book figures into three-dimensional (3D) images, access high-yield videos and view pertinent digital media. More on how AR technology works can be found on page 2.

Second, *Gunner Goggles* provides a plethora of tips on how to manage time efficiently when studying for the shelf. Mnemonics and strategies for how to approach difficult concepts can be found in the blue "Gunner Column" to the right of each page. We also tell you how to *think* about these concepts so that surgery never feels like a laundry list of items you simply have to memorize.

Third, this review book is written and organized optimally for shelf exam test prep. Each chapter is organized according to the NBME Clinical Science Subject Examination and USMLE Course Content outlines. In addition, a concise summary of how topics are tested prefaces each chapter.

As experts on the shelf exam, we understand how difficult it is to carve out time to study while juggling clinical responsibilities during your clerkship rotation. We also know that each student's learning curve is different based on timing of the rotation (first block vs. last block), year in medical school (MS3 vs. MD/PhD returning after graduate school), and future career interests (e.g., an aspiring orthopedic surgeon learning about obstetrics and gynecology). However, we believe that any student can perform well on the shelf with the right strategy and study resources.

We created this book anticipating the needs of all types of students, and hope that *Gunner Goggles* will be the most comprehensive, authoritative shelf exam review book that you ever use. We are confident that *Gunner Goggles* will enable you to achieve your test performance goals and stick it to your "gunner" classmates, whose advice, or lack thereof, you won't be needing after all.

II. Augmented Reality: A New Paradigm for Shelf Exam Test Prep

Think of AR as your best friend.

To use it, download the free *Gunner Goggles Surgery* application on your iPad or iPhone and create your own optional profile. Now with the application open, point your smart mobile camera at this page.

Notice how on your camera, there are now links you can click on, 3D figures you can rotate, and a video you can watch. You have just unlocked the AR features for this page!

Take a moment to play around with these AR features on your smart mobile device. The way this works is anytime you see the *Gunner Goggles* icon **gg** in the blue Gunner Column to the right or left, there is an AR feature accompanying the text with which you have the opportunity to interact with.

Still not convinced? Here are three reasons why AR is your ideal study companion.

Presentation

AR breaks the boundaries of how information can be presented in this textbook.

gg AR
Introduction Video

gg AR
Gunner Goggles email

Traditionally, if you wanted to learn about a disease in a review book, you would be expected to read and memorize a block of text similar to the following:

Huntington disease (HD) is a GABAergic neurodegenerative disorder that is caused by an autosomal dominant mutation leading to CAG repeats on chromosome 4. Patients typically present in the fourth and fifth decade of life with chorea, memory loss, caudate atrophy on neuroimaging, and motor impairment, depending on the variant. Although there is no cure for Huntington's, the movement disorders associated with the disease, such as chorea, can be treated with drugs like tetrabenazine and reserpine to decrease dopamine release.

Having read (or most likely glazed) through that last paragraph, do you feel comfortable enough to answer questions about the genetics, presentation, and treatment of Huntington's right now? A week from now? Three weeks from now when you have to take your shelf exam?

Here's where AR comes in. Use your *Gunner Goggles* app to check out how we're able to present HD in different, memorable ways.

For visual learners, here's a video of an effective HD mnemonic →

If you are an audio learner, here's a link to key points about Huntington's for the shelf →

Forgot your neuroanatomy? Here's where the caudate is →

What's the difference between chorea, athetosis, and ballismus again? Chorea looks like this →

Now write a one-line description of Huntington's in your own words in the margins of this page for future reference. It's much easier with AR right? Like we said, your best friend.

gg AR
Huntington's Disease Mnemonic

gg AR
Huntington's Podcast

gg AR
The caudate nucleus is part of the basal ganglia

gg AR
Chorea patient example

Evaluation

The GG Surgery app has the potential to exponentially enhance how you can evaluate your own understanding of the material. Although not available with the first edition, we are in the process of developing a personalized question bank as well as a flashcards feature. Our vision is to allow you to scan a topic on the page for immediate access to relevant practice questions and flashcards. In future versions, you will also be able to create your own flashcard deck and track your mastery.

In addition the GG app can keep track of the AR Targets scanned and the Learning links viewed. These links are saved to a Link Library which you can view at any time. You can also like or dislike a Learning Link with an opportunity to provide us feedback for better resources available.

As development of the GG Surgery app is an ongoing process, we encourage and welcome your feedback. If you like the idea of having a personalized question bank and flashcard feature or have an idea for how we can improve the GG app to better serve your studying needs, please provide us feedback through an in-app message. You can also email us at GunnerGoggles@gmail.com.

Community Engagement

Studying for the shelf can be isolating. Our vision is to develop a feature in the GG Surgery that would allow you to connect with chapter authors and fellow readers. We are in the process of developing a medium in which shelf-related inquiries can be discussed among authors and readers through an optional short message system (SMS) feature.

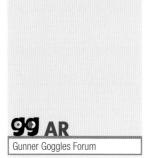

Given that the community engagement feature is in development and unavailable for the first edition, we welcome your input on how we can connect you with the people who will enable your test day success.

To provide feedback, please scan the page and vote. You can also email us GunnerGoggles@gmail.com for any comments or suggestions.

Augmented Reality Frequently Asked Questions

"Since augmented reality is integrated into *Gunner Goggle Surgery*, does this mean I have to pull out my iPad of iPhone for every page of the book?"

No, only if you need it. Some may use AR more than others depending on background and level of comfort with surgery. For instance, you may already have a solid understanding of Huntington's and only need to read the text as a refresher. On the other hand, if you are less comfortable with Huntington's, the AR features are there just in case.

"Can't I just look up everything I don't know on my own? Why do I have to use the *Gunner Goggles* app?"

You can absolutely look things up on your own. But that takes time. And sometimes, you can't find the best reference or mnemonic. Our team of experts has already gone through the trouble of identifying potential sources of confusion for you and found the perfect resources. In the *Gunner Goggles* app, we have compiled the slickest and most concise resources one can use to better understand a topic. Videos, audio files, and images are first vetted by subject experts for accuracy of content. They are then evaluated by students like yourself for utility of content to enhance test performance. Only resources with the most Gunner votes are embedded into each page.

"What if a link doesn't work or I want something on the page to change?"

Please tell us! Another advantage of AR is that we can immediately receive and implement your feedback. Just use the *Gunner Goggles* app to text us your concerns and our tech support team will respond ASAP!

III. Study Smart: Mnemonics and Gunner Study Tips

Even with incredible AR features at your disposal, you won't be able to optimize exam performance unless you know how to study. Below are the four most important things one can do to study for the Surgery shelf under the time restraints imposed by clerkships.

Understand the Organizing Principle

The easiest way to save time and perform well on the shelf is to understand how a specific disease or concept fits into the big picture. For instance, knowing the buzz words, diagnostic steps, and treatment plan for ulcerative colitis will likely lead to only one correct answer on the test. However, understanding that ulcerative colitis (UC) is a disease of hindgut and midgut, and knowing how to differentiate gastrointestinal (GI) disorders based on location in the gut can help you quickly identify any GI complaint.

Create Effective Mnemonics

If you have photographic memory, skip this section. For the rest of us mere mortals, below outlines the organizing principles (OP) of what constitutes a Gunner mnemonic.

Mnemonics are important when:

1. You have to learn a lot of material.
2. You want to teach something to your colleagues during morning rounds. Attendings and residents are always impressed when they can learn something from a medical student.
3. You want to remember something 15 years from now when you are working the 30th hour of a busy call day.
   OP for mnemonics are as follows:
1. Use the spelling of a name to your benefit (**Spell**)
   Example:
   a. "8urk14tt's" lymphoma (Burkitt lymphoma), lep"thin" (leptin), "supraoptiuretic" nuclei

(supraoptic nuclei that produces antidiuretic hormone)

   b. Tenofovir is the only NRTI nucleoTide

   c. We"C"ener's granulomatosis (GPA) for C-ANCA and Cyclophosphamide tx

2. Create an acronym that contains distinguishing syllables or letters of names (**Distinguish**)
   Example:

   a. Chronic alcoholics Steal PhenPhen and Never Refuse Greasy Carbs (<u>Chronic alcohol</u> abuse + <u>St</u> John's wort + <u>phen</u>ytoin + <u>phen</u>obarb + <u>neva</u>ripine + <u>rif</u>ampin + <u>grise</u>ofulvin + <u>carb</u>amazepine)

   - reinforce mnemonic by spelling name of item-to-be-memorized accordingly
   - e.g., "Refus"ampin, "Never"apine, "Greasy"ofulvin, "Carb"amazepine, etc.
   - This ties mnemonic OP 1 with mnemonic OP 2

3. Drawings help (**Draw**)
   Example: Trisomy 13 looks like polydactyly + cleft lip when the number 13 is rotated 90 degrees clockwise (the horizontal 1 is the extra digit, and the cleft of the horizontal 3 is the cleft lip)

Trisomy 13 mnemonic

4. Counting the letters of a word (**Count**)
   Example: Patau syndrome = 13 letters = Trisomy 13

5. Arrange acronym in alphabetical order (**Arrange**)
   Example: ABCDEF for diphtheria (ADP ribosylation, beta prophage, C Diphtheria, elongation factor 2)

   Examples of instructors who practice this concept well are Dr. John Barone of Kaplan and Dr. Husain Sattar of Pathoma.

   On the flip side, here are examples of poor mnemonics (although you may remember them now given how they were highlighted in this text):

1. Blind as a bat, mad as a hatter, red as a beet, hot as Hades, dry as a bone, the bowel and bladder lose their tone, and the heart runs alone = poor mnemonic for anticholinergic syndrome:

   - This mnemonic forces you to memorize extra and extraneous things (like bat, beet, hare, and desert) which have nothing to do with anticholinergic syndrome.

2. WWHHHHIMP (withdrawal + wernicke + hypertensive crisis + hypoxia + hypoglycemia + hypoperfusion + intracranial bleed + meningitis/encephalopathy + poisoning) = poor mnemonic for causes of delirium:

   - Wait how many H's does this mnemonic have again?

   A good rule of thumb: if you can still remember a mnemonic under a high-pressure situation (attending pimps you) or after a 7-day period, then you have a winner.

Ultimately, the best mnemonics are the ones you invent and apply repeatedly. So use these mnemonic principles to give yourself a solid head start.

Devise a Study Schedule and Stick to It

The third most important piece of advice for the shelf is to create a study schedule at the beginning of the rotation and follow it. Rotations such as Surgery are particularly draining. Oftentimes you may find yourself coming home after a 12-hour shift not wanting to study, especially when pre-rounds are the next day at 5 a.m. However, if you are mentally committed to following a schedule, you will find creative ways to get studying done. For example, some students wake up an hour early to read before pre-rounds. Other students fit study material into their white coat and read during downtime. Surgery is unique because you are almost guaranteed to have downtime in between cases. Take that opportunity to peruse notes and do shelf practice questions on your cell phone.

Distinguish Rotation-Knowledge From Shelf-Knowledge

Most things you learn on rotation do not apply to the shelf exam and vice versa. For example, you may be able to impress your surgery attending by committing the names of all the surgical instruments to memory. However, with only 150 minutes to answer 100 lengthy questions on the shelf, details like that have no real utility.

Thus, be able to compartmentalize. Know exactly what is needed for your surgery rotation and what is expected on the shelf to save yourself precious study time. Also, be aware of the differences amongst surgical specialties. Transplant surgeons are very different from trauma surgeons who are very different from neurosurgeons. If your surgery clerkship allows you to do a sub-specialty rotation, keep in mind what material you can learn from your attendings that would help you for the shelf (e.g., the algorithm trauma surgeons go through to conduct primary/secondary/tertiary surveys and rule out life-threatening emergencies).

IV. Intro to the National Board of Medical Examiners Clinical Science Surgery Subject Exam

The Clinical Science Surgery NBME Shelf Exam is a 110-question computerized exam administered over a recommended course of 2 hours and 45 minutes, typically at

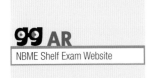

NBME Shelf Exam Website

the conclusion of one's surgery clerkship rotation. The test questions come from either retired step 2 CK questions or are written by a committee of faculty across the country. Thus, it is important to master shelf exam-style questions to set yourself up nicely for step 2 CK.

Unlike step 1, shelf exam questions focus almost exclusively on disease processes rather than normal processes. That being said, the most high-yield principles to know for the medicine shelf are normal lab values. Knowing what values to expect for the basic metabolic panel will help you quickly identify abnormal processes, such as hyper/hyponatremia, anion gap metabolic acidosis, or acute kidney injury.

According to the NBME, the exams are curved to a mean of 70 with a standard deviation of 8. The curve does not take into account timing of rotation. For instance, students who take the exam during their first block will be held to the same statistical standard as students who take the exam during their fourth clerkship block. However, the NBME does release "quarterly norm information" to medical schools in order to make clerkship directors aware of the relationship between exam score and rotation timing. Importantly, as of now, shelf exam scores are sent to the school directly; students cannot request their shelf exam score independent of their school.

Although different surgery clerkships have different standards for determining grades, in general, each program has its own internally generated shelf exam cutoff score one needs to achieve in order to be eligible for the highest clerkship grade (e.g., honors). If this is the case, confirm the cutoff score with your clerkship director so that you have a reasonable performance goal to shoot for.

Students are expected to master content organized into these following categories:

General Principles	1%–5%
Organ Systems	
Immunologic Disorders	1%–5%
Diseases of the Blood and Blood-Forming Organs	5%–10%
Diseases of the Nervous System and Special Senses	5%–10%
Cardiovascular Disorders	10%–15%
Diseases of the Respiratory System	10%–15%
Nutritional and Digestive Disorders	25%–30%
Gynecologic Disorders	5%–10%
Renal, Urinary, and Male Reproductive System	5%–10%
Disorders of Pregnancy, Childbirth, and the Puerperium	1%–5%

Surgery Outline

Disorders of the Skin and Subcutaneous Tissues	1%–5%
Diseases of the Musculoskeletal System and Connective Tissue	5%–10%
Endocrine and Metabolic Disorders	5%–10%

Currently, the NBME Surgery Content Outline breaks down question types into these categories:

- Applying Foundational Science Concepts (8%–12%)
- Diagnosis: Knowledge Pertaining to History, Exam, Diagnostic Studies, and Patient Outcomes (50%–60%)
- Health Maintenance, Pharmacotherapy, Intervention and Management (30%–35%)

However, devising a study plan from these three categories can be confusing. "Applying Foundational Science Concepts," for instance, is vague and difficult to prepare for. Instead, many students prefer to study according to Physician Tasks provided in older content outlines. Since every subject exam question asks about one of four things – 1) protocol for promoting health maintenance (Prophylaxis [**PPx**]), 2) the mechanism of disease (**MoD**), 3) steps to establishing a diagnosis (**Dx**), and 4) steps of disease management (**Tx/Mgmt**) – we recommend studying according to Physician Tasks from the 2016 Content Outline.

Physician Tasks (from 2016 Content Outline)

Promoting Health and Health Maintenance	1%–5%
Understanding Mechanisms of Disease	20%–25%
Establishing a Diagnosis	45%–50%
Applying Principles of Management	25%–30%

In addition, the NBME breaks down questions by Site of Care, including

- Ambulatory (35%–40%)
- Emergency Department (25%–35%)
- Inpatient (30%–35%)

Our recommendation is to not worry about site of care and focus on studying content related to Physician Tasks.

Gunner Goggles Surgery presents material to reflect how the NBME structures its shelf exams. Each chapter that follows falls into the main testable categories of General Principles (see Chapter 2) or Organ Systems (see Chapters 3–14). Each disease will also be presented in a "PPx, MoD, Dx and Tx/Mgmt" format, which represents the four physician tasks the NBME can test you on. Since establishing a diagnosis is weighted especially heavily (45%–50%), a "Buzz Words" category has been added to show readers how to quickly identify the disease process from just a few key words. A "Clinical Presentation" section has also been added to more thoroughly describe the disease. However, it is important to note that Buzz Words are sufficient in correctly identifying the corresponding disease on the shelf. The detail provided in the Clinical Presentation section is only meant to augment your understanding, particularly if it is your first pass. However, by the end of studying, the focus should primarily be on Buzz Words.

Finally, here are six things to keep in mind when studying for the Surgery shelf:

1. If pressed for time, practice identifying disease processes only through "Buzz Words." For instance, patients with sclerosing cholangitis on the shelf exam always have underlying ulcerative colitis. Petechial rash after fracture of a long bone is fat emboli.

2. In contrast, "Promoting Health and Maintenance" is only going to be one to five questions on the test. Thus, if in a rush, ignore the PPx material and jump straight into the Buzz Words, Clinical Presentation, Mechanism of Disease, Diagnostic Steps, and Treatment/Management. The most important prophylactic measures to know are those for cancer screening. Make sure to know the prophylactic measures for breast cancer and cervical cancer.

3. Know your medicine! One of the biggest mistakes that people make when studying for the Surgery shelf is assume that only diseases with surgical management can be tested. In fact, many of the questions on the Surgery shelf are taken from the Medicine shelf. The highest yield medicine topics seen on the Surgery shelf, such as which heart murmurs correspond to which cardiac disorders, make sure to do pertinent medicine questions from your question bank of choice. Advice for what types of medicine questions to do are included in Chapter 15.

4. Make sure to begin doing questions early (e.g., 10 questions a day starting from day 1). Ideally you should make a second pass of the most high-yield questions before test day.

5. For each question, write a one-line take-home-point in an Excel spreadsheet. This makes for quick and easy review in the days leading up to the exam.

6. Make sure you know your solid tumors for each discipline (e.g., Wilms Tumors in Renal, Atrial myxoma for Cards, VIPoma for GI). As long as it can be surgically removed, the neoplasm is fair game.

If any questions arise while studying, use the *Gunner Goggles* app to access the AR features embedded on each page.

Good luck and happy hunting.

—The Gunner Goggles Team

General Principles

Rachel Dillinger, Kaitlyn Barkley, Hao-Hua Wu, Leo Wang, Rebecca Gao, and Sean Harbison

Introduction

Although the Surgery shelf focuses on surgical topics, to say that it is "medicine heavy" would be an understatement. The medical management of surgical patients is a big focus for this exam and will additionally aid you in both subjects for the boards.

The organizing principle for this chapter is categorical due to its broad nature. It will examine several aspects of caring for surgical patients as well as infectious and genetic topics that have been known to appear from time to time. When studying, pay closer attention to nutrition, fluids and electrolytes, acid-base disorders, and multisystem failure. Genetic disorders and abuse are lower yield for this exam but still important for boards.

The chapter is divided into (1) Nutrition; (2) Fluid, Electrolyte, and Acid-Base Balance Disorders; (3) Abuse; (4) Multisystem Failure; (5) Genetic, Metabolic, and Developmental Disorders; (6) Ethics; and (7) Gunner Practice (application of the material learned).

Nutrition

Protein-Calorie Malnutrition

Protein-calorie malnutrition is a form of malnutrition that has two distinct yet related subtypes: kwashiorkor and marasmus. Both result from inadequate energy intake that cannot meet the demands for proper growth and maintenance of tissues. Although not common in the western world, it globally represents a main cause of mortality in developing countries. The two subtypes are distinguished by the presence or absence of edema.

Buzz Words:

- **Marasmus:** Inadequate caloric intake + muscle *and* fat wasting + irritable affect + apparently large head and "staring eyes" + absence of edema
- **Kwashiorkor:** Inadequate **protein** intake + muscle wasting with *normal or increased* body fat + apathetic affect + moon facies + presence of edema

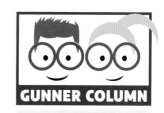

GUNNER COLUMN

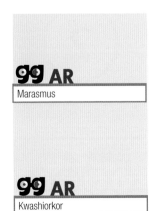

Marasmus

Kwashiorkor

Clinical Presentation:

Marasmus: in addition to the Buzz Words above, children suffering from marasmus present with severe constipation, decreased height and weight, bradycardia, hypotension, hypothermia, and extra skin folds caused by the depletion of the underlying subcutaneous fat. It is the more common of the two.

Kwashiorkor: in addition to the Buzz Words above, children suffering from kwashiorkor present with anorexia, organomegaly, normal weight, pitting edema that includes the extremities, presacral area, genitalia, and periorbitally, areas of the skin with hyperkeratosis and hyperpigmentation, a distended abdomen (2/2 distended loops of bowel, *not* ascites), and hypothermia.

Treatment/Management Steps (Tx/Mgmt):

Three phases:

1. Initial stabilization—correct hypoglycemia and dehydration with fluids and formula feeding, address possible infection with antibiotics
2. Rehabilitation—supplement iron, folate, vitamin A, and other nutrients, and advance diet
3. Follow up—monitor patient's physical, mental, and emotional well-being

Vitamin Deficiencies and/or Toxicities

Vitamin A

Buzz Words: Night blindness + teratogenic

Clinical Presentation:

- **Deficiency:** night blindness, scaly rash, xerophthalmia, bitot spots (debris on conjunctiva), increased rate of infections
- **Toxicity:** Increased ICP, bone thickening, teratogenic

Tx/Mgmt: Vitamin A supplementation

Vitamin B1 (Thiamine)

Buzz Words: Beri-beri + Korsakoff syndrome + Wernicke syndrome

Clinical Presentation:

Deficiency: Wet beri-beri (high-output cardiac failure), dry beri-beri (peripheral neuropathy), Wernicke and Korsakoff syndromes (confusion, ophthalmalgia, ataxia, confabulations)

Tx/Mgmt: Vitamin B1 supplementation (give B1 before giving an alcoholic glucose!)

Vitamin B3 (Niacin)

Buzz Words: Pellagra + tryptophan + glossitis + increases HDL

Clinical Presentation: Deficiency—pellagra (dementia, dermatitis, diarrhea), stomatitis

Pellagra

Tx/Mgmt: Vitamin B3 supplementation

Vitamin B6 (Pyridoxine)

Buzz Words: Transamination reactions + neurotransmitter synthesis

Clinical Presentation:
- **Deficiency:** peripheral neuropathy, stomatitis, convulsions in infants, microcytic anemia, seborrheic dermatitis
- **Toxicity:** peripheral neuropathy

Tx/Mgmt: Vitamin B6 supplementation

Vitamin B9 (Folic Acid)

Buzz Words: "Tea and toast diet" + anemia + short period of time since lifestyle change

Clinical Presentation: Deficiency—megaloblastic anemia WITHOUT neurologic symptoms

Mechanism of Disease (MoD):
- Dietary—most common, takes 3 months to deplete stores
- Alcoholism
- Pregnancy and increased demand
- Folate antagonist medications like methotrexate

Dx:
1. Peripheral blood smear
2. Elevated homocysteine levels
3. No change in methylmalonic acid levels (unlike B12 deficiency)

Tx/Mgmt: Daily PO folate supplementation

Vitamin B12 (Cobalamin)

Buzz Words: Pernicious anemia + glossitis + neuropathy

Clinical Presentation: Megaloblastic anemia with neurologic symptoms

Prophylaxis (PPx): Adequate diet with or without B12 supplementation

MoD:
- Iatrogenic—status post gastrectomy (loss of parietal cells → loss of intrinsic factor) or ileal resection (site of dietary absorption of B12)
- Autoimmune—antibodies against parietal cells result in their destruction and subsequent loss of intrinsic factor
- Dietary—takes years; seen in strict vegans and alcoholics

Dx:
1. Peripheral blood smear (megaloblastic anemia)
2. Low serum B12 levels

99 AR

B12 Deficiency

QUICK TIPS

As compared to folate deficiency, timing, and elevated MMA differentiates

3. Elevated serum MMA and homocysteine levels
4. Schilling test

Tx/Mgmt: Parenteral B12 IM once per month is preferred

Vitamin C
Buzz Words: No fruits/vegetables + bleeding
Clinical Presentation: Hemorrhages, skin petechiae, gums bleeding, loose teeth, gingivitis, poor wound healing, hyperkeratotic hair follicles, bone pain (2/2 periosteal hemorrhages)
Tx/Mgmt: Vitamin C supplementation

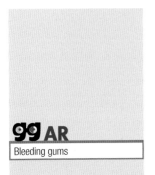
Bleeding gums

Vitamin D
Buzz Words: Rickets + osteomalacia + helps with calcium homeostasis
Clinical Presentation:
- **Deficiency:** rickets, osteomalacia, hypocalcemia
- **Toxicity:** hypercalcemia, nausea, renal toxicity

Tx/Mgmt: Vitamin D supplementation

Vitamin E
Buzz Words: Anemia + normocytic + neurologic symptoms
Clinical Presentation:
- **Deficiency:** anemia, peripheral neuropathy, ataxia
- **Toxicity:** necrotizing enterocolitis (infants)

Tx/Mgmt: Vitamin E supplementation; surgery if indicated for infantile necrotizing enterocolitis

Vitamin K
Buzz Words: Prolonged PT + bleeding
Clinical Presentation:
- **Deficiency:** hemorrhage, prolonged thrombin time
- **Toxicity:** hemolysis (kernicterus)

Tx/Mgmt: Vitamin K supplementation

Mineral Deficiencies and/or Toxicities

Iron
Buzz Words: Microcytic anemia
Clinical Presentation:
- **Deficiency:** microcytic anemia, koilonychias
- **Toxicity:** hemochromatosis

Tx/Mgmt: Iron supplementation

Zinc
Buzz Words: Loss of taste + slow wound healing

Clinical Presentation:
- **Deficiency:** hypogeusia, rash, slow wound healing

Tx/Mgmt: Zinc supplementation

Special Nutritional Considerations

Obesity

Buzz Words: Excessive body habitus

Clinical Presentation: Patients will present with a body mass index (BMI) greater than 25 if they are overweight and a BMI greater than 30 if they are obese.

Dx: Height and weight used to calculate BMI

Tx/Mgmt: Address comorbid health conditions (e.g., joint pain and OA, insulin resistance, cardiovascular disease), and encourage diet and exercise. If lifestyle modifications fail, surgical procedures may be a viable option. Surgical procedures also carry higher risk in obese patients 2/2 comorbidities and increased peak pressures when ventilating.

Total Parenteral Nutrition

Buzz Words: Critically ill patient + inability to feed PO or by G/J tube

Clinical Presentation: Patients who are critically ill and unable to feed enterally may use TPN via a central venous catheter or PICC line. Insertion of G/J tube is preferred to allow natural digestion.

Tx/Mgmt:
1. Supplement nutrients that may not be included in TPN, including vitamins and trace elements
2. Monitor labs to assess for electrolyte imbalances

Fluid, Electrolyte, and Acid-Base Balance Disorders

Fluid Volume Disorders

Dehydration/Hypovolemia

Buzz Words: Hypotension + tachycardia + poor skin turgor + oliguria + acute renal failure

Clinical Presentation: The patient will present with all the signs and symptoms of volume depletion, including the above as well as decreased pulse pressure, central venous pressure, and pulmonary capillary wedge pressure.

PPx: Adequate fluid intake (~1500 mL PO per day)

MoD: Causes range from gastrointestinal (GI) losses (2/2 vomiting, nasogastric suction, or diarrhea), third-spacing, inadequate fluid intake, DKA, sepsis, trauma induced losses, and insensible losses via the GI tract and skin

Dx:

1. Daily urine output less than ~500 mL
2. Increased hematocrit (3% increase for every liter of fluid lost), BUN/Cr ratio of greater than 20/1

Tx/Mgmt: Bolus isotonic IV fluids to achieve euvolemia, with a urine output goal of 0.5–1.0 mL/kg per hour

Volume Overload/Hypervolemia

Buzz Words: Weight gain + peripheral edema + JVD with elevated PCWP

Clinical Presentation: The patient will present with edema and the above features with possible pulmonary rales on auscultation and, 2/2 pulmonary edema, and labs will show dilution via low hematocrit and albumin.

PPx: In hospitalized patients, avoiding fluid overload

MoD: Iatrogenic or 2/2 fluid retaining states like nephrotic syndrome, cirrhosis, ESRD, and CHF

Dx: Clinical diagnosis: aided by presence of pulmonary rales and/or respiratory distress and dilution of labs

Tx/Mgmt: Fluid restriction with or without diuretics (e.g., furosemide)

Electrolyte and Ion Disorders

Hyponatremia

Buzz Words: Serum sodium <135 mmol/L + increased ICP + AMS + seizures + coma + HTN + oliguria

Clinical Presentation:

There are several varieties of hyponatremia:

1. Hypertonic hyponatremia—elevated serum osmolality (>295 mmol/L), 2/2 presence of osmotic substances
2. Pseudohyponatremia—normal serum osmolality (280–295 mmol/L), 2/2 increase in triglycerides or proteins
3. True hyponatremia—low serum osmolality (<280 mmol/L) requires assessing volume status:
   - Hypovolemic with high urine sodium (>20 mmol/L) indicates salt loss from renal causes.
   - Hypovolemic with low urine sodium (<10 mmol/L) indicates salt loss from non-renal causes.
   - Euvolemic indicates several causes such as psychogenic polydipsia, SIADH, and hypothyroidism.
   - Hypervolemic indicates causes like CHF, nephrotic syndrome, and liver disease.

FOR THE WARDS
4-2-1 rule: 4 mL/kg for first 10 kg, 2 mL/kg for next 10 kg, 1 mL/kg for every 1 kg over 20

Tx/Mgmt:
1. Hypertonic hyponatremia—identify and treat underlying disorder
2. Pseudohyponatremia—identify and treat underlying
   disorder
3. True hyponatremia
   • Hypotonic:
   • Mild (sodium 120–130 mmol/L)—fluid restriction
     and close monitoring to goal of normal sodium
     levels
   • Moderate (sodium 110–120 mmol/L)—loop
     diuretics
   • Severe (sodium <110 mmol/L)—hypertonic
     saline to correct no more than 8 mmol/L dur-
     ing the first 24 hours to prevent central pontine
     demyelination

gg AR
Hyponatremia flowchart

Hypernatremia

Buzz Words: Serum sodium >145 mmol/L + AMS + seizures
  + coma + dry membranes and decreased salivation
Clinical Presentation:
There are several varieties of hypernatremia:
1. Hypovolemic hypernatremia (water loss > sodium
   loss)—points to renal loss or extra renal water loss
2. Isovolemic hypernatremia (water loss with normal
   sodium stores)—points to diabetes insipidus
3. Hypervolemic hypernatremia (sodium excess)—
   points to exogenous steroids, iatrogenic
   causes like TPN, Cushing syndrome, or primary
   hyperaldosteronism
Dx: Urine osmolarity should be more than 800 mOsm/kg
  to qualify
Tx/Mgmt:
1. Hypovolemic—give isotonic NaCl to achieve hemodynamic stability before replacing free water deficit.
2. isovolemic—for patients with DI, administer vasopressin, and encourage oral fluid intake.
3. hypervolemic—diuretics to remove excess sodium;
   if ESRD, dialysis to remove excess sodium.
GG: Free water deficit = Total body weight × (1 − measured sodium/desired sodium)

gg AR
Hypernatremia flowchart

Hypokalemia

Buzz Words: Flattened T waves/presence of U waves on
  EKG + arrhythmias + muscle weakness/cramps/fatigue
  + decreased DTRs

Clinical Presentation: Patients with hypokalemia present with the above features in addition to prolonged cardiac conduction, polyuria and polydipsia, and nausea and vomiting. On the Surgery shelf, it is unlikely that you will have to read an EKG to ascertain the appropriate findings. However, the question stem may contain a Buzz Word from the EKG (i.e., "Patient's EKG shows flattened T waves").

PPx: Adequate dietary intake, management of medications that can predispose to hypokalemia

MoD: GI losses (either as contents of vomitus or diarrhea or 2/2 microbiome disruption by antibiotics), renal losses (diuretics or genetic diseases such as Bartter syndrome—increases renin and aldosterone levels—and renal disease), inadequate dietary intake, 2/2 insulin use, and in trauma patients.

Dx: Serum potassium of less than 3.5 mEq/L

Tx/Mgmt:
1. Identify and treat underlying etiology
2. Administer PO potassium chloride (10 mEq for every 0.1 increase in serum potassium desired) if mild or moderate
3. IV potassium chloride if severe and/or arrhythmias are present

Hyperkalemia

Buzz Words: Peaked T waves on EKG + muscle weakness + decreased DTRs + respiratory distress

Clinical Presentation: Patients will present with the above symptoms in addition to nausea, vomiting, diarrhea, and if severe, flaccid paralysis.

PPx: Management of underlying medical conditions

MoD: Etiologies include: renal failure, medications (potassium-sparing diuretics, ACE inhibitors), Addison disease, insulin deficiency (insulin shifts potassium intracellularly), acidosis (increased H+ redistributes K+ extracellularly), rhabdomyolysis and crush injury (K+ leaks from injured cells into the extracellular environment), and blood transfusion (older cells that lyse release K+ extracellularly).

Dx: Serum potassium of more than 5.0 mEq/L

Tx/Mgmt:
1. Insulin with glucose (to avoid hypoglycemia)
2. Kayexelate (to bind potassium in the GI tract, takes longer)
3. If severe hyperkalemia, administer IV calcium to stabilize myocardial resting membrane potential
4. Hemolysis if hyperkalemia is intractable.

99 AR

Peaked t waves

QUICK TIPS

Both hyperkalemia and hypokalemia present with loss of DTRs and weakness, so EKG and lab findings are key to distinguishing the two.

Hypocalcemia

Buzz Words: Tetany (Chvostek sign/Trousseau sign) + rickets/osteomalacia + numbness/tingling + prolonged QT interval

Clinical Presentation: Patients can present asymptomatically or with the features listed above, and in extreme cases may have seizures. Hypocalcemia may be associated with hypomagnesemia. Primary hypomagnesemia for instance, decreases PTH secretion, leading to secondary hypocalcemia.

PPx: Maintaining an adequate diet, intake of vitamin D, and managing medications

MoD: There are a variety of etiologies, most commonly hypoparathyroidism, that usually follows thyroid surgery (loss of parathyroids producing PTH → decreased bone calcium resorption and decreased kidney reabsorption). Other causes include acute pancreatitis (calcium deposition), renal insufficiency (decreased vitamin D conversion to 1,25), hyperphosphatemia, pseudohypoparathyroidism, hypomagnesemia (decreases PTH secretion), vitamin D deficiency, malabsorption from the intestine, hypoalbuminemia (albumin is a carrier for calcium), and DiGeorge syndrome.

Dx: Labs to order include PTH, phosphate, BUN, creatinine, magnesium, albumin, and ionized calcium (not affected by albumin levels); calcium greater than 8.5 mg/dL

Tx/Mgmt:
1. Symptomatic patients → IV calcium gluconate
2. Maintenance includes daily PO calcium and vitamin D supplementation
3. Check for and correct hypomagnesemia

Hypercalcemia

Buzz Words: "Stones, bones, groans, and psychiatric overtones" + shortened QT interval

Clinical Presentation: Patients can present asymptomatically or with nephrolithiasis, bone aches, osteitis fibrosis cystica with subsequent fractures, 2/2 weakened bone, muscle pain and weakness, constipation, depression, fatigue, anorexia, anxiety, and other psychiatric symptoms, along with polydipsia and polyuria, HTN, and other constitutional symptoms.

PPx: Avoidance of excessive vitamin D

MoD: Based on the etiology: hyperparathyroidism (increased PTH increases bone and kidney resorption), malignancy (PTHrP and osteoclastic activity), vitamin D intoxication (increases GI absorption of

99 AR

Video: Chvostek's sign = twitching of facial muscles in response to tapping of ipsilateral facial nerve; Trousseau's sign = spasm of hand in response to inflation of BP cuff at or above systolic pressure for 3 minutes

99 AR

Article about hypomagnesemia and hypocalcemia

calcium), milk-alkali syndrome (2/2 excessive calcium supplementation, calcium carbonate, or milk), medications (thiazide diuretics inhibit renal calcium excretion), and diseases like sarcoidosis (increases GI absorption).

Dx:

1. Labs to order include PTH, phosphate, BUN, creatinine, magnesium, albumin, and ionized calcium (not affected by albumin levels).
2. Tests can include bone scans to look for malignancy and osteolytic lesions.

Tx/Mgmt:

1. IV fluids and loop diuretics increase urinary excretion of calcium.
2. In patients with osteoclastic disease, bisphosphonates can help.
3. Sarcoidosis and multiple myeloma hypercalcemia respond well to steroids.
4. In patients with ESRD → dialysis.

Hypophosphatemia

Buzz Words: Altered mental status + signs of hyperparathyroidism + blood cell dysfunction + myocardial depression with or without cardiac arrest + anorexia

Clinical Presentation: If mild, it is typically asymptomatic, but severe deficiency results in the aforementioned signs and symptoms and is a contraindication to surgery.

MoD: Can result from decreased intestinal absorption (alcohol, vitamin D deficiency, antacids, TPN, starvation), states with increased PTH (hyperparathyroidism), anabolic steroids, DKA, and respiratory alkalosis.

Dx: Serum phosphate less than 3.0 mg/dL

Tx/Mgmt: PO phosphate supplementation if mild, and IV if severe

Hyperphosphatemia

Buzz Words: Metastatic and soft tissue calcification + consequent hypocalcemia and its features

Clinical Presentation: Largely based on the rise in serum calcium triggered by increased PTH production.

MoD: Typically the result of renal insufficiency, but can also arise 2/2 bisphosphonates, hypoparathyroidism, vitamin D intoxication, acidosis, and rhabdomyolysis.

Dx: Clinical picture and serum phosphate levels greater than 4.5 mg/dL

Tx/Mgmt: If renal failure is the cause, hemodialysis is the treatment. Otherwise, administer antacids to bind the excess phosphate (carbonate or aluminum hydroxide).

Hypomagnesemia

Buzz Words: Muscle twitching/tremors + weakness + **coexisting hypocalcemia** and **hypokalemia** + prolonged QT + torsade de pointes

Clinical Presentation: The above features are present in addition to mental status changes, coexisting hypocalcemia and hypokalemia (T wave flattening on EKG). Hypomagnesemia is associated with hypokalemia due to increased potassium wasting at the level of the kidney.

Article about hypomagnesemia and hypokalemia

PPx: Avoid aggravating factors like alcohol

MoD: GI causes (malabsorption, TPN without magnesium supplementation), alcoholism, SIADH, medications (diuretics, gentamicin, cisplatin, amphotericin B, cisplatin), surgical (post parathyroidectomy), medical conditions (DKA, burns, thyrotoxicosis, pancreatitis)

Dx: Clinical picture and serum magnesium less than 1.8 mg/dL

Tx/Mgmt: Magnesium PO or IV

Hypermagnesemia

Buzz Words: Magnesium levels >2.5 mg/dL + facial paresthesias + nausea + loss of DTRs + somnolence progressing to coma + pre-eclamptic pregnant patient

Clinical Presentation: The first sign is typically a loss of DTRs, followed by the more severe symptoms of lethargy and coma. If untreated, death results from cardiac arrest or respiratory failure.

PPx: Manage underlying conditions, especially renal failure, and avoid excessive use of laxatives

MoD: While renal failure is the most common cause, it also results from burns, severe acidosis, rhabdomyolysis, adrenal insufficiency, and iatrogenically, 2/2 obstetric use of magnesium to prophylax and treat pre-eclampsia and eclampsia.

Dx: Clinical picture and serum magnesium levels greater than 2.5 mg/dL

Tx/Mgmt:
1. If magnesium is being administered, stop the infusion.
2. IV saline and furosemide to clear the excess.
3. If severe, IV calcium gluconate for cardioprotection.
4. Intubation if there is impending respiratory distress.
5. Dialysis for ESRD patients.

Video example of Kussmaul breathing

Acid-Base Balance Disorders

Metabolic Acidosis

Buzz Words: Decreased blood pH + decreased plasma bicarbonate + Kussmaul respirations

Clinical Presentation: Patients will present with hyperventilation (Kussmaul respirations) to compensate by blowing off CO_2, along with decreased cardiac output, 2/2 decreased tissue responsiveness to catecholamines.

MoD: The mnemonic for increased anion gap acidosis is MUDPILES: Methanol, Uremia, DKA, Paraldehyde, Iron/INH, Lactic acidosis, Ethylene glycol, Salicylates. The mnemonic for non-anion gap acidosis is HARD UP: Hyperalimentation, Acetozolamide, RTA, Diarrhea, Uretoenteric fistula, Pancreatoduodenal fistula.

Dx:
1. Basic metabolic panel (BMP)
2. Arterial blood gas (decreased blood pH and decreased plasma bicarbonate):
   - Remember Winter's formula: Expected $PaCO_2$ = 1.5 (measured bicarbonate) + 8 ± 2

Tx/Mgmt:
1. Identify and treat underlying cause
2. Sodium bicarbonate
3. Intubate is respiratory distress, 2/2 exhaustion from hyperventilation

Metabolic Alkalosis

Buzz Words: Increased blood pH + increased plasma bicarbonate + hypoventilation

Clinical Presentation: As there are few obvious signs or symptoms, the history is key to determining if a patient may have metabolic alkalosis.

MoD: Metabolic alkalosis generally results from either loss of H+ with ECF volume contraction or from ECF volume expansion. Triggering events for loss of H+ with ECF contraction include vomiting, NG suction, and diuretics. Triggering events for ECF expansion include adrenal disorders such as primary hyperaldosteronism, as well as Cushing syndrome.

Dx:
1. BMP (hypokalemia from renal losses 2/2 increased aldosterone release)
2. ABG (elevated bicarbonate and blood pH)

Tx/Mgmt:
1. If the urine chloride level is less than 10 mEq/L, it is saline responsive → IV saline and potassium.

2. If the urine chloride level is greater than 20 mEq/L, it is saline-nonresponsive → address the underlying cause of the metabolic alkalosis.

Respiratory Acidosis

Buzz Words: Reduced blood pH + $PaCO_2$ > 40 mm Hg + somnolence + myoclonus

Clinical Presentation: Patients will present with the above symptoms and can be separated into acute or chronic based on bicarbonate level. In acute, there will be 1 mmol/L increase for every 10 mm Hg increase in $PaCO_2$. In chronic, there will be a 4 mmol/L increase for every 10 mm Hg increase in $PaCO_2$.

MoD: Alveolar hypoventilation from various causes: chronic obstructive pulmonary disease (COPD), airway obstruction, myasthenia gravis, respiratory muscle fatigue, narcotic or sedative-induced hypoventilation, as well as brainstem injury.

Dx:
1. BMP
2. ABG

Tx/Mgmt:
1. If PaO_2 < 60 mm Hg → supplemental oxygen, remove obstruction if present, reverse drug-induced causes, and administer bronchodilators.
2. Mechanical ventilation may be necessary (severe acidosis, unresponsive to supplemental O_2, severe respiratory muscle fatigue).

Respiratory Alkalosis

Buzz Words: Increased blood pH + decreased $PaCO_2$ + lightheadedness + periorbital numbness

Clinical Presentation: Increased pH, decreased $PaCO_2$, and decreased cerebral blood flow result in the signs and symptoms above. These patients can also be separated into acute and chronic based on bicarbonate level. In acute, there is a 2 mEq/L decrease in bicarbonate for every 10 mm Hg decrease in $PaCO_2$. In chronic, there is a 5–6 mEq/L decrease in bicarbonate for every 10 mm Hg decrease in $PaCO_2$.

MoD: Alveolar hyperventilation results from: anxiety, sepsis, pneumonia, pulmonary embolism (PE), mechanical ventilation, cirrhosis, pregnancy (2/2 increased progesterone levels), and medications.

Dx:
1. BMP
2. ABG

Tx/Mgmt: Identify and treat the underlying cause.

Abuse

Buzz Words: Avoiding eye contact + unexplained or poorly explained injuries

Clinical Presentation:
- **Child:** spiral fractures, burns, subdural hematomas, posterior rib fractures, retinal detachment, genital/anal/oral trauma, STDs, and behavioral problems
- **Sexual:** Genital/anal/oral trauma, withdrawal from normal activities
- **Elder:** bruises, broken bones, burns, pressure marks, and unexplained withdrawal from normal activities

Tx/Mgmt: Encourage patients to seek help and develop a safety plan. Give them information about available resources. Report child or elder abuse as per individual state guidelines (i.e., Child Protection Services).

Multisystem Failure

Bacteremia

Buzz Words: Bacteria in the bloodstream → bacteremia

Clinical Presentation: Patients typically have an identifiable risk factor like recent catheterization, surgical treatment of a wound, IV access, dental procedures, and many more. They could be asymptomatic or have mild fever. If other symptoms are present, the bacteremia has likely progressed to either sepsis or septic shock. Bacteremia itself is often transient and can spontaneously resolve.

PPx: Some procedures that can predispose to bacteremia require prophylactic antibiotics, whereas others do not.

MoD: Procedures can introduce bacteria into the body that would not typically be found there, with local spread to blood supply resulting in spread of the bacteria.

Dx: Blood culture

Tx/Mgmt: Antibiotics tailored to culture sensitivities

Systemic Inflammatory Response Syndrome

Buzz Words: Fever + hyperventilation + tachycardia + increased or decreased WBCs → systemic inflammatory response syndrome (SIRS)

Clinical Presentation: Any two of the above Buzz Words qualifies a patient as having SIRS.

PPx: Identify and treat infections or other conditions (e.g., pancreatitis)

MoD: Abnormal regulation of cytokines resulting in a systemic inflammatory response
Dx: Fulfilling any two of the four criteria above
Tx/Mgmt: Treat the cause of the inflammatory response

Sepsis

Buzz Words: SIRS + positive blood cultures
Clinical Presentation: Often hospitalized patients who present with persistent SIRS symptoms
MoD: Bacteremia (positive blood cultures) results in a systemic inflammatory response
Dx: SIRS criteria with two positive blood cultures drawn from two different sites before antibiotics are administered
Tx/Mgmt: Broad-spectrum antibiotics; fluid resuscitation with IV saline

Shock

Buzz Words: Life-threatening circulatory failure + tissue and cellular hypoxia + elevated lactate levels
Clinical Presentation:
- **Distributive:** severe peripheral vasodilation (septic, neurogenic, or anaphylactic) → hypotension, moist membranes, and flushing of the skin. Bronchospasms and increased airway resistance are present in anaphylactic shock.
- **Cardiogenic:** decreased cardiac output → respiratory distress, cold clammy skin, dry mucous membranes, weak pulse, and tachycardia.
- **Hypovolemic:** loss of intravascular volume → collapsed neck veins, dry mucous membranes, decreased skin turgor, tachycardia, delayed capillary refill, and low CVP.
- **Obstructive:** extra-cardiac pump failure → chest pain, weak pulse, tachycardia, and cold and clammy skin.

MoD:
- **Distributive:** sepsis (TNF-alpha and IL-1), anaphylaxis (IgE-mediated hypersensitivity), and neurogenic (severe TBI/spinal cord injuries interrupt autonomic pathways) causes all decrease vascular tone, shifting blood away from the vasculature and inducing a state of shock.
- **Cardiogenic:** MI, valvular insufficiency, and aortic retrograde dissection causes depressed cardiac function and output leading to tissue hypoperfusion.
- **Hypovolemic:** loss of intravascular volume via loss of IVF or blood (trauma, hemorrhage, etc.) leads to tissue hypoperfusion.

99 AR
Types of shock

99 AR
Videos on shock (parts 1, 2, 3)

99 AR
Table showing CV effects of subtypes of shock

- **Obstructive:** extra-cardiac causes of cardiac pump failure (pulmonary hypertension, PE, poor RV function, tension pneumothorax, pericardial tamponade, constrictive pericarditis) lead to pulmonary or mechanical obstruction of blood flow and a decrease in preload resulting in tissue hypoperfusion.

Dx: Clinical diagnosis

Tx/Mgmt: In general, supplemental O_2, venous access, and IV fluids should be procured:

1. **Distributive:** septic → IV fluids and vasopressors; anaphylaxis → epinephrine, diphenhydramine, and hydrocortisone; neurogenic → stimulate vasoconstriction
2. **Cardiogenic:** Aspirin (ASA), heparin, vasopressors (norepinephrine or dopamine); avoid negative ionotropic agents
3. **Hypovolemic:** replace losses with IV fluids, if necessary PRBCs and control source of blood loss if 2/2 hemorrhagic shock
4. **Obstructive:** treat underlying cause of obstruction

QUICK TIPS

Multiorgan Dysfunction Syndrome (MODS) is the feared endpoint of the sepsis continuum.

gg AR

Keeping them straight SIRS through MODS video

Genetic, Metabolic, and Developmental Disorders

Beckwith-Wiedemann Syndrome

Buzz Words: Hemihypertrophy + macroglossia + embryonal tumors + chromosome 11

Clinical Presentation: A chromosomal disorder that affects children and predisposes to the development of embryonal tumors such as Wilms tumor, hepatoblastoma, neuroblastoma, and rhabdomyosarcoma. Affected patients will have the features described in the Buzz Words section in addition to variable visceromegaly, midface hypoplasia with infraorbital creases, and oomphalocele or abdominal wall defects.

PPx: 85% of cases are sporadic, so no prophylaxis exists. If a familial form is identified, genetic counseling is recommended.

MoD: Methylation of chromosome 11, usually sporadic

Dx: Genetic testing

Tx/Mgmt: Mostly surgical to correct whichever features are present, from oomphalocele to the various tumors

Down Syndrome

Buzz Words: Upslanting palpebral fissures + epicanthal folds + low set ears + flat nasal bridge + transverse palmar crease + chromosome 21

Clinical Presentation: Patients with Down syndrome will have varying degrees of cognitive impairment, early-onset Alzheimer's (2/2 the location of APP on Chapter 21), and varying heart defects with CAVSD and VSD being most common.

PPx: N/A

MoD:

- Meiotic nondisjunction (most common)—incidence increases with increasing maternal age
- Robertsonian translocation
- Mosaicism—post-fertilization mitotic error with typically less severe phenotype

Dx: Second trimester quad screen will show increased B-hCG and inhibin A and decreased alpha-fetoprotein and estriol.

Tx/Mgmt: Surgical repair of cardiac anomalies, along with monitoring of medical conditions like Alzheimer's

Alpha-1 Antitrypsin Deficiency

Buzz Words: Panacinar emphysema + cirrhosis

Clinical Presentation: Signs and symptoms of both emphysema and cirrhosis occur at a younger age than expected (<45 years old) in the absence of risk factors for both.

PPx: Genetic identification

MoD: A misfolded protein aggregates in hepatocellular endoplasmic reticulum to result in cirrhosis. Alpha-1-antitrypsin (AAT) deficiency in the lung results in uninhibited elastase destroying elastic tissue leading to panacinar emphysema and a bibasilar obstructive lung pattern.

Irregular Emphysema

Dx: Elevated serum AAT levels: liver biopsy will show PAS positive globules.

Tx/Mgmt: Lung and liver transplants in advanced disease

Antitrypsin Deficincy

Hemochromatosis

Buzz Words: "Bronze diabetes"

Clinical Presentation: Patients will present with a tan skin tone, diabetes, HF, testicular atrophy, and eventually HCC, 2/2 chronic cirrhosis.

PPx: Genetic identification and repeated phlebotomy or chelation

MoD: Mutations of C28Y or H63D on the HFE gene lead to increased iron absorption in the GI tract and deposition in various tissues

Dx:

1. Increased ferritin and iron levels in the blood
2. Liver biopsy and Prussian blue stain

Tx/Mgmt:
1. Phlebotomy and chelation
2. Liver transplantation with advanced cirrhosis

Ethics

Patient Nonadherent to Treatment or Test

Action: Ask why patient is nonadherent and be respectful
Avoid: Referring patient to another physician

Patient Nonadherent to Total Lifestyle Change, Behavior

Action: Ask about patient's willingness to change behavior. If patient is not willing, then provider cannot move on to next step why and issue needs to be addressed.
Avoid: Forcing patient to change if not willing to or scaring patient. Remember, D.A.R.E. does not work.

Patient Who Is Seductive

Action: Set limits, define tolerable behavior, see patient with chaperone
Avoid: Refusing to care for patient, asking open-ended questions, referring patient to another physician, entering into relationship with patient (never the right answer)

Patient Who Is Angry

Action:
NURSE: Name the emotion (e.g., "You appear angry."). Understand why and thank patient for sharing. Recognize what patient is doing right. Show support for the patient. Explore emotion.
Avoid: Taking patient's anger personally. Blaming others.

Patient Who Is Sad and Tearful

Action:
NURSE: Name the emotion (e.g., "You appear angry."). Understand why and thank patient for sharing. Recognize what patient is doing right. Show support for the patient. Explore emotion.
Avoid: Using patronizing statements such as "do not worry," rushing patient, and stating "I understand." Instead, further explore emotion to better understand where patient is coming from.

Patient Who Complains About Another Doctor

Action: Recommend patient speak to other doctor directly

Avoid: Saying anything to disparage the other doctor, intervening with care unless emergent need

Patient Who Complains About You or Your Staff

Action: Verify complaint, speak to staff member who was named in complaint

Avoid: Blaming patient, being defensive

Patient Who You Need to Break Bad News To

Action:

SPIKES: Set-up patient encounter by making sure patient is sitting in a chair with social support nearby. Ask about patient perception of what is going on. Ask patient for an invitation or permission to share the bad news. Explain your own knowledge of the bad news; make sure to preface by statements that convey the gravity of the situation (e.g., "I'm worried" or "I have bad news"). Manage patient's emotion after bad news is shared. Summarize situation and suggest concrete next steps.

Avoid: Sharing bad news when patient is in a vulnerable position (e.g., standing up while on the phone), breaking bad news without warning

Patient Being Evaluated for Decision-Making Capacity

Action: Patients with adequate decision-making capacity can refuse labs, imaging (e.g., CT scans), and treatment. Determine if patient meets criteria for being a legally competent decision-maker, including:

- Patients ≥18 or legally emancipated through marriage, military, or financial independence
- Patient makes and communicates a choice
- Patient knows and understands benefit and risks
- Patient decision stable over time
- Decision congruent to patient value system
- Decision not a result of mood disorder, hallucinations, or delusions

Avoid: Assuming patient lacks decision-making capacity if less than 18 (remember marriage, military, and financial independence from parents)

QUICK TIPS

If patient has decision-making capacity and refuses a surgical intervention, respect this patient's wish, even if the condition is life-threatening.

Patient Who Is a Jehovah's Witness and Needs Blood Transfusion

Action: Determine if patient meets criteria for not needing informed consent (e.g., legally incompetent, implied consent in emergency with no ability for communication, patient waived right to informed consent)

Avoid: Giving blood if patient does not give consent but not meet one of the exceptions

Patient With Meningitis Refusing Treatment

Action: Determine if patient has right to refuse treatment; in this case, patient does not have a right because doing so would pose a threat to the health and welfare of others

Avoid: Consulting hospital ethics committee unless there is a dilemma with no clear way to proceed

QUICK TIPS

Pediatric patient + emergent condition + no parental approval → proceed with treatment anyway
    Pediatric patient + non-emergent condition + no parental approval → proceed with treatment only after legal approval granted

Pediatric Patient With Nonemergent, Potentially Fatal Medical Condition and Parents Refuse Treatment

Action: Seek a court order mandating treatment
Avoid: Complying with parents' demand

Patient With HIV Diagnosis Refuses to Share With Significant Other

Action: Assess confidentiality rules; in this case, significant other needs to be legally notified to prevent harm from transmission. Encourage patient to discuss health and medical conditions with loved ones. Share patient results with local health department.

Avoid: Allowing patient to avoid disclosing potentially fatal communicable disease

GUNNER PRACTICE

1. A 28-year-old male arrives to the trauma center following a motorcycle accident in which he collided with a truck. He denies any loss of consciousness. He is agitated, denies any symptoms, and wants to go home. He has a GCS of 15. His vital signs are T 36.6, HR 126, BP 88/62, RR 29, and O_2 is 98% on room air. The physical exam is remarkable for ecchmyoses in the right and left upper quadrant of the abdomen. Urine drug screen is negative. Which is the most appropriate first step in the management of this patient?
   A. CT scan of abdomen and pelvis
   B. Intubation
   C. FAST ultrasound exam of the abdomen and pelvis
   D. Fluid resuscitation via 2 large bore IV's
   E. Discharge without further work-up
2. A 54-year-old woman with a past medical history of COPD is on her third hospital day for an episode of pneumonia. This morning's BMP comes back with Na^+ 138,

K^+ 3.2, Cl^- 106, CO_2 24, BUN 12, creatinine 0.9, and glucose 95. She has no complaints and reports improving shortness of breath. How would you address her metabolic abnormality?

A. IV potassium chloride 50 mEq
B. IV potassium chloride 30 mEq
C. PO potassium chloride 10 mEq
D. PO potassium chloride 20 mEq

3. A 25-year-old college student comes to your office for evaluation of easy bruising for the past semester. He states he has had no issues with school and is quite happy with his grades, and has not noticed any increased clumsiness or injuries that he can recall. You note several petechiae on his extremities as well as scattered bruising. He also notes that his gums have been bleeding easily when brushing his teeth. What would you recommend he increase intake of?

A. Vitamin A
B. Vitamin C
C. Vitamin D
D. Thiamine
E. Cobalamin

ANSWERS: What Would Gunner Jess/Jim Do?

1. WWGJD? A 28-year-old male arrives to the trauma center following a motorcycle accident in which he collided with a truck. He denies any loss of consciousness. He is agitated, denies any symptoms, and wants to go home. He has a GCS of 15. His vital signs are T 36.6, HR 126, BP 88/62, RR 29, and O_2 is 98% on room air. The physical exam is remarkable for ecchmyoses in the right and left upper quadrant of the abdomen. Urine drug screen is negative. Which is the most appropriate first step in the management of this patient?

Answer: D, Fluid resuscitation via 2 large-bore IVs

Explanation: His BP and tachycardia are concerning for hypovolemia and impending hypovolemic shock. Fluid resuscitation should be first priority with NS or LR. Further diagnostic workup to locate the source of blood loss can be delayed until after administration is begun.

A. CT scan of abdomen and pelvis → Incorrect. Although an important diagnostic step, his BP necessitates fluid resuscitation first.

B. Intubation → Incorrect. The question stem gives no indication of impending respiratory failure or current need for intubation.

C. FAST ultrasound exam of the abdomen and pelvis → Incorrect. This is an important diagnostic step but fluid resuscitation should be first.

E. Discharge without further workup → Incorrect. Unstable vital signs such as his BP along with ecchymoses concerning for internal bleeding necessitate further workup.

2. WWGJD? A 54-year-old woman with a past medical history of COPD is on her third hospital day for an episode of pneumonia. This morning's BMP comes back with Na^+ 138, K^+ 3.2, Cl^- 106, CO_2 24, BUN 12, Creatinine 0.9, and Glucose 95. She has no complaints and reports improving shortness of breath. How would you address her metabolic abnormality?

Answer: D, PO potassium chloride 30 mEq

Explanation: As the patient has no reports of symptoms from hypokalemia (arrhythmias, weakness, etc.), there is no need for IV administration, which also causes a burning sensation upon administration. PO potassium chloride supplementation will be adequate. The rule is 10 mEq for every 0.1 increase in serum potassium required. From 3.2 → 3.5, it would

require 30 mEq. A. IV potassium chloride 50 mEq →
Incorrect. IV administration is not indicated, and 50
mEq would overcorrect.

B. IV potassium chloride 30 mEq → Incorrect. IV
administration is not indicated.

C. PO potassium chloride 10 mEq → Incorrect. 10 mEq
would only correct the serum potassium to 3.3,
which is still deficient.

3. WWGJD? A 25-year-old college student comes to your
office for evaluation of easy bruising for the past semester. He states he has had no issues with school and is
quite happy with his grades, and has not noticed any
increased clumsiness or injuries that he can recall. You
note several petechiae on his extremities as well as
scattered bruising. He also notes that his gums have
been bleeding easily when brushing his teeth. What
would you recommend he increase intake of?

Answer: B, Vitamin C

Explanation: This patient is presenting with typical
signs and symptoms of scurvy. This is common
in college-age students 2/2 poor dietary habits.
Supplementation with vitamin C will resolve his
symptoms over time.

A. Vitamin A → Incorrect. Symptoms such as night
blindness and a scaly rash were absent from this
vignette.

C. Vitamin D → Incorrect. There was no mention of
consequences like osteomalacia or rickets, or calcium disequilibrium.

D. Thiamine → Incorrect. Mention of neuropathy, cardiac problems, or cognitive problems were absent.

E. Cobalamin → Incorrect. Deficiency in this would
result in neuropathy and anemia.

3

Immunologic Disorders

Hao-Hua Wu, Kaitlyn Barkley, Leo Wang, Rebecca Gao, and Sean Harbison

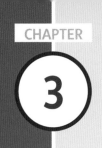

GUNNER COLUMN

QUICK TIPS

USMLE Content Outline Immune System Abnormal Processes, Page 5

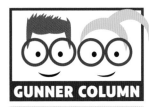

99 AR

Immunology terminology, video series

Introduction

Five to ten questions on the shelf will be directly related to immunologic disorders, defined as abnormal processes that arise from a defective immune system. This chapter will be organized according to the USMLE Content Outline, which categorizes immunologic disorders into four sections: (1) disorders associated with immunodeficiency, (2) human immunodeficiency virus/acquired immunodeficiency syndrome (HIV/AIDS), (3) immunologically mediated disorders, and (4) adverse effects of drugs on the immune system.

Unlike step 1, the Surgery shelf will not test you directly on the normal immune system; you will not get questions on the difference between mast cells versus macrophages or the function of specific interleukins. However, a basic understanding of terminology associated with the immune system, such as MHC complexes or innate versus adaptive immunity, would be helpful.

As in other chapters, the diseases below are presented in the following format: (1) Buzz Words, (2) Clinical Presentation, (3) Prophylaxis (PPx), (4) Mechanism of Disease (MoD), (5) Diagnostic Steps (Dx), and (6) Treatment and Management Steps (Tx/Mgmt).

Human Immunodeficiency Virus/Acquired Immunodeficiency Syndrome

HIV/AIDS is the most high-yield subsection of the immunologic disorders for the Surgery shelf. This is because it is a disease that primarily affects adults, is well publicized, and is very well studied. Thus, it is important to understand the clinical presentation, PPx, MoD, Dx, and Tx/Mgmt of HIV/AIDS.

Human Immunodeficiency Virus Infection and Acquired Immunodeficiency Syndrome

Buzz Words:
- **Acute Phase:** Sexually active male or female + IV-drug user + enlarged inguinal lymph nodes (or generalized lymphadenopathy) + fever/recent sickness + sore throat + unspecified rashes

- **AIDS:** *Toxoplasma* infection + *Cryptosporidium* infection, *Mycobacterium avium* infection, fungal infections *(Candida, Cryptococcus, Pneumocystis jirovecii, Histoplasma, Coccidioides)* + CMV + Kaposi sarcoma + lymphomas + encephalopathy + wasting syndrome

Clinical Presentation: HIV is a double-stranded RNA virus that infects immune cells (e.g., CD4) by embedding themselves into DNA through reverse transcription. On the Surgery shelf, patients can either present in the acute phase of illness (e.g., sore throat, generalized lymphadenopathy, fever) or late stage of illness, aka with AIDS. AIDS is diagnosed if patient has a CD4 cell percentage ≤14%, CD4 count less than 200/µL, and presence of AIDS-defining condition. For the Surgery shelf, you will only encounter adults with HIV; congenital HIV Buzz Words will only be needed for Pediatrics. Be prepared to recognize the classic signs of acute illness as well as a few frequently tested AIDS-defining conditions, such as Kaposi sarcoma. You may also be tested on prevention techniques, diagnostic steps as well as treatment/management steps, although, unlike Step 1, you do not have to know the exact details of mechanism of disease and or drug target of action (although we do encourage you to learn this for your patients and to impress your attendings!).

PPx: To understand prophylactic measures, know the common modes of HIV transmission: (1) sexual intercourse through genital, rectal, or oral fluids; (2) use of contaminated instruments or needles (e.g., IV drug users sharing needles); (3) maternal to fetus through breastfeeding or childbirth; and (4) blood transfusion. Thus, to prevent HIV transmission: condom use, avoidance of dirty needles, treat pregnant patient to reduce HIV viral load and chance of vertical transmission, screen blood donors for HIV, HIV antibody testing for sexually active patients.

MoD: HIV Env (envelope glycoprotein) binds to CD4 and chemokine coreceptors (CXCR4, CCR5) → HIV RNA w/ reverse transcriptase release into cell → HIV integration into genome and replication within cell → lysis of infected cell to release of HIV and propagate infection.

HIV infection leads to immunodeficiency by (1) loss of CD4 cells 2/2 direct cytotoxic effect; (2) infection of macrophages, dendritic cells, and follicular dendritic cells; (3) decreased immune response 2/2 depletion of CD4 T cells.

FOR THE WARDS

Notable AIDS-Defining Conditions frequently seen on the shelf: Kaposi's sarcoma + salmonella septicemia + toxoplasmosis of brain >1 month old + **Pneumocystis jirovecii** pneumonia + *Candida* infection of the esophagus + encephalopathy 2/2 HIV

99 AR

Full list of AIDS-Defining Conditions, CDC

99 AR

To counsel your patients on HIV Transmission Risk through sexual activities, refer to the CDC

NIH treatment guidelines for HIV/AIDS

QUICK TIPS

Immune reconstitution inflammatory syndrome (IRIS) occurs when there is an immune reaction to sub-clinically detectable infection, even though CD4 count and HIV viral load improve. Self-limited and improve with steroids. Make sure to think of IRIS in a patient who appears to be getting sicker even though lab values paint a healthier picture.

99 AR

Introduction to vasculitis

Dx:
1. HIV antibody testing
2. Nucleic acid amplification assays for HIV RNA level
3. ELISA ± Western blot to confirm diagnosis

To monitor HIV, order CD4 count (e.g., complete blood count [CBC] with diff), plasma HIV RNA level, PPD or quantiferon gold to r/o concomitant tuberculosis (TB)

Tx/Mgmt:
1. Combination treatment with antiretroviral therapy, for example, highly active antiretroviral therapy (HAART).
2. If AIDS (CD4 < 200/μL), TMP/SMX or dapsone to PPxx against *Pneumocystis jirovecii*.
3. If AIDS (CD4 < 50), azithromycin/clarithromycin to PPx against *Mycobacterium avium-intracellulare* (MAI).
4. If HIV + suspicion of TB, start patient on isoniazid and pyridoxine (vitamin B6 to counter isoniazid side effects).

Vasculitides

Vasculitis refers to a set of disorders where the blood vessel wall is inflamed and is a high-yield topic on the Surgery shelf for three reasons. First, while rare from an epidemiological standpoint, many of the vasculitides have unique Buzz Words and interesting Clinical Presentations that attending physicians love to test students about (e.g., giant cell arteritis in an old lady with headache and visual disturbances). Second, vasculitis is a disease process that affects many different organ systems and can thus present with many different chief complaints. Third, vasculitis can affect folks of all different age groups; thus, be prepared to run into this set of diseases on the Pediatrics, Neurology, Medicine, and Family Medicine shelves as well. The MoD of all vasculitides tested on the shelf is unclear. That being said, these disorders are considered part of the Immunological Disorder category since inflammation is a hallmark of disease. Overall, the vasculitides can be divided into three categories: small-vessel, medium-vessel, and large-vessel vasculitis.

Small Vessel

Behçet Syndrome

Buzz Words: Oral ulcers + genital ulcer + skin lesions + anterior uveitis + dementia/blindness + past viral infection

Clinical Presentation: Often included as an answer choice for patients who present with oral ulcers. Behçet syndrome is technically a small-vessel vasculitis, but not much is known about its etiology. Its defining characteristic is the recurring ulcers but patients can also present with uveitis. PPx, MoD, Dx, and Tx/Mgmt for this disease will not be tested.

Churg-Strauss Syndrome

Buzz Words: Asthma + eosinophils + elevated serum p-ANCA + fatigue/myalgias

Clinical Presentation: Churg-Strauss syndrome is a small-vessel vasculitis that is notable for inflammation filled with eosinophils and associated with asthma. Most commonly, the vessels inflamed supply/drain the lung and the heart, but can also affect the blood supply of peripheral nerves (e.g., wrist drop). This is one of two vasculitides to use serum p-ANCA (the other being microscopic polyangiitis) as a measure of disease activity.

Dx:
1. Serum P-ANCA (e.g., antibodies against PMN myeloperoxidase)
2. Biopsy (shows eosinophilia)

Tx/Mgmt:
1. Steroids
2. Cyclophosphamide

Granulomatosis With Polyangiitis (Wegener Granulomatosis)

Buzz Words: Pneumonitis + hematuria/hemoptysis + necrotizing arteritis + epithelioid histiocytes

Clinical Presentation: Granulomatosis with polyangiitis (GPA) is a small-vessel vasculitis that used to be known as Wegener granulomatosis. Patients with GPA will present with dysfunction of the tissues primarily affected by cigarette smoke: nasopharynx, lung, and kidney (from clearing cigarette metabolites).

Dx:
1. Serum C-ANCA
2. Biopsy (large necrotizing granulomas w/ necrotizing vasculitis)

Tx/Mgmt:
1. Steroids
2. Cyclophosphamide

MNEMONIC

The C's of We"c"ener's granulomatosis: C-ANCA, Cyclophosphamide, Cigarette-smoking-symptoms (e.g., affects nasopharynx, lung, and kidney, similar to the organs affected by smoking cigarettes). GPA patients can also concomitantly present with immunofluorescent negative RPGN.

QUICK TIPS

C-ANCA = cytoplasmic antineutrophil cytoplasmic antibodies; obtained by adding patient serum to slide with neutrophil → aggregation of antibodies around cytoplasm = C-ANCA vs. aggregation of antibodies around nucleus = P-ANCA

Microscopic Polyangiitis

Buzz Words: Palpable purpura + muscle pain + fatigue + weight loss + lung pathology + kidney pathology

Clinical Presentation: Similar to GPA but without the nasopharyngeal involvement

Dx:
1. P-ANCA (activation of neutrophils and monocytes by perinuclear antinuclear cytoplasmic antibodies (MPO-ANCAs/p-ANCAs)
2. Biopsy

Tx/Mgmt:
1. Steroids
2. Cyclophosphamide

Henoch-Schonlein Purpura

HSP Review

Buzz Words: Palpable purpura + joint pain + immunoglobulin (Ig)A immune complex deposition in kidney **and** skin/gastrointestinal (GI) tract + normal-elevated platelets + hematuria + GI bleed/pain + recent upper respiratory tract infection

Clinical Presentation: Henoch-Schonlein purpura (HSP) is a small-cell vasculitis that is associated with palpable purpura, IgA immune complex deposition in both the kidney and organs outside the kidney (e.g., skin or GI tract), and normal-elevated platelets. Often presents after an upper respiratory tract infection.

If IgA deposition only found in kidney, the disease is likely IgA nephropathy. If platelets are low in patient with palpable purpura, suspect TTP. Given its penchant for affecting multiple organ systems and mimicking pathology, HSP is frequently tested on the Surgery, Medicine, and Pediatrics shelves.

Other disorders that mimic HSP include:
- Purpura fulminans: Associated with neisseria meningitides/strep pneumo and presents with hypotension and DIC
- Leukemia: Bone marrow infiltration → purpura → elevated WBC and decreased platelet count
- Viral exanthems (vesicular/macular/maculopapular rather than purpuric)
- Rocky Mountain spotted fever + atypical measles
- Von Willebrand disease (vWD) deficiency
- Hemophilia A/B

MoD: Palpable purpura 2/2 bleeding from IgA immune complex-mediated inflammation; hematuria 2/2 IgA immune complex deposition in the mesangium of the glomerulus

Dx:
1. CBC (normal platelets)
2. Coags (normal)
3. BMP (Nl to mildly elevated Cr)
4. UA (hematuria + red cell casts + mild proteinuria)
5. Skin exam to look for palpable purpura
6. Renal biopsy → immunofluorescence IgA IC deposition in the kidney; mesangial deposition of IgA

Tx/Mgmt:
1. Supportive management (hydration/pain control with nonsteroidal anti-inflammatory drugs [NSAIDs])
2. Hospitalization indicated for severe abdominal pain + renal insufficiency + AMS + poor PO intake
3. Glucocorticoids (e.g., steroids) in patients with severe abdominal pain unresponsive to NSAIDs

Medium Vessel

Kawasaki Disease

Buzz Words: Young adult with coronary artery aneurysms/MI + no cocaine use + history of fever >5 days, conjunctivitis, strawberry tongue, rash, erythema/fissured lips, edema, erythema, desquamation of hands and feet, cervical LAD

Clinical Presentation: Kawasaki disease is a medium-vessel vasculitis that affects children (e.g., more common on Pediatrics shelf) but may present on the Surgery shelf as patient who survived and is dealing with complications of Kawasaki's. Complications include coronary artery aneurysms, MI, and myocarditis. Classically, Kawasaki's is associated with an Asian child with a ≥5-day fever with a strawberry tongue and desquamation of the hands/feet (Fig. 3.1). This is not as high yield on the Surgery shelf but will be sure to appear when you are on Peds.

PPx: Monitor with echocardiogram and EKG to avoid cardiovascular sequelae (such as coronary vessel thrombosis/aneurysmal rupture)

Dx:
1. CBC → leukocytosis with neutrophilia, thrombocytosis
2. CRP and ESR (both elevated)
3. UA (sterile pyuria)

Tx/Mgmt:
1. Aspirin (prevents coronary thrombosis)
2. Substitute aspirin with clopidogrel if there is flu or varicella infections
3. IVIG
4. Usually will self-resolve in 12 days but treat to prevent cardiac issues

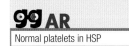

99 AR

Normal platelets in HSP

QUICK TIPS

Scarlet fever, a toxin-mediated illness caused by group A beta hemolytic strep, can also present with strawberry tongue and desquamation. However, unlike Kawasaki's, can be resolved with penicillin.

QUICK TIPS

Strawberry tongue
1. CBC leukocytosis with neutrophilia, thrombocytosis
2. CRP and ESR (both elevated)
3. UA (sterile pyuria)

QUICK TIPS

Aspirin is typically contraindicated as a treatment for children because it may cause **Reye syndrome**, acute liver failure with characteristic microvesicular fatty infiltration. Treatment of Kawasaki disease is the one exception.

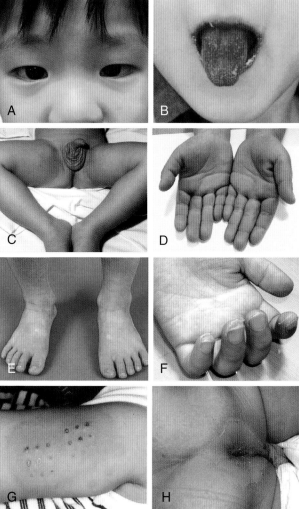

FIG. 3.1 Clinical presentation of Kawasaki disease. A, Bilateral conjunctival erythema; B, strawberry tongue; C, erythematous rash involving perineum; D, palmar erythema and edema; E, erythema of the soles and edema of the dorsal feet; F, desquamation of fingertips; G, erythema at the site of a previous Bacille Calmette-Gurin vaccination; H, perianal desquamation and erythema. (From Kim DS: Kawasaki disease. *Yonsei Med J* 47(6):759–772, 2006.)

Buerger Disease (Thromboangiitis obliterans)

Buzz Words: Calf pain + painful foot ulcers + painful fingers with cold weather + cyanosis of distal extremities + reaction to intradermal tobacco extract + smoking

Clinical Presentation: Buerger disease is a medium-vessel vasculitis known for its classic association with smoking. Buerger disease is also associated with Reynaud's and ulceration of the distal extremities. It can be characterized as a segmental vasculitis that extends into contiguous veins and nerves. This disease is not high yield on the Surgery shelf, but be sure to know the Buzz Words/Treatment in order to rule it out as an answer choice.

Polyarteritis Nodosa

Buzz Words: Young adult + hypertension + abdominal pain + dark stools + altered mental status + hepatitis B + "string-of-pearls" on angiogram

Clinical Presentation: Polyarteritis nodosa is a medium-vessel vasculitis that can be fatal if not treated. The chief complaint can range from high blood pressure (2/2 renal artery involvement), abdominal pain/bloody stools (2/2 mesenteric artery involvement), skin lesions, or altered mental status. The distinguishing feature of this vasculitis is that it is associated with the hepatitis B antigen (HBsAg), which may likely be shown in the question stem to differentiate from other vasculitides. Imaging of the vessels affected by PAN may exhibit a strong-of-pearls sign due to the pattern of inflammation and fibrosis.

Dx:
1. CBC/BMP
2. Hepatitis panel
3. Angiogram
4. Biopsy of inflamed vessels (segmental ischemic necrosis)

Tx/Mgmt:
1. Steroids
2. Cyclophosphamide

Large Vessel

Temporal (Giant Cell) Arteritis

Buzz Words: Older woman + ischemic optic neuropathy + temporal headache + vision change + ESR elevated + polymyalgia rheumatica

Clinical Presentation: Temporal arteritis is a large-vessel vasculitis that is extremely high yield on the shelf for two reasons. First, it is easy to treat and identification of giant cell arteritis in an individual can save her/his eyesight. Second, it can present with a variety of chief complaints in real life and has been associated with multiorgan syndromes such as polymyalgia rheumatica, making it a popular test question on the Surgery, Medicine, Neurology, and Psychiatry shelves. The most common complaint patients present with is headache. Usually the patient is an older woman who has associated vision changes/jaw pain with the headache as

> **QUICK TIPS**
>
> Buerger disease is the only vasculitis that is associated with smoking. Do not get confused with We"c"ener mnemonic, where one of the C's was Cigarette-like-symptoms (e.g., Wegener's affects the organs most commonly diseased in smokers → nasopharyngeal tract, lungs and kidney).

well as muscle pain. Make sure to order an ESR in these individuals immediately, which, if elevated, suggests temporal arteritis. Biopsy of the affected temporal artery makes the definitive diagnosis and gold standard of treatment remains steroids.

MoD: Blindness can be caused by ophthalmic artery involvement

Dx:
1. CBC/BMP
2. ESR (elevated)
3. Biopsy (inflamed vessel wall with fibrosis/giant cells)

Tx/Mgmt: Steroids

Takayasu Arteritis

Buzz Words: Less than 50 years old + Asian female + headache and vision changes + weak/absent upper extremity pulse + elevated ESR

Clinical Presentation: Takayasu arteritis is a large-vessel vasculitis that can be thought of as the "younger variant" of temporal arteritis because of its similar presentation (e.g., headache/vision changes) but only affects women less than 50 years old. Aside from age, the biggest differences are that the inflamed vasculature are typically closer to the branch points off the aorta and the upper extremity pulse can be weaker in Takayasu arteritis.

Dx:
1. CBC/BMP
2. ESR (elevated)
3. Biopsy

Tx/Mgmt: Steroids

Autoimmune Disorders

Autoimmune disorders are characterized by damaged tissues from aberrant attacks from one's own immune system. These typically affect multiple organ systems and thus are high yield on the Surgery shelf. In addition, many of these autoimmune disorders, such as systemic lupus erythematosus (SLE), are known as great imitators and should be on the differential for most chief complaints. When studying autoimmune disorders, keep two organizing principles in mind. First, there typically is an environmental trigger that sets off the immune system to attack one's own cells. For instance, in lupus, ultraviolet rays from the sun can damage exposed skin and release intranuclear contents into the bloodstream, whereby they are recognized and attacked by the humoral immune

QUICK TIPS

Older patients exhibiting symptoms of polymyalgia rheumatica (e.g.) should strongly increase your suspicion of temporal arteritis on the shelf. Treat early to avoid blindness.

system. Second, disease activity of autoimmune disorders can wax and wane. Treatment aims to reduce disease activity during flares and prevent future flares from occurring.

Systemic Lupus Erythematosus (aka Lupus)

Buzz Words: RPR and VDRL positive + elevated PTT + recurrent abortions + malar rash → antiphospholipid antibody in s/o SLE

Presents with recurrent pregnancy loss, stroke, and venous thrombosis. Treat with anticoagulation. Can be primary d/o or associated with SLE.

Antihistone antibody + malar rash + new drug/medication → drug-induced lupus

IgG + malar rash + discoid rash + ANA + mucositis (mouth ulcers) + neuro dysfunction + serositis (pleuritis/pericarditis) + hematologic d/o (pancytopenia) + arthritis + renal d/o (wire loops) + photosensitivity + psychosis → SLE

Clinical Presentation: SLE is an autoimmune disorder that can present as nearly any chief complaint and is thus often kept somewhere on the differential. It is thus very easy to get lost when thinking about SLE. Here are two organizing principles to guide your study.

First, be clear on how SLE presents on the shelf. Although, SLE is the "great imitator," there are only a handful of Buzz Words or clinical vignettes that can be used to describe SLE. First, be on the lookout for a (most likely) female patient with a malar (e.g., "butterfly") rash over the bridge of her nose (Fig. 3.2) who presents with constitutional symptoms, such as fatigue, fever, and night sweats.

On the shelf, these patients typically have been recently exposed to sun (e.g., beach trip) or perhaps forgot to put on sunscreen. The shelf may try to trick you by showing either (1) lab results that falsely suggest syphilis (e.g., VDRL and RPR positive) or (2) lab results that falsely suggest a hematologic disorder (e.g., elevated PTT). Be very suspicious that these findings are due to antiphospholipid antibodies (e.g., lupus anticoagulant). For the Ob/Gyn shelf, these findings may present as a woman with a history of recurrent spontaneous abortions, a sequelae of having circulating lupus anticoagulant.

Anytime someone is positive anti-dsDNA or anti-Sm antibodies, know that it is pathognomonic for SLE. SLE patients are also ANA positive, but ANA is not specific for the disease. Finally, patients with anti-histone

QUICK TIPS

Antiphospholipid antibodies include (1) lupus anticoagulant (elevates PTT), (2) anticardiolipin (false-positive VDRL and RPR), (3) anti-beta 2-glycoprotein

QUICK TIPS

Antiphospholipid d/o characterized by hypercoagulable state 2/2 antiphospholipid antibodies

QUICK TIPS

Agents (e.g., slow acetylators in the liver) that lead to drug-induced lupus: SLE caused by Sulfa HIPP-E's (Sulfa drugs, Hydralazine, Isoniazid, Procainamide, Phenytoin, Etanercept)

99 AR

Oral ulcers in SLE

99 AR

Lupus presentation video

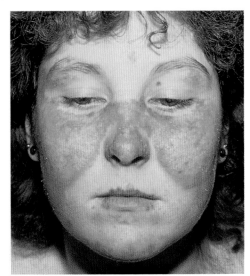

FIG. 3.2 Malar rash. (From Elsevier Lupus Image Bank. www.lupusimages.com/browser/detail/129/mucocutaneous-sle-malar-rash.)

antibodies have drug-induced lupus. Knowing these Buzz Words will help you avoid confusion and immediately sniff out what the NBME examiners are up to.

Second, for your clerkship rotation, remember that SLE can affect every organ system due to deposition of immune complexes. Make sure you have a systematic way to think through how the disease may present, such as telling a story from head to toe.

- Face/sun-exposed skin → malar or discoid rash, photosensitivity
- Brain → seizures, psychosis
- Respiratory tract → inflammation of lung pleura
- Heart → pericarditis, Libman-Sacks endocarditis
- GI tract → oropharyngeal ulcers
- Renal → diffuse proliferative glomerulonephritis with deposits on subendothelium, membranous glomerulonephritis with deposits on the subepithelium, kidney failure
- MSK → inflammatory arthritis (usually at least 2 joints)
- Heme → leukopenia (more susceptible to infection), anemia, thrombocytopenia, hypercoagulability (more susceptible to CAD, thrombosis to placenta during pregnancy)
- Reproductive → mucositis, recurrent pregnancy loss due to thrombosis
- Endocrine → thyroid autoimmunity

Lastly, remember that most SLE patients die from renal failure (most commonly from DPGN), so keep a keen eye on renal function.

99 AR

Libman-Sacks endocarditis is a form of nonbacterial endocarditis mediated by vegetations and associated with SLE.

99 AR

Thyroid autoimmunity associated with SLE

PPx: Sunscreen (avoid sun exposure)

MoD: Mostly considered type 3 hypersensitivity because damage is mediated by antigen-antibody immune complexes. Sun damage → apoptotic debris → activation and production of antibodies that target antigens from patient cell nucleus → immune complex formed → immune complex deposited in body tissues and upregulates immune responses (using up complement proteins leading to deficient C1, C2, and C4).

In pregnancy, **Lupus anticoagulant** leads to thrombus development within the placenta → spontaneous abortion/pregnancy loss.

Pancytopenia in SLE is mediated by direct antibody attack on RBCs, WBCs, and platelets (type 2 hypersensitivity).

Dx:

1. CBC/BMP
2. ANA
3. Anti-Smith and anti-dsDNA antibodies (specific/gold standard for diagnosis)
4. Complement levels (may show decrease C1, C3, C4)

Tx/Mgmt:

1. NSAIDs
2. Steroids
3. Anticoagulation (e.g., warfarin, heparin) if antiphospholipid antibody syndrome
4. Methotrexate
5. Biologics (e.g., TNF-alpha inhibitors)

Sjogren Syndrome

Buzz Words: Enlarged parotid glands (like a chipmunk) + dry eyes + dry mouth + anti-Ro (SSA) and anti-La (SSB) antibodies + RA

Clinical Presentation: Sjogren syndrome is an autoimmune disorder characterized by lymphocytic damage to salivary and lacrimal glands. Patients are usually older women who present with enlarged parotid glands, dry mouth (perhaps as recurrent dental infections), and dry eyes. Like many autoimmune disorders, Sjogren's can be associated with other autoimmune pathology. Folks with Sjogren's often present with rheumatoid arthritis, SLE, systemic sclerosis, or primary biliary cirrhosis. Diagnosis is made by anti-SSA or anti-SSB antibodies, although a biopsy of the salivary/lacrimal glands can also be used to confirm. Complications of Sjogren's include marginal zone lymphoma and acute interstitial nephritis.

> **QUICK TIPS**
> PTT is artificially elevated in lupus. RPR and VDRL are falsely positive in lupus as well.

> **QUICK TIPS**
> Sjogren = dry

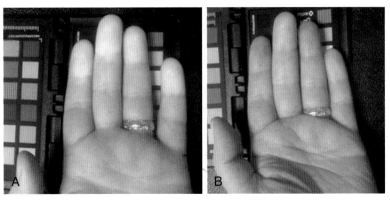

FIG. 3.3 Raynaud phenomenon. A, Raynaud phenomenon; B, normal. (From *Best Practice & Research: Clinical Rheumatology*, 30(1):112–132, 2016.)

MoD: Damage in Sjogren's is mediated by lymphocytes and is therefore considered a type 4 hypersensitivity reaction. Lymphocytes attack lacrimal and salivary glands → dry mouth and dry eyes → dental infections and eyes susceptible to abrasion.

Dx:

1. CBC/BMP
2. ANA (positive)
3. Rheumatoid factor (RA, which is often concomitant)
4. Anti-SSA (anti-ro) and anti-SSB (anti-La) antibodies
5. Biopsy of salivary glands (lymphocytic infiltration)

Tx/Mgmt: Supportive

Systemic Sclerosis (aka Scleroderma)

Buzz Words:

- **Diffuse:** anti-scl-70 + tightening of skin all over body + GERD + Raynaud's (Fig. 3.3) + pulmonary hypertension
- **Limited (CREST):** Anti-centromere antibody + sclerodactyly + tightening of skin on hand/face only + Raynaud phenomenon + esophageal dysmotility + telangiectasias + calcinosis

Clinical Presentation: Scleroderma is an autoimmune disorder that is characterized by fibrosis of skin and internal organs. Like other autoimmune disorders, it more commonly is seen in females (middle aged). It is divided into two types of disease: diffuse and limited. Diffuse scleroderma means the fibrosis characteristic of the disease can occur anywhere in the body, and

QUICK TIPS

Raynaud Phenomenon: When arterioles of distal extremities vasospasm 2/2 cold exposure → white/blue hands and feet. Treatment is to keep distal extremities warm (e.g., move to warm climate, gloves) and CCBs.

frequently leads to death through pulmonary hypertension. Limited scleroderma is known as CREST syndrome due to the mnemonic: **C**alcinosis/anti**C**entromere antibody; **R**aynaud phenomenon; **E**sophageal dysmotility; **S**clerodactyly; **T**elangiectasia. For the shelf, the easiest way to distinguish the two entities is through the presence of antibodies: Anti-scl-70 = diffuse scleroderma; anti-centromere = limited scleroderma. Unlike SLE and Sjogren's, you will mainly be responsible for identifying the clinical presentation rather than knowing the diagnostic and treatment steps.

Dx: Anti-scl-70 and anti-centromere antibody
Tx/Mgmt: Supportive

Mixed Connective Tissue Disease

Buzz Words: Anti-U1 ribonucleoprotein antibodies + ANA + features of SLE, scleroderma and polymyositis

Clinical Presentation: Mixed connective tissue disease (MCTD) combines features of three prominent autoimmune disorders (e.g., polymyositis, SLE, and scleroderma). On the shelf, the only thing you will be tested on is disease recognition or the ability to eliminate this as an answer choice. Recognize that anti-U1 ribonucleoprotein antibodies are associated with MCTD and move on.

GUNNER PRACTICE

1. A 35-year-old IV-drug abuser presents to the hospital complaining of abdominal pain. She has been using IV heroin for 5 years, more frequently over the past 10 months. The pain is associated with a decreased frequency of bowel movements and a 5-pound weight loss. Prior to examining her abdomen, the physician notices the following lesion on the patient's nose. Which of the following pathogens is most likely?
   A. MRSA
   B. MSSA
   C. *P. acnes*
   D. HHV4
   E. HHV8
2. A 62-year-old female complains of headaches for 2 weeks. The headache has been waxing and waning and is a 3–8/10 in severity. It is located just superior to her right TMJ and is sharp in quality. The pain is better with

rest and NSAIDs and nothing makes it worse. On exam, CN II–XII are intact except for poor distance vision. There is a bilateral carotid bruit. Heart and lungs are normal except for a faint systolic murmur. What is the next best step?

A. Start sumtriptan
B. Start valproic acid
C. Start methylprednisolone
D. Obtain CBC
E. Obtain ESR
F. Biopsy

3. A 28-year-old female with history of SLE presents to her PCP 3 months post-partum from her first child. She is G4P1031. She states that after having her child, she has been breastfeeding regularly and the baby is doing great. Her mood has been a bit low and she is feeling anxious but she is not having any uncontrolled crying spells and is still able to care for herself, her husband, and her child. On physical exam her BMI is 29. Her pulse is 122/min, respirations 20/min, and blood pressure 90/58. Her skin is without rash or jaundice. Heart sounds without m/r/g and lungs CTAB. Which of the following is the next best step?

A. Follow up in 6 months
B. Duplex bilateral lower extremities
C. Chest x-ray
D. CTA chest
E. VQ scan
F. D-dimer

Notes

ANSWERS: What Would Gunner Jess/Jim Do?

1. WWGJD? A 35-year-old IV-drug abuser presents to the hospital complaining of abdominal pain. She has been using IV heroin for five years, more frequently over the past 10 months. The pain is associated with a decreased frequency of bowel movements and a 5-pound weight loss. Prior to examining her abdomen, the physician notices the following lesion on the patient's nose. Which of the following pathogens is most likely?

Answer: E, HHV8.

Explanation: The abdominal pain is a red herring. It is probably caused by constipation due to opiate use but it is irrelevant to the question. This is typical of Kaposi's sarcoma. Often these lesions are described as reddish violacious papules without surrounding swelling, erythema, or fluctuance. Answers A and B are both possible infections in an IV drug user but they would be more likely at injection sites. *P. acnes* is associated with acne but these lesions lack the pustule appearance more consistent with acne. HHV4 is EBV which can cause a morbilliform rash and is associated with some lymphomas but is not associated with a rash like this. HHV8 is associated with Kaposi sarcoma in patients with HIV.

2. WWGJD? A 62-year-old female complains of headaches for 2 weeks. The headache has been waxing and waning and is a 3–8/10 in severity. It is located just superior to her right TMJ and is sharp in quality. The pain is better with rest and NSAIDs and nothing makes it worse. On exam, CN II–XII are intact except for poor distance vision. There is a bilateral carotid bruit. Heart and lungs are normal except for a faint systolic murmur. What is the next best step?

Answer: C, start methylprednisolone.

Explanation: The scenario describes giant cell arteritis, the treatment for which is methylprednisolone. Answers A and B are both treatments for migraines. Onset of migraines in the 60s is very uncommon. There is no reason to believe the patient has history of headaches. Do not assume things that are not stated in the question. Answer C is the treatment for giant cell arteritis, which should be immediately suspected in an elderly patient with unilateral headache. Answers D, E, and F are helpful in the diagnosis of giant cell arteritis but not the *best next* step. It is often hard to know if treating or diagnosing a disease is more important. In the case of giant cell arteritis, treatment should be started immediately to prevent blindness which may be developing in this patient since she has poor distance vision.

3. WWGJD? A 28-year-old female with history of SLE presents to her PCP three months post-partum from her first child. She is G4P1031. She states that after having her child, she has been breastfeeding regularly and the baby is doing great. Her mood has been a bit low and she is feeling anxious but she is not having any uncontrolled crying spells and is still able to care for herself, her husband, and her child. On physical exam her BMI is 29. Her pulse is 122/min, respirations 20/min, and blood pressure 90/58. Her skin is without rash or jaundice. Heart sounds without m/r/g and lungs CTAB. Which of the following is the next best step?

Answer: D, CTA chest.

Explanation: If it was not clear in the question, the answer choices should have clued you in that this patient may have a pulmonary embolism. A test-taking tip is to always read each answer choice and quickly decide why the question writer chose to include it. If the answer seems completely absurd, you may have missed something in the question. Answer A is incorrect because the patient has many signs of a PE and should be further evaluated. The patient has a history of SLE with three early-term miscarriages. This is highly suggestive of having lupus-anticoagulant, which is a hypercoagulable state due to antibodies to phospholipids such as cardio-lipin. In the post-partum period (as well as during pregnancy), women are in a prothrombotic state. Anxiety, tachycardia, and tachypnea are all other signs of pulmonary embolism. The gold standard for diagnosis of PE is CTA chest, so answer D is the best answer. Answer B is too simple—checking the lower extremities for DVT using ultrasound cannot rule out PE. Answer C would likely be uninformative. Most chest x-rays are not diagnostic for PE. Answer E is an alternative to answer D but VQ is not the gold standard for diagnosing PE. Answer F is a common trick on shelf exams. A D-dimer can be used to rule out PE when clinical suspicion is low. In this patient, our clinical suspicion is very high. Additionally, her hypercoagulable state would likely cause the D-dimer to be positive even if she did not have a PE so the test would be uninformative.

Notes

Diseases of the Blood and Blood-Forming Organs

Diana Kim, Drake Lebrun, Leo Wang, Hao-Hua Wu, Rebecca Gao, and Sean Harbison

Introduction

This chapter covers the hematology/oncology that you will face on the Surgery shelf. Heme/onc disorders, especially as related to coagulation, are extremely relevant to any procedural intervention, making this the most important topic in this section. Despite the length of this chapter, you will only get 5–10 questions on this chapter on the Surgery shelf, making it relatively lower yield than chapters on major organ systems. If you are short on time, focus specifically on coagulation disorders and particularly the hypercoagulable states.

This chapter is divided into subsections that highlight the various pathologies that can occur in the blood, ranging from infections to clotting problems to cancer. As a rule, complete blood counts (CBCs) and peripheral blood smears play major diagnostic roles in the work-up of many of these diseases. As such, recognizing normal CBC values and what peripheral blood smears look like can go a long way. Bone marrow aspirates are used for many blood disorders, and it will be helpful but not absolutely mandatory to also have a sense of what normal marrow looks like. For specific diseases such as coagulopathies, understanding principles behind prothrombin (PT) and activated partial thromboplastin time (aPTT) (discussed later) will be helpful.

Infections of the Blood

Bacterial Infections of the Blood

Buzz Words: High/low temp + high heart rate, resp rate + high leukocyte count

Clinical Presentation: Sepsis is a spectrum that exists between bacteremia, ranging all the way to septic shock. Bacteremia is defined as the presence of bacteria in the bloodstream. It can have no accompanying symptoms and is diagnosed based on the presence of bacteria from blood cultures. Bacteria in the bloodstream can lead to systemic inflammatory response

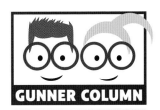

GUNNER COLUMN

syndrome (SIRS), which is the presence of two or more of the following:

1. Temp >38 or <35
2. HR >90
3. RR >20 or PCO_2 <32
4. Leukocytes >12,000 or <4000 or >10% immature

Sepsis is defined as the presence of SIRS with a documented source of infection (such as pneumonia, meningitis). Severe sepsis is defined as the additional presence of end-organ damage from hypoperfusion or hypotension. Septic shock (SBP < 90) is defined as the presence of the aforementioned with refractory hypotension that does not respond to fluids.

Infections of Lymphoid Tissue

Lymphadenitis

Buzz Words: Red, tender skin over lymph node + swollen or tender lymph nodes + tender red streaks

Clinical Presentation: This is an infection of the lymph nodes. In most situations, this term is used interchangeably with lymphadenopathy, although they are functionally different. Lymphadenopathy is a disease process that increases the size or consistency of the lymph nodes, whereas lymphadenitis refers to an inflammatory disease process from underlying infection. Unlike lymphadenopathy, lymphadenitis spreads quickly and can become lymphangitis. It can also lead to complications like abscess formation, cellulitis, and sepsis.

Prophylaxis (PPx): Proper hygiene

Mechanism of Disease (MoD): Infection from various agents that causes infection/inflammation of one or more lymph nodes

Diagnostic Steps (Dx):

1. Physical exam
2. Lymph node biopsy
3. Blood cultures

Treatment and Management Steps (Tx/Mgmt):

1. Treat underlying infection
2. Analgesics
3. Nonsteroidal antiinflammatory drugs (NSAIDs)
4. Surgical drainage if abscess formation

Lymphangitis

Buzz Words: Reddening of skin + warmth/swelling + inflammation of lymph gland + raised border over affected area + fever + history of trauma

Clinical Presentation: This is an inflammation of the lymphatic system, including bone marrow, spleen, and thymus. Typically caused by an infected wound and invasion of lymph system, most commonly caused by *Streptococcus pyogenes*, *Staphylococcus aureus*, and *Sporothrix schenckii*.

PPx: Treat precipitating infection

MoD: Infection of wound site leading to lymphoid spread to lymphatic organs like bone marrow, spleen, thymus

Dx:
1. Physical exam
2. Biopsy of affected area
3. Culture of affected area
4. Blood culture

Tx/Mgmt:
1. Antibiotics
2. Analgesics
3. NSAIDs

Immunologic and Inflammatory Disorders

These concepts are low yield on the Surgery shelf.

Autoimmune Hemolytic Anemia

Buzz Words: Anemia symptoms (fatigue, pallor, jaundice) + jaundice from hemolysis →

Clinical Presentation: This is a disease caused by production of autoantibodies (immunoglobulin [Ig]G or IgM) toward red blood cells (RBCs). It is separated into **warm,** which is more common than **cold.** Warm occurs with **IgG** and only at 37°C—it leads to **extravascular** hemolysis and **splenic** sequestration of RBCs. Cold occurs with IgM and only at 0°C—it leads to **intravascular** hemolysis and **liver** sequestration of RBCs.

MoD:
- **Warm AIHA:** primary—idiopathic, secondary—lymphomas, leukemias, malignancies, collagen vascular diseases, methyldopa
- **Cold AIHA:** idiopathic, infectious mononucleosis, *Mycoplasma pneumoniae*

In both cases, they elevate IgG or IgM, respectively, binding to RBC membranes, which leads to hemolysis and sequestration of RBCs.

Dx:
1. Coombs test (Fig. 4.1)
   a. Coating with IgG → warm AIHA; coating with complement → cold AIHA

2. Positive cold agglutinin titer
3. Spherocytes in warm AIHA

Tx/Mgmt:

1. No tx necessary in most cases
2. Warm AIHA:
   a. Glucocorticoids
   b. Splenectomy
   c. Immunosuppressants
   d. Tx anemia—RBC transfusions, folic acid supplementation
3. Cold AIHA:
   a. Avoid cold exposure
   b. Tx anemia—RBC transfusions
   c. Immunosuppressants

QUICK TIPS

Glucocorticoids are never indicated in cold AIHA

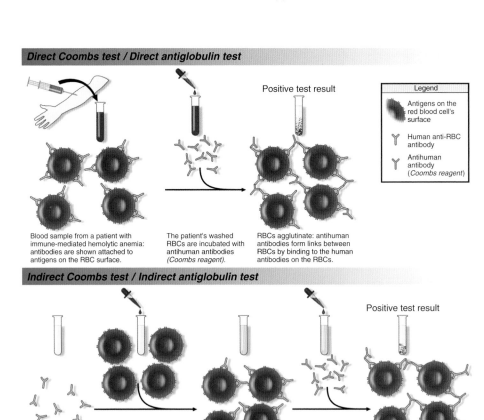

FIG. 4.1 Coombs test. (From Wikimedia Commons. https://commons.wikimedia.org/wiki/File:Coombs_test_schematic.png. Used under GNU Free Documentation License: https://en.wikipedia.org/wiki/GNU_Free_Documentation_License.)

Thrombotic Thrombocytopenia Purpura

Buzz Words: Fever + anemia + thrombocytopenia + renal dysfunction + neurologic dysfunction + schistocytes

Clinical Presentation: Thrombotic thrombocytopenia purpura (TTP) is a rare disease that causes small blood clots to form in the circulation. Microthrombi can shear RBCs, which can lead to hemolytic anemias and schistocytes.

MoD: TTP is caused by a deficiency in ADAMTS13, a metalloprotease that cleaves von Willebrand factor (vWF). In its absence, vWF builds up, leading to spontaneous activation and aggregation of platelets, leading to thrombosis and thrombocytopenia from consumption of platelets during this thrombotic process. Most cases are idiopathic but can be linked to autoantibodies to ADAMTS13.

Dx:
1. CBC (platelets low)
2. PT/aPTT (normal)
3. Bleeding time (prolonged)
4. ADAMTS13 activity testing

Tx/Mgmt:
1. Plasmapheresis
2. Rituximab
3. Caplacizumab (vWF-blocking antibody)
4. LDH levels to measure disease progression (hemolysis)

Hemolytic Uremic Syndrome

Buzz Words: Hemolytic anemia (jaundice, fatigue, pallor) + thrombocytopenia + renal dysfunction + shistocytes + child

Clinical Presentation: This is a medical emergency consisting of a triad of hemolytic anemia, thrombocytopenia, and renal dysfunction and is usually associated with previous infection, especially from EHEC O157:H7, *Campylobacter*, or *Shigella* (Shiga toxin). Toxins damage kidneys and can activate platelets, leading to microthrombi that can shear RBCs leading to shistocytes and a hemolytic anemia.

PPx: Hygiene to prevent food-borne illness

MoD: Toxins damage kidney/activate platelets → kidney damage, platelet activation, and microthrombi formation

Dx:
1. CBC/BMP
2. UA/UCX
3. Blood culture
4. Rule out TTP via ADAMTS13 levels

MNEMONIC

FATRN (fever, anemia, thrombocytopenia, renal dysfunction, neurologic dysfunction)

99 AR

Distinguishing TTP, DIC, HUS

Tx/Mgmt: Supportive, do not administer antibiotics because they can elevate Shiga toxin

Neoplasms

Neoplasms of the blood are infrequently tested on the Surgery shelf; however, neoplasms including solid tumors of vascular tissue including hemangiomas are extremely high yield (see Chapter 6).

Neoplasms in the blood are organized into leukemias versus lymphomas. Leukemias are cancers of the blood, whereas lymphomas are cancers of the lymph. Leukemias will NOT be tested on the Surgery shelf. Lymphomas will be because they can infiltrate solid organs, necessitating surgery. Lymphomas are typically broken down into Hodgkin versus non-Hodgkin lymphoma (NHL). Hodgkin lymphoma carries a significantly better prognosis. Leukemias are also broken down as chronic or acute. Remember that chronic leukemias involve mature cells, whereas acute leukemias tend to involve immature cells. Leukemias are also myelogenous or lymphoid in origin, indicating their origin cell line in hematopoiesis. For the Surgery shelf, focus specifically on Buzz Words for this section. Surgical management in these cases is minimal.

Hodgkin Lymphoma

Buzz Words: Painless lymphadenopathy + spread to adjacent nodes + B symptoms (fever, night sweats, weight loss) + hepatomegaly + splenomegaly

Clinical Presentation: Burkitt occurs in individuals between the age of 15 and 30 and in individuals over the age of 50. There are four subtypes (in order of prevalence):
- Nodular sclerosis: Reed-Sternberg cells in collagen envelope pools (tumor nodules)
- Mixed cellularity: Reed-Sternberg cells among many pleomorphic cells
- Lymphocyte predominant: primarily B cells, few Reed-Sternberg cells
- Lymphocyte depleted: no reactive cells, worst prognosis

Hodgkin lymphoma is further staged based on lymph node spread:
- Stage I—single lymph node
- Stage II—two or more lymph nodes on same side of diaphragm
- Stage III—lymph nodes on both sides of diaphragm
- Stage IV—presence in extralymphatic organs

MoD: Unclear, acquired mutation → proliferation of B cells
Dx:
1. Lymph node biopsy for Reed-Sternberg cell (B cell phenotype) (Fig. 4.2):
   a. Inflammatory cell infiltrate must be present—these are lymphocytic reaction to Reed-Sternberg cells
2. Chest x-ray (CXR), computed tomography (CT) scan—lymph node involvement
3. Bone marrow biopsy—bone marrow infiltration
4. CBC—leukocytosis and eosinophilia
Tx/Mgmt:
1. Radiation therapy for stages I, II, and IIIA
2. Chemotherapy for stages IIIB and IV

Non-Hodgkin Lymphoma

Buzz Words: Painless lymphadenopathy + B symptoms (fever, chills, night sweats)
Clinical Presentation: NHL is a cancer of lymphoid cells that causes proliferation of T cells, B cells, or NK cells, often with extranodal involvement. It usually presents as a rapidly growing, painless mass that is associated with autoimmune disorders. This mass can sometimes compress on surrounding vasculature, causing problems like SVC syndrome, facial plethora, or respiratory distress. It is overall much more common than Hodgkin lymphomas.
MoD: Acquired mutation in lymph cells that causes proliferation of T cells, B cells, or NK cells that invade surrounding lymph tissue.
Dx: Lymph node biopsy
Tx/Mgmt:
1. Chemotherapy
2. Radiation therapy (except in pediatric populations)

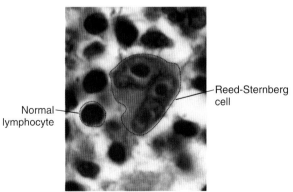

FIG. 4.2 Reed-Sternberg cell. (From National Cancer Institute, http://www.cancer.gov.)

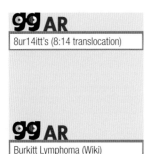

GG AR
8ur14itt's (8:14 translocation)

GG AR
Burkitt Lymphoma (Wiki)

Burkitt Lymphoma

Buzz Words: EBV exposure + rapidly growing mass in jaw + "starry sky appearance"

Clinical Presentation: Burkitt is a lymphoma of B cells causing their proliferation within germinal centers of lymph nodes. Burkitt affects children and young adults, leading to a very typical enlarging jaw mass. It is associated with immunodeficiencies, which can precipitate EBV infection leading to Burkitt.

MoD: EBV infection stimulates translocation of chromosomes 8 and 14 in B cells and leads to a constitutively active c-Myc oncogene. Other less common translocations all include chromosome 8 for c-Myc.

Dx: Tumor biopsy with "starry sky" appearance (Fig. 4.3)

Tx/Mgmt: Chemotherapy with rituximab

T-Cell Lymphoma

Buzz Words: Rash + generalized lymphadenopathy + lytic bone lesions

Clinical Presentation: This is a cancer of CD4+ T cells occurring in elderly individuals from the Caribbean or Japan. It presents with lytic bone lesions, a rash, and generalized lymphadenopathy. It is associated with HTLV-1.

PPx: N/A

MoD: Acquired mutation → proliferation of mature CD4+ T cells

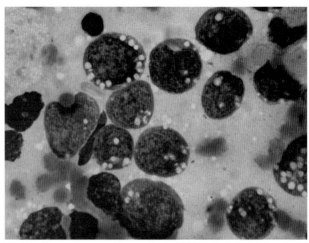

FIG. 4.3 Starry sky appearance in Burkitt lymphoma. (From Wikimedia Commons. https://commons.wikimedia.org/wiki/File:Burkitt_lymphoma,_touch_prep,_Wright_stain.jpg. In the public domain.)

Dx:
1. Lymph node biopsy
2. Flow cytometry (CD4+ T cell proliferation)

Tx/Mgmt: Chemotherapy

Anemia

Anemia should be approached systematically as microcytic (MCV < 80), macrocytic (MCV > 100), and normocytic anemias, corresponding to small-, large-, and normal-sized RBCs, respectively. Causes of microcytic anemia include: iron deficiency, thalassemias, sideroblastic anemia/lead poisoning. Causes of macrocytic anemia include B12 and folate deficiency, alcoholism/liver failure, kidney disease, and certain drugs. Normocytic anemia is further classified into hemolytic versus nonhemolytic anemias and on the basis of whether these hemolytic processes occur extravascularly or intravascularly. They can also be caused by intrinsic or extrinsic processes, respectively. A hemolytic anemia can easily be recognized by a few key features: elevated bilirubin, decreased haptoglobin, increased LDH. Clinical features will include jaundice and pallor (Fig. 4.4).

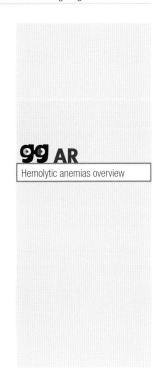

99 AR

Hemolytic anemias overview

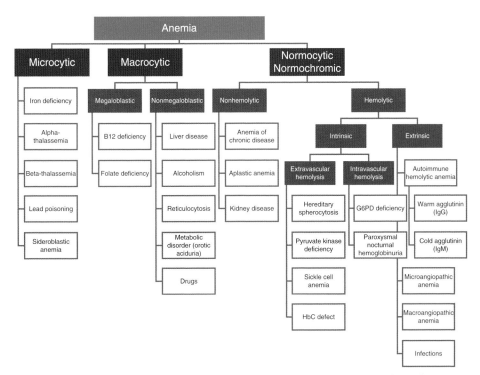

FIG. 4.4 Major types of anemia. (From https://www.youtube.com/watch?v=z2Wd3pQsnKg.)

Anemia of Chronic Disease

Buzz Words: Microcytic anemia + elevated ferritin + decreased Fe/TIBC + malignancy + autoimmune conditions

Clinical Presentation: Microcytic anemia presents with elevated ferritin (storage form of iron) but decreased serum iron levels. TIBC is decreased. Can be seen in the setting of malignancy and autoimmune conditions. Patients will present with fatigue, weakness, pallor in setting of autoimmune disorders, endocarditis, malignancy.

MoD: Chronic disease state → elevated acute phase reactants (hepcidin) → hepcidin pushes iron into storage form in order to prevent bacterial access to iron → decreased free iron causes decreased hemoglobin production → microcytic anemia

Dx:

1. CBC
2. Peripheral blood smear (microcytic anemia)
3. Iron studies (elevated ferritin, decreased serum iron, decreased TIBC)
4. Acute phase reactants (elevated hepcidin)

Tx/Mgmt:

1. Treat underlying cause, otherwise, no treatment for asymptomatic anemia
2. EPO if symptomatic
3. Transfusion if severely decreased hemoglobin

G6PD Deficiency

Buzz Words: Hemolysis and jaundice after fava bean ingestion or use of sulfa antibiotics in African Americans

Clinical Presentation: G6PD deficiency is the most common red cell enzymopathy. It is inherited in an X-linked recessive pattern, and females only get it from lyonization (X-chromosome inactivation). There are two common variants:

- G6PD A → present in 10% of AA males, decreased activity only in aged RBCs (less severe disease)
- G6PD B → present in 5% of Mediterranean and Asians, decreased activity in all RBCs

PPx: G6PD is precipitated by an acute event that induces oxidant stress; such events include acute illness, exposure to certain drugs or chemicals (naphthalene, sulfa antibiotics), or fava bean ingestion.

MoD: Glutathione is responsible for reducing oxidant free radicals in RBCs; generation of glutathione requires G6PD. In G6PD deficiency, there is decreased glutathione, rendering hemoglobin (Hb) susceptible to oxidant free radicals. This denatures Hb and form

99 AR

G6PD management

intracellular Heinz bodies; macrophages in the spleen remove Heinz bodies and form "bite cells" causing hemolysis

Dx:
1. CBC
2. G6PD biochemical assay, tested several months after acute event; don't measure during acute event, because those with the disease may have "normal" levels due to selective destruction of older cells

Tx/Mgmt: RBC transfusions for acute episodes

Pyruvate Kinase Deficiency

Buzz Words: Anemia + cholelithiasis + splenomegaly + jaundice precipitated by stress/illness + Northern European/ Japanese

Clinical Presentation: Pyruvate kinase (PK) deficiency occurs in both autosomal dominant and recessive inheritance patterns, although recessive is more common. This leads to hemolysis, which will cause anemia. Breakdown of RBCs can lead to cholelithiasis, splenomegaly, and jaundice.

PPx: Prevent precipitating factors

MoD: PK deficiency is caused by a mutation in the PKLR gene, which is important in glycolysis. This causes less ATP in RBCs and as a result leads to cell death and extravascular hemolysis under conditions in which high levels of ATP are needed.

Dx:
1. CBC (elevated reticulocytes)
2. Bilirubin levels

Tx/Mgmt:
1. Monitoring for most patients
2. In severe cases, blood transfusions/splenectomy

Hereditary Spherocytosis

Buzz Words: Jaundice + pallor + fatigue + familial pattern + spherocytes on blood smear

Clinical Presentation: This is a commonly tested disease and cause of anemia and extravascular hemolysis. The unique shape of RBCs in hereditary spherocytosis is very characteristic, and it is this unique shape that causes them to be targeted by the spleen.

MoD: Autosomal dominant disease is caused by defect in **spectrin** or other RBC structural proteins. As a result, RBCs lose surface area but NOT volume, leading to spherical shape. Spherical RBCs are destroyed in the spleen, leading to extravascular hemolysis.

Dx:

1. Osmotic fragility test (test ability for RBCs to swell in hypotonic solutions; spherocytes have less membrane integrity and rupture more easily)
2. CBC (elevated MCHC, reticulocyte count)
3. Peripheral blood smear (spherocytes [Fig. 4.5])
4. Coombs test (rule out warm AIHA)

Tx/Mgmt: Splenectomy

Hereditary Elliptocytosis (Ovalocytosis)

Buzz Words: Hemolytic anemia (pallor, jaundice) + elliptocytes on blood smear + splenomegaly + gallstones

Clinical Presentation: This is the baby brother of hereditary spherocytosis. It is a relatively benign inherited disease that gets passed down in various patterns of inheritance. In this disease, RBCs take on a spheroid shape and get cleared by the spleen, leading to a hemolytic anemia.

PPx: Folate supplementation

MoD: Various mutations (most common is Spectrin) in the RBC cytoskeleton destabilize them. Of note, ALL RBCs assume an ellipsoid shape when they pass through capillaries. However, they can rearrange themselves to a normal configuration once outside. In hereditary elliptocytosis, these RBCs never rearrange themselves and retain that shape permanently and are later removed by the spleen.

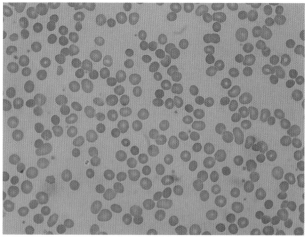

FIG. 4.5 Spherocytes on blood smear. (From Wikimedia Commons. https://commons.wikimedia.org/wiki/File:Hereditary_Spherocytosis_ smear_2010-03-17.JPG. Created by Paulo Henrique Orlandi Mourao. Used under Creative Commons Attribution-Share Alike 3.0 Unported license: https://creativecommons.org/licenses/by-sa/3.0/deed.en.)

Dx:
1. CBC
2. Blood smear (>25% of RBCs are ellipsoid)
3. Osmotic fragility testing
4. Bilirubin levels

Tx/Mgmt:
1. Monitoring, most patients are asymptomatic
2. Tx cholelithiasis with cholecystectomy if pain is problematic
3. Splenectomy in severe cases
4. Folate supplementation

Sickle Cell Disease

Sickle cell is arguably the single most commonly tested hematologic disease on every standardized exam available, including the Surgery shelf. This is a disease worth knowing cold.

Sickle cell overview

Buzz Words: Painful fingers and toes in young African-American child + fatigue, pallor + shortness of breath (acute chest) + familial pattern + splenic atrophy

Clinical Presentation: Sickle cell is an autosomal recessive trait that causes the formation of hemoglobin S. Hemoglobin S is prone to "sickling" under low oxygen states, which leads to a plethora of complications that arise from hemolysis and sickling in inappropriate places. Vasoocclusion can occur when sickled RBCs obstruct capillary beds and lead to ischemia, infarction, and necrosis of organs.

One of the most commonly infarcted organs is the **spleen**, which will lead to splenic atrophy. Many sickle cell patients are therefore functional asplenics. Lack of spleen function renders these patients susceptible to encapsulated organisms, most commonly *S. pneumoniae* and *H. influenzae*. In some cases, splenic sequestration can occur, where sickled cells get sequestered in the spleen, leading to huge falls in hemoglobin and eventual circulatory failure.

Acute chest syndrome is a common finding in patients with sickle cell disease (SCD), where sickled RBCs occlude the capillaries in the lungs, leading to respiratory compromise and hypoxemia. Dactilytis is an early finding in patients with sickle cell, which is characterized by painful fingers and toes due to sickled RBC occlusion of their vasculature. Sickle cell patients can also have aplastic crises, where an infection by parvovirus B19 (or other agents) leads to rapid degradation of RBCs, leading to abrupt declines in RBC count that can be life threatening.

Other complications of sickle cell include priapism, cholelithiasis (bilirubin breakdown → gallstones), stroke, renal papillary necrosis, ulcers, osteomyelitis pulmonary hypertension → right heart failure, and opioid tolerance and addiction. Frequently ask yourself why each of these complications happen as a means to better learn them. The precipitant behind everything anyone can get from sickle cell is **vasoocclusion and hemolysis.**

PPx: (1) Daily penicillin prophylaxis as child for *Streptococcus pneumoniae*. (2) Vaccination for *S. pneumoniae*, *Haemophilus influenzae*, *Meningococcus*. (3) Antimalarial chemoprophylaxis in areas endemic. (4) Counseling for parents with sickle trait/disease.

MoD: Glutamic acid (hydrophilic) to valine (hydrophobic) substitution of the beta-globin gene leads to sickling (hydrophobic amino acids like to aggregate) inherited in autosomal recessive fashion. Oxygen tension normally leads to high elasticity, allowing RBCs to pass through capillary beds. In sickled states, oxygen tension is unable to enhance RBC elasticity due to the aggregated, sickled beta-globin. This leads to hemolysis and vasoocclusive crises.

Dx:

1. CBC; low Hb, high reticulocyte count
2. Sodium metabisulfite–induced RBC sickling
3. Hb electrophoresis
4. UA, UCx, CXR, blood cultures for infection work-up

Tx/Mgmt:

1. Folic acid
2. Patient-controlled analgesia for vasoocclusion
3. Oxygen supplementation, transfusion for acute chest crisis
4. **Hydroxyurea** → elevated HbF production (fetal hemoglobin has higher affinity for O_2)
5. Blood transfusions
6. Bone marrow transplant (curative)

Anemia From Blood Loss

Buzz Words: Normocytic anemia + source for bleeding (heavy menstrual bleeding)

Clinical Presentation: Normocytic anemia is the **most common cause of anemia overall.** May see spoon-shaped nails or diminished attention. Occurs in setting of recent trauma or surgery. Bleeding into the retroperitoneal space or the thigh is often missed. If iron deficiency from chronic blood loss, will appear as microcytic anemia. This is an extremely important concept for the Surgery shelf since blood loss can occur following surgery.

MoD: Blood loss → increased reticulocyte formation + decrease in iron levels necessary to produce new RBCs → iron deficiency leads to worsening anemia

Dx:
1. CBC
2. Iron studies (low ferritin if chronic blood loss)
3. Identify bleeding source via imaging

Tx/Mgmt:
1. Management of the source
2. Iron supplementation for several months if there was evidence of iron deficiency on iron studies
3. Transfusion if Hb < 7 with symptoms (dyspnea, dizziness, severe fatigue)

Cytopenias

Aplastic Anemia

Buzz Words: Pancytopenia + low reticulocyte count

Clinical Presentation: Varies based on severity. Common manifestations include fatigue, bleeding, and infection. Can be precipitated by recent parvovirus B19 infection, which likes to infect the bone marrow. Fanconi anemia is an autosomal recessive congenital aplastic anemia with renal dysfunction, absent thumb and radius, short stature, and hyperpigmentation

MoD: Injury to hematopoietic stem cells caused by infection, autoimmune damage, inherited disorders, or drugs → pancytopenia

Dx:
1. CBC (low reticulocyte count)
2. Bone marrow biopsy (empty)

Tx/Mgmt:
1. Remove causative agents
2. Marrow-stimulating factors including GM-CSF, G-CSF, and EPO may be used
3. Transfusion if severe

Leukopenia

Buzz Words: Decreased white blood cell (WBC) count + recurrent infection

Clinical Presentation: Leukopenia is an isolated decrease in WBC count.

MoD: Leukopenia occurs secondary to a number of conditions, including radiation therapy, myelofibrosis, aplastic anemia, autoimmune conditions (lupus), infections, or HIV. Drugs can also cause leukopenia, and some examples include immunosuppressants or chemotherapeutic agents. Agranulocytosis is the isolated decrease in neutrophils and will be tested as this is a common manifestation of the antipsychotic clozapine.

Dx: CBC

Tx/Mgmt: Treat underlying cause

Immune Thrombocytopenic Purpura

Buzz Words: Petechiae/purpura + thrombocytopenia + s/p viral infection/immunization + increased megakaryocytes on biopsy + easy bruising/bleeding

Clinical Presentation: This is a disease characterized by low platelet counts that leads to petechiae/purpura. Immune thrombocytopenic purpura (ITP) typically is an autoimmune process that occurs secondary to infection or immunization. One characteristic finding is large numbers of megakaryocytes (platelet precursor) on bone marrow biopsy.

MoD: Various conditions like infection/immunization cause antibodies to form against platelets toward GPIIb-IIIa (fibrinogen receptor) or GPIb-Ix (vWF receptor); these antibodies cause platelets to be cleared by splenic macrophages and Kupffer cells in the liver.

Dx:

1. CBC (low platelet count)
2. PT/aPTT (normal)
3. Bleeding time (elevated)
4. Rule out secondary causes of low platelets (leukemia, cirrhosis, lupus, HIV, vWF deficiency, etc.)

Tx/Mgmt:

1. Steroids
2. Rho(D) immune globulin
3. Immunosuppressants (azathioprine, mycophenolate), IV IG
4. Thrombopoietin receptor agonists (stimulate platelet production):
   a. Romiplostim, eltrombopag
5. Splenectomy

Coagulation Disorders

Coagulation disorders are some of the highest yield concepts on the Surgery shelf, and you will likely get at least two to three questions. This is only because coagulation

99 AR

ITP vs. TTP vs. HUS vs. DIC Video

QUICK TIPS

ITP gets confused with TTP a lot. The biggest difference is the lack of anemia, renal, or neurologic findings in ITP.

disorders are everywhere and every kind of doctor, in and outside of surgery, will deal with these at some time in his or her life. Every operative procedure requires a firm understanding of all of these problems. Mastering coagulation disorders requires an understanding of the coagulation cascade but is not absolutely necessary if you are short on time. At the least, a minimum understanding should include which coagulation factors prolong PT, which prolong PTT, and which prolong both.

Next, recognize an important distinction between platelet function and clotting cascade—together, these terms come together to form coagulation. Platelets are important in forming an initial platelet plug. Platelets are activated by biomolecules released from sites of injury like ADP, thromboxane A2, vWF, and collagen. Platelets are then bound to each other by fibrinogen through the GPIIb-IIIa receptor. Remembering these steps will help you in both identifying pathologies and drug targets. Unfortunately, platelet plugs are very weak and require the support of the fibrin mesh that forms from the coagulation cascade. Thus, after platelet plug formation, the coagulation cascade is activated and forms a cross-linked fibrin clot that is much stronger to support the entire wound healing process (Fig. 4.6). Bleeding time is a measure of how long it takes to form this platelet plug and is strictly a measure of platelet activity or amount. PT/aPTT are tests of the clotting factors themselves and do not tell you anything about platelets.

99 AR
Easy way to memorize the coagulation cascade (PPT)

99 AR
Hemostasis

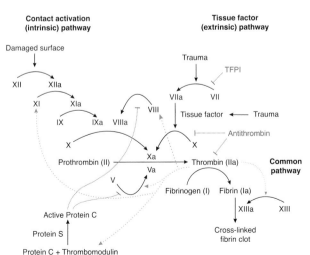

FIG. 4.6 Coagulation cascade. (From Wikimedia Commons. https://commons.wikimedia.org/wiki/File:Coagulation_full.svg. Used under GNU Free Documentation License: https://en.wikipedia.org/wiki/GNU_Free_Documentation_License.)

Recognizing these fundamental differences between platelet activation and clotting are vital to understanding how deficiencies in either are tested. Platelet activation is required only in areas where a weak plug would be sufficient to stop bleeding. Thus low-pressure venous sites tend to exhibit deficiencies in platelets to a greater degree. This will manifest with mucosal bleeding from more outward sites prominent with easily damaged venous vasculature such as the GI tract, nasal or gingival mucosa, or the uterus. Oppositely, arterial sites tend to exhibit deficiencies in clotting factors to a greater degree. This is because platelets are already insufficient for maintaining a blood clot in the high-pressure arterial system. As such, injury depends on the clotting cascade. Resultantly, deficiencies in members of the clotting cascade such as in hemophilia lead to more serious deep bleeds such as in the joints or brain.

As an organizing principle, most coagulopathies are diagnosed from CBC, PT, aPTT, and bleeding times. Treatments should be commensurate with the underlying pathologies, which should be anticoagulants in hypercoagulable states, and procoagulants in hypocoagulable states. This should be intuitive.

Hypocoagulable States

The following diseases cause hypocoagulable states, which means the coagulation system is NOT functioning and leads to bleeding. These diseases will be characterized by low levels or dysfunction of components within the coagulation cascade. This can range from the factors themselves to platelets to fibrinogen to vWF. The work-up for these diseases will always begin with a CBC, PT/aPTT, and bleeding times based on an initial clinical suspicion, and further testing is available for specific genetic abnormalities. Remember that deficiencies in platelets will lead to decreased bleeding times, whereas deficiencies in clotting factors will decrease PT/aPTT. Deficiencies in platelets (vWF, Bernard-Soulier, Glanzmann thrombasthenia) tend to lead to bleeding from mucosal surfaces, where platelet activation plays a more important role. Deficiencies in coagulation factors (hemophilia A, B) tend to lead to bleeding in deeper, more serious sites such as the joints and brain. See the previous paragraph for a more detailed explanation for why this phenomenon occurs. Treatment for the majority of these diseases is usually to replace missing procoagulation components.

Disseminated Intravascular Coagulation

Buzz Words: Ecchymoses, petechiae, purpura + bleeding from mucosal surfaces (GI tract, gingival, oral mucosa) + surgical procedure bleeding + current infection, malignancy or obstetric complication + elevated PT/aPTT + increased bleeding time/low platelets + increased fibrin split products/D-dimers

Clinical Presentation: Disseminated intravascular coagulation (DIC) is a condition in which microthrombi are formed in your body, consuming all your platelets and coagulation factors, leading to bleeding. This is usually occurring secondary to infection. Although DIC is characterized as a hypocoagulable process, it is caused by a transient hypercoagulable induced by some precipitating factor.

MoD: DIC causes pathologic, transient activation of the coagulation cascade leading to microthrombi that disseminate throughout the circulation, consuming platelets, fibrin, and coagulation factors. The absence of these factors leads to hypocoagulability and eventual hemorrhage. This is a paradoxical disease in which bleeding and thrombosis are **occurring at the same time.** This pathologic activation that starts these sequelae can be caused by infection (most common), obstetric complications, major tissue injury, malignancy, shock, or rattlesnake venom.

Dx:
1. CBC, PT/aPTT:
   a. Platelet count is decreased
   b. PT/aPTT are elevated
   c. Bleeding is elevated
2. Fibrin split products (elevated)
3. D-dimers (elevated)
4. Fibrinogen levels (decreased)
5. Peripheral blood smear (schistocytes from shearing of RBCs by microthrombi)

Tx/Mgmt:
1. Manage precipitating condition
2. Supportive measurements for severe hemorrhage (transfusions, heparin)

Hemophilia A

Buzz Words: Knee joint bleeding at early age + intracranial bleeding + hematuria + familial pattern

Clinical Presentation: It is an X-linked recessive disorder from missing factor VIII. The most common sign is joint

> **QUICK TIPS**
> The diagnostic findings from DIC should be intuitive. If too many microthrombi are forming, there should be evidence of elevated D-dimers and fibrin split products. As a result of these microthrombi, coagulation factors, fibrinogen and platelets are consumed, leading to elevated PTT, aPTT, decreased fibrinogen, decreased platelet count, and resultant elevated bleeding time.

bleeding, also known as hemarthrosis, which can lead to joint destruction. However, bleeding can occur in other areas, and the most common cause of death in these patients is intracranial bleeding.

PPx: Prevent trauma

MoD: Deficiency in factor VIII leads to defect in intrinsic pathway → hypocoagulability.

Dx:

1. CBC
2. Prolonged PTT
3. Low VIII levels and normal vWF

Tx/Mgmt:

1. Analgesia and immobilization for acute hemarthrosis
2. FVIII replacement
3. DDAVP → leads to endothelial secretion of vWF, which is a carrier for FVIII and protects it

Hemophilia B

Buzz Words: Knee joint bleeding at early age + intracranial bleeding + hematuria + familial pattern

Clinical Presentation: It is an X-linked recessive disorder; rarer than hemophilia A but presents identically. Caused by deficiency in factor IX.

PPx: Prevent trauma

MoD: Deficiency in factor IX leads to defect in intrinsic pathway → hypocoagulability.

Dx:

1. CBC
2. Prolonged PTT
3. Low VIII levels

Tx/Mgmt:

1. Analgesia and immobilization for acute hemarthrosis
2. FVIII replacement

Hypofibrinogenemia/Afibrinogenemia (Factor I Deficiency)

Buzz Words: Umbilical cord bleeding at birth + surgical bleeding (GI, oral mucosa) + splenic rupture + intracranial hemorrhage

Clinical Presentation: There is a defect in factor I (fibrinogen) that is required to become activated during the coagulation cascade. This leads to a hypocoagulable state.

PPx: Prevent trauma, avoid antiplatelets, aspirin/NSAIDs

MoD: Fibrinogen is important for both forming fibrin during the cascade and for cross-linking platelets during initial platelet plug formation. Thus this is a defect in both coagulation cascade and platelet activation. Defects in fibrinogen can also be acquired during diseases like cirrhosis.

Dx:
1. CBC
2. Fibrinogen levels
3. PT/aPTT/bleeding times (all elevated)
4. Thrombin time (elevated)

Tx/Mgmt:
1. Cryoprecipitate
2. Factor I concentrate
3. Antifibrinolytics (tranexamic acid, aminocaproic acid)

von Willebrand Disease

Buzz Words: Recurrent nosebleeds + cutaneous bleeding + gingival bleeding + bleeding after surgical procedures + menorrhagia + GI bleeding + elevated bleeding time

Clinical Presentation: vWF disease is a common, autosomal dominant disease leading to deficiency in vWF. vWF plays two roles; it binds to platelets to allow them to adhere to vessel walls and is a carrier for factor VIII that prevents it from degradation. Thus vWF plays two procoagulant roles that when missing leads to a hypocoagulable state. There are three kinds in order from most to least common:
- Type 1—decreased levels
- Type 2—dysfunctional, but normal levels
- Type 3—missing vWF (severe)

PPx: Avoid aspirin/NSAIDs → overbleeding

MoD: vWF is secreted from megakaryocytes and endothelial cells that protect FVIII in the blood from degradation and is also part of aggregating platelets by allowing them to adhere to endothelial cells after injury. In vWF disease, vWF is missing or defective, leading to an inability for platelets to aggregate and for FVIII to partake in the coagulation cascade. This leads to problems primarily with mucosal bleeding, where the most common sign is recurrent nosebleeds (epistaxis).

Dx:
1. CBC
2. PT/aPTT (normal)
3. Bleeding time (prolonged)
4. Decreased vWF and factor VIII activity
5. Ristocetin platelet aggregation (platelets will not aggregate)

Tx/Mgmt:
1. DDAVP—causes endothelial cells to secrete vWF
2. Factor VIII concentrates

Bernard-Soulier Syndrome (Hemorrhagiparous Thrombocytic Dystrophy)

Buzz Words: Bleeding after surgical procedures + easy bruising + nosebleeds + menorrhagia

Clinical Presentation: This is a rare deficiency in platelets that causes large platelets, and another name for this is giant platelet disorder. Like vWF disease and Glanzmann thrombasthenia, this disease leads to mucosal bleeding that is characteristic of platelet problems.

PPx: Avoid aspirin/NSAIDs or antiplatelet drugs

MoD: This is caused by a defect in GPIb-Ix on platelets caused by mutations in GP1BA, GP1BB, or GP9 that prevents the GPIb-IX receptor from forming. This is the receptor for vWF that allows vWF to activate platelets and for platelets to adhere to vWF on the endothelium.

Dx:
1. CBC (low platelet count)
2. PT/aPTT (normal)
3. Bleeding time (prolonged)
4. Blood smear (platelets are abnormally large)
5. Ristocetin platelet aggregation (do not aggregate)

Tx/Mgmt:
1. Platelet transfusion
2. Tranamexic acid for mucosal bleeding

Glanzmann Thrombasthenia

Buzz Words: Excessive bleeding after surgical procedure OR mucosal membrane bleeding (frequent nosebleeds, GI bleeding, menorrhagia) + petechiae + prolonged bleeding time + normal platelet count + normal PT/aPTT + autosomal inheritance pattern → Glanzmann thrombasthenia

Clinical Presentation: This is an autosomal recessive disease causing a defect in fibrinogen receptor on platelets (GPIIb-IIIa) leading to platelet hypoactivity.

PPx: Do not take antiplatelet drugs or NSAIDs

MoD: GPIIb-IIIa is required to bind to fibrinogen and cross-links platelets into a platelet plug, stabilizing initial thrombus formation. The absence of functional GPIIb-IIIa leads to a deficit in the ability to form the initial platelet plug and therefore leads to failure to form a thrombus upon injury which is most prominent in mucosal vasculature.

Dx:
1. Examine for petechiae/ecchymoses
2. CBC

3. PT/aPTT
4. Bleeding time
5. Flow cytometry
6. Antibody levels to GPIIb-IIIa
7. Ristocetin platelet aggregation:
    a. Platelets will not aggregate

Tx/Mgmt:
1. Avoid antiplatelets
2. If actively bleeding → platelet transfusions (leukocyte depleted)
3. Vaccinate against Hep B (due to multiple transfusions)
4. Oral contraceptives to control menorrhagia
5. Recombinant factor VII:
    a. Children refractory to platelet transfusions

Hypercoagulable States

The following diseases cause hypercoagulable states, which means the coagulation system is functioning and **working in overdrive**. These diseases will be characterized by high levels of components that can induce the coagulation cascade OR low levels/dysfunction in components that inhibit the coagulation cascade. The workup for these diseases will always begin with a CBC, PT/aPTT, and bleeding times based on an initial clinical suspicion, and further testing is available for specific genetic abnormalities. In most of these diseases, prophylaxis, treatment, and management will consist of anticoagulation with heparin and warfarin. This section is **extremely high yield** for the Surgery shelf. Deep vein thrombosis (DVT) and pulmonary emboli (PEs) are some of the most common complications of these diseases and are managed by surgeons frequently.

Heparin-Induced Thrombocytopenia/Thrombosis
Buzz Words: Low platelets 4–5 days following heparin administration + enlargement of clots or formation of new clots (DVTs)

Clinical Presentation: This is a disease where heparin-platelet complexes are recognized by autoantibodies, leading to platelet activation and clot formation. Resultantly, it is another disease where platelet levels are LOW while there is an overall hypercoagulable state. This is an extremely high-yield disease for the Surgery shelf.

MoD: Heparin binds to platelet factor 4 (PF4) on platelets. This complex is recognized by autoantibodies in circulation that form immune complexes that can do two things:

(1) activates platelets, leading to microthrombi and (2) platelet removal by macrophages in the spleen, leading to thrombocytopenia.

Dx:
1. CBC (low platelets)
2. ELISA for heparin/PF4 complexes
3. Doppler sonography to detect DVTs

Tx/Mgmt:
1. Discontinue heparin:
   a. Avoid warfarin because of increased risk of warfarin-induced skin necrosis
2. Switch to other anticoagulants (argatroban, danaparoid, fondaparinux, bivalirudin)

Homocysteinemia

Buzz Words: High homocysteine + recurrent thrombosis

Clinical Presentation: This is a disease caused by abnormally high levels of homocysteine in the blood and urine. This can lead to thrombosis and a hypercoagulable state but can also lead to neuropsychiatric illness and fractures.

PPx: Prevent deficiency in B6, B9, and B12; alcohol consumption can precipitate homocysteinemia

MoD: Can be caused by deficits in B6, B9, and B12 or deficiency in 5-MTHF reductase → these all elevate homocysteine levels; homocysteinemia is also related to a rare disease called homocystinuria, an autosomal recessive deficiency in cystathionine beta synthase. Elevated homocysteine levels damage endothelial lining of blood vessels, leading to thrombosis and coagulation.

Dx:
1. CBC
2. B6, B9, B12 levels
3. Complete medical evaluation

Tx/Mgmt:
1. Supplement B6, B9, B12
2. Taurine supplementation

Hypoplasminogenemia

Buzz Words: Recurrent DVT/PE + low plasminogen + family history

Clinical Presentation: This is an extremely rare disease characterized by plasminogen deficiency and impaired fibrinolysis leading to hypercoagulability and fibrin-rich membranes forming at sites of wound healing. It can also be acquired secondary to conditions that consume plasminogen, including DIC, malignancy, or trauma.

PPx: Warfarin anticoagulation

MoD: Plasminogen gets activated into plasmin, which cleaves fibrin from clots into fibrin degradation products. When plasminogen is missing, clots cannot get broken down, leading to a hypercoagulable state.

Dx:
1. CBC
2. PT/aPTT
3. Plasminogen levels (decreased)

Tx/Mgmt:
1. Treat underlying cause or acute DVT/PE, if applicable
2. Warfarin for recurrent DVT/PE

Antithrombin III Deficiency

Buzz Words: Recurrent DVT/PE + repetitive intrauterine death + requiring higher doses of heparin or heparin resistance

Clinical Presentation: Autosomal dominant deficiency occurs in ATIII, which is an inhibitor of thrombin. A deficiency leads to thrombin hyperactivity and hypercoagulability. A common finding is heparin resistance or requiring high doses of heparin because heparin requires active ATIII to work.

PPx: Screen family members

MoD: Mutation 1q23–q25 causes low or dysfunctional ATIII

Dx:
1. CBC + ATIII levels
2. Rule out liver/kidney disease

Tx/Mgmt: IV ATIII replacement

Protein C/S Deficiency

Buzz Words: Recurrent DVT or PE at young age + family history

Clinical Presentation: Protein C and S are two major cofactors that downregulate the clotting cascade. Protein C cleaves activated FV and FVIII. Protein S is a cofactor for protein C. Their absence promotes a recurrent hypercoagulable state that presents with venous thromboembolisms.

PPx: Heparin to prevent recurrent DVTs

MoD:
1. Protein C deficiency:
   a. Congenital (autosomal dominant)
   b. Acquired:
      i. Warfarin, DIC, liver disease
2. Protein S deficiency:
   a. Congenital
   b. Acquired (OCPs, pregnancy, nephrotic syndrome)

QUICK TIPS

Protein S deficiency is an underlying cause of DIC (see above).

Dx:
1. CBC
2. PT/aPTT
3. Protein C/S activity/antigen assays

Tx/Mgmt:
1. Tx DVT/PE with heparin
2. Protein C and S replacement
3. Liver transplant in severe cases

Warfarin-Induced Skin Necrosis

Buzz Words: Skin necrosis 3+ days after warfarin administration + hypercoagulability + obese, middle-aged woman + underlying protein C/S deficiency

Clinical Presentation: This is a disease in which an usually obese, middle-aged woman on anticoagulants (warfarin) for any number of reasons presents with pain and redness in some area of her skin, leading to petechiae and then purpura. The most common sites are breasts, thighs, and buttocks, all of which are surrounded with a lot of subcutaneous fat.

PPx: Prevent large loading doses of warfarin and bridge with heparin

MoD: Warfarin inhibits vitamin K–dependent factor synthesis, which includes factor II, factor VII, factor IX, factor X, and protein C and S. Protein C and S have the shortest half-lives (3–6 hours, 30 hours, respectively) and are depleted the fastest of all the factors. Therefore, during early warfarin administration, patients actually exhibit a procoagulant state due to the fact that they have lost anticoagulant factors and have not yet lost their procoagulants. This will manifest in hypercoagulability in the skin, leading to ischemia and necrosis. Patients with undiagnosed protein C and S deficiency may present with warfarin-induced skin necrosis.

Dx:
1. CBC
2. PT/aPTT, INR

Tx/Mgmt:
1. Discontinue warfarin (reverse with vitamin K)
2. Administer heparin to prevent further clotting
3. FFP, activated protein C

Factor V Leiden

Buzz Words: Recurrent episodes of DVT (leg pain after long periods of immobility) or PE (shortness of breath) + occurring before age of 40 + thrombosis in unusual sites + family history

---

QUICK TIPS

In one-third of cases, patients who get warfarin-induced skin necrosis actually have an underlying protein C deficiency.

Clinical Presentation: Factor V Leiden is a hypercoagulable state that causes recurrent thromboembolic events, thrombosis in weird sites, and usually occurs in younger individuals who have a family history of such events.

PPx: Warfarin in individuals with 2+ thromboembolic events

MoD: This is a disease caused by a mutation in the factor V gene that renders factor V unable to be inactivated by protein C—therefore factor V is always activated and leads to a hypercoagulable state that presents with DVT, PE, or thromboses in sites like the mesentery.

Dx:
1. Coagulation testing with APC resistance assay (patient cannot be on anticoagulants)
2. Genetic testing for factor V Leiden

Tx/Mgmt:
1. Tx for DVT/PE (heparin)
2. 2+ thromboembolic events → lifetime warfarin anticoagulation

Antiphospholipid Syndrome (Lupus Anticoagulant, Anticardiolipin)

Buzz Words: Repeat arterial and venous thromboses + stroke/TIA + lupus + intrauterine death or intrauterine growth restriction + placental infarctions

Clinical Presentation: Antiphospholipid antibodies lead to recurrent venous/arterial thromboses, presenting with complications like recurrent DVT/PE, stroke, and other conditions. A common presenting finding is a pregnancy complication, such as intrauterine death. APLS is categorized into primary versus secondary. Primary APLS is idiopathic in nature. Secondary APLS is caused by conditions like lupus.

MoD: Phospholipids are part of all cell membranes. Antiphospholipid antibodies are antibodies made against these components of all cell membranes. Sometimes, these phospholipids take on specific names, like cardiolipin. Anticardiolipin antibodies are antibodies toward a specific phospholipid in the mitochondrial (and hence they are also antimitochondrial) and are elevated in diseases including SLE and syphilis. These bind to ApoH, activating it and leading to inhibition of protein C. Protein C is then unable to exert its anticoagulant effect on the clotting cascade. Lupus anticoagulant is an antiphospholipid that binds to prothrombin, activating it to form thrombin leading to a procoagulant state. They also target beta2-microglobulin, which also leads to thrombosis. The lupus anticoagulant is a PROcoagulant in vivo despite its name. It receives its name for its function in vitro, where it increases PTT.

Dx:
1. CBC
2. PT/aPTT
3. Mixing test:
   a. Lupus anticoagulant will inhibit clotting in normal plasma
4. Serologic testing (ELISA)

Tx/Mgmt:
1. Observation
2. Lifelong anticoagulation

Prothrombin G20210A Mutation

Buzz Words: Caucasian/European + recurrent DVT + PE + elevated plasma prothrombin

Clinical Presentation: Common

PPx: Test family members, women should not take OCPs

MoD: It is caused by a single nucleotide polymorphism of guanine to adenine in the noncoding region of the prothrombin gene. This mutation stabilizes the mRNA of prothrombin, leading to improved synthesis and hypercoagulability.

Dx: Polymerase chain reaction (PCR) for G to A polymorphism

Tx/Mgmt:
1. Tx acute DVT/PE
2. Most patients do not require treatment
3. Lifetime anticoagulation with heparin/warfarin in serious cases

Reactions to Blood Components

Blood transfusions are listed as Tx/Mgmt for various complications listed in this chapter. Recognizing the various processes that can go wrong during a blood transfusion can go a long away (Table 4.1).

Traumatic, Mechanical, and Vascular Disorders

This section includes miscellaneous disorders involving mechanical and vascular disorders that affect the blood and lymph.

TABLE 4.1 Common Transfusion Reactions

Reaction	Signs and Symptoms	Mechanism	Treatment	Comments
Febrile nonhemolytic transfusion reaction	Fever, chills, headache, malaise, flushing	Host antibodies against donor MHC antigens or due to cytokines from leukocytes in donor blood	May need to discontinue transfusion, but usually fever resolves in 15–30 min without specific treatment. Acetaminophen may be used.	Most common transfusion reaction. Can be prevented with leukocyte filters or irradiation.
Hemolytic transfusion reaction	Fever, chills, pain at the infusion site, dark urine, nausea, shock	ABO incompatibility with host antibodies against antigens on donor RBCs	Immediately discontinue transfusion and administer fluids	Most severe reaction
Allergic transfusion reaction	Urticaria, pruritus	Allergic reaction to plasma proteins in transfused blood	Symptomatic treatment with antihistamines. Does not require discontinuing the transfusion.	Can be prevented with antihistamine pretreatment
Anaphylactic transfusion reaction	Urticaria, angioedema, wheezing, laryngeal edema, abdominal pain, hypotension, shock	Host antibodies against IgA antibodies in the donor plasma	Immediately discontinue transfusion and administer epinephrine	Usually seen in patients with IgA deficiency. Can be prevented by administering washed or IgA deficient products.
TRALI (transfusion-related acute lung injury)	Dyspnea, hypoxemia, bilateral chest infiltrates	Donor antibodies to MHC class I or class II or human neutrophil antigens. Activated neutrophils cause endothelial damage.	Immediately discontinue transfusion and provide airway support	Most common cause of transfusion-associated death
TACO (transfusion-associated circulatory overload)	Dyspnea, pulmonary edema, hypertension, peripheral edema	Rapid volume expansion	Supportive, diuretics can be used	Seen in elderly patients with heart failure or anemia. Can be prevented with slower transfusions and diuretics.

Cardiac Valve Hemolysis

Buzz Words: RBC fragmentation (schistocytes) + previous cardiac valve replacement + anemia (fatigue, pallor) + increased indirect bilirubin

Clinical Presentation: Cardiac valve hemolysis leads to a hemolytic anemia that will elevate bilirubin and LDH and decrease haptoglobin. It will also present with traditional symptoms of anemia such as jaundice, fatigue, and pallor.

PPx: Valve replacement for malfunctioning valves

MoD: Intravascular RBC shearing due to malfunctioning heart valves or VADs, platelet microthrombi in TTP, or fibrin shearing across vessels as seen in DIC.

Dx:
1. CBC
2. Peripheral smear with fragmented RBCs

Tx/Mgmt:
1. Treat underlying defect
2. In the case of prosthetic valve damage replace the valve
3. Folic acid or iron supplementation to optimize RBC production

Splenic Rupture/Laceration

Buzz Words: Pain radiating to the left shoulder (Kehr sign) + hypotension and signs of blood loss + LUQ pain + splenomegaly

Clinical Presentation: Splenic rupture/laceration can occur in the history of recent trauma or sports injury and is more likely to occur in setting of history of malaria or recent mononucleosis infection. Malaria can also cause nontraumatic splenic rupture.

MoD: Direct impact to spleen leading to rupture/laceration and bleeding.

Dx:
1. CT if stable
2. Surgery

Tx/Mgmt:
1. Surgical intervention
2. Hemodynamic stabilization
3. Transfusions

Splenic Infarct

Buzz Words: Fibrotic spleen in sickle cell patients + acute onset + LUQ abdominal pain

Clinical Presentation: It is often accompanied by fever, nausea/vomiting, leukocytosis, and splenomegaly. Suspect in patient with history of Gaucher disease (marked splenomegaly), SCD, hypercoagulability, embolic disease.

PPx: N/A

MoD: Occlusion of one or more branches of the splenic artery results in infarction of splenic tissue.

Dx: CT abdomen with contrast

Tx/Mgmt:

1. Pain management
2. If rupture or abscess formation may require surgical intervention or transfusion

Splenic Abscess

Buzz Words: LUQ pain + persistent fever (despite antibiotics) + splenomegaly

Clinical Presentation: It may also be accompanied by left pleural effusions or splenic infarcts due to septic emboli. Suspect in setting of endocarditis, recent infection with antibiotic treatment.

MoD: Splenic infection occurs secondary to septic emboli, most commonly from endocarditis.

Dx: CT abdomen with contrast

Tx/Mgmt:

1. Antibiotics
2. Splenectomy

Effects/Complications of Splenectomy

Buzz Words: Sepsis secondary to encapsulated organisms + splenectomy/functional asplenia (sickle cell patients) + fever

Clinical Presentation: Be especially wary of splenectomies in patients with inherited RBC disorders. Although these diseases are NOT tested on the Surgery shelf, they are tested if they lead to splenectomy, a surgical intervention.

PPx: Pneumococcal, meningococcal, and *H. influenzae* type b vaccines

MoD: The spleen plays an important role in humoral immunity and bacterial clearance. As such, asplenia results in increased risk of severe bacterial sepsis secondary to encapsulated organisms most notably *S. pneumoniae*, *H. influenzae*, and *Neisseria meningitides*. Physicians should have a high suspicion for encapsulated bacteria in these patients.

Dx: Blood culture if febrile

Tx/Mgmt: Broad coverage with ceftriaxone and hospital admission if febrile

Hypersplenism

Buzz Words: Splenomegaly (LUQ mass) + thrombocytopenia, anemia, neutropenia

Clinical Presentation: Hypersplenism is an overactive spleen. It can be caused by a number of things, but some of the most common are cirrhosis, lymphoma, and TB. In most cases, this will accompany splenomegaly, a large spleen. The consequence of hypersplenism is **pancytopenia.** Be wary of hypersplenism in patients with sickle cell, for whom hypersplenism can induce a sickle cell crisis.

MoD: The spleen clears the blood of circulating RBCs, platelets, and neutrophils. Hyperactivity of the spleen will lead to anemia, thrombocytopenia, and neutropenia, respectively, with associated symptoms of fatigue/pallor, easy bleeding, and recurrent infections.

Dx:
1. CBC
2. Consider liver, bone marrow, or lymph node biopsy for precipitating conditions

Tx/Mgmt:
1. Supportive
2. Transfusions
3. Splenectomy (prophylactic vaccination afterward)

GUNNER PRACTICE

1. A 62-year-old male who underwent total hip arthroplasty 2 weeks ago presents to the emergency room with difficulty breathing. He had been doing well postoperatively until earlier in the day when he developed pleuritic chest pain and shortness of breath. His temperature is 99.0°F, pulse is 110/min, blood pressure is 135/80 mm Hg, respiratory rate is 26/min, and SpO_2 is 95% on room air. A spiral CT reveals a pulmonary embolus in the left segmental pulmonary artery. The patient is admitted, and an infusion of unfractionated heparin is started. Three days later, the patient's white blood cell count is 10,000 and platelet count is 90,000. On admission, his platelet count was 340,000. Which of the following is the next best step in the management of this patient?

   A. Replace unfractionated heparin with Coumadin

   B. Replace unfractionated heparin with lepirudin

C. Replace unfractionated heparin with enoxaparin
D. Platelet transfusion
E. Whole blood transfusion

2. A 21-year-old male presents to the emergency room following a motor vehicle accident. He is complaining of severe left upper quadrant abdominal pain and left shoulder pain. His temperature is 98.9°F, blood pressure is 95/55 mm Hg, pulse is 115 bpm, respiratory rate is 18/min, and SpO$_2$ is 97% on room air. On exam, his abdomen is rigid and exquisitely tender to palpation in all quadrants with rebound tenderness. He has ecchymoses over his left 9th and 10th ribs. Bedside ultrasound reveals fluid in the peritoneal space. Multiple saline boluses are given. The patient's new vital signs are: temperature 98.9°F, blood pressure 85/50 mm Hg, pulse 118 bpm, respiratory rate 20/min, SpO$_2$ 97% on room air. What is the next best step in the management of this patient?
A. Abdominal radiograph
B. Ultrasound of the kidneys, ureter, and bladder
C. CT of the abdomen and pelvis
D. Exploratory laparotomy
E. Continue saline boluses and add phenylephrine

3. A 17-year-old male is discharged from the hospital after undergoing a laparoscopic splenectomy for a splenic rupture he sustained when he was tackled at a rugby game. His postoperative course was uneventful. He was scheduled to follow-up with his surgeon and a hematologist in 1 week for normal postoperative care. However, following discharge he did not show up for his follow-up visits. Which of the following complications will this patient be at increased risk for without appropriate follow-up?
A. Infection with members of the herpes virus family
B. Idiopathic thrombocytopenic purpura
C. Thrombotic thrombocytopenic purpura
D. Hereditary spherocytosis
E. Meningococcemia

ANSWERS: What Would Gunner Jess/Jim Do?

1. WWGJD? A 62-year-old male who underwent total hip arthroplasty 2 weeks ago presents to the emergency room with difficulty breathing. He had been doing well postoperatively until earlier in the day when he developed pleuritic chest pain and shortness of breath. His temperature is 99.0°F, pulse is 110/min, blood pressure is 135/80 mm Hg, respiratory rate is 26/min, and SpO$_2$ is 95% on room air. A spiral CT reveals a pulmonary embolus in the left segmental pulmonary artery. The patient is admitted and an infusion of unfractionated heparin is started. Three days later, the patient's white blood cell count is 10,000 and platelet count is 90,000. On admission, his platelet count was 340,000. Which of the following is the next best step in the management of this patient?

Answer: B, replace unfractionated heparin with lepirudin

Explanation: This patient develops thrombocytopenia following initiation of heparin for a pulmonary embolus. This presentation is consistent with **heparin-induced thrombocytopenia (HIT)**, a disorder caused by antibodies against the heparin-platelet factor 4 complex. The management of HIT involves stopping heparin and replacing it with a direct thrombin inhibitor such as lepirudin or argatroban.

A. Replace unfractionated heparin with Coumadin → Incorrect. Coumadin is an appropriate long-term anticoagulant but is not appropriate as an immediate replacement of heparin because it takes several days for Coumadin to become effective.

C. Replace unfractionated heparin with enoxaparin → Incorrect. Enoxaparin is a form of low-molecular-weight heparin (LMWH). HIT can be caused by unfractionated and low-molecular-weight forms of heparin. All heparin products must be stopped in the case of HIT.

D. Platelet transfusion → Incorrect. Additional platelets will still be subject to antibody-mediated platelet destruction. Heparin must be discontinued and replaced with a direct thrombin inhibitor.

E. Whole blood transfusion → Incorrect. Whole blood transfusion will not address the underlying cause of HIT. Heparin must be discontinued and replaced with a direct thrombin inhibitor.

2. WWGJD? A 21-year-old male presents to the emergency room following a motor vehicle accident. He is complaining of severe left upper quadrant abdominal pain and left shoulder pain. His temperature is 98.9°F, blood pressure is 95/55 mm Hg, pulse is 115 bpm, respiratory rate is 18/min, and SpO_2 is 97% on room air. On exam, his abdomen is rigid and exquisitely tender to palpation in all quadrants with rebound tenderness. He has ecchymoses over his left 9th and 10th ribs. Bedside ultrasound reveals fluid in the peritoneal space. Multiple saline boluses are given. The patient's new vital signs are: temperature 98.9°F, blood pressure 85/50 mm Hg, pulse 118 bpm, respiratory rate 20/min, SpO_2 97% on room air. What is the next best step in the management of this patient?

Answer: D, exploratory laparotomy

    Explanation. This patient presents with acute left upper quadrant abdominal pain and physical exam and imaging findings consistent with hemoperitoneum. He has likely sustained a **splenic laceration** leading to fluid in the peritoneal space and referred pain to the shoulder via diaphragmatic irritation (Kerr sign). This patient has an acute abdomen and is hemodynamically unstable. Exploratory laparotomy is urgently indicated to identify the source of bleeding.

    A. Abdominal radiograph → Incorrect. This patient is hemodynamically unstable and requires immediate intervention. Additional imaging is not needed at this time.

    B. Ultrasound of the kidneys, ureter, and bladder → Incorrect. This patient is hemodynamically unstable and requires immediate intervention. Additional imaging is not needed at this time.

    C. CT of the abdomen and pelvis → Incorrect. This patient is hemodynamically unstable and requires immediate intervention. Additional imaging is not needed at this time.

    E. Continue saline boluses and add phenylephrine → Incorrect. This patient remains hypotensive despite multiple fluid boluses. Definitive intervention is needed to identify the source of the bleed. Vasoconstrictive agents such as phenylephrine are not indicated in this case.

3. WWGJD? A 17-year-old male is discharged from the hospital after undergoing a laparoscopic splenectomy for a splenic rupture he sustained when he was tackled at a rugby game. His postoperative course was uneventful. He was scheduled to follow-up with his surgeon and a hematologist in 1 week for normal postoperative care. However, following discharge he did not show up for his follow-up visits. Which of the following complications will this patient be at increased risk for without appropriate follow-up?

Answer: E, meningococcemia

Explanation: Patients who have undergone splenectomy are at increased risk for infection with encapsulated bacteria. These patients should receive vaccinations against the encapsulated bacteria *S. pneumoniae*, *H. influenzae*, and *N. meningitidis* to prevent these infections. This patient will be at increased risk of infection by all of these bacteria unless he receives the appropriate preventive measures.

A. Infection with members of the herpes virus family → Incorrect. There is no increased risk for viral infections among splenectomized patients.

B. Idiopathic thrombocytopenic purpura → Incorrect. Splenectomy is the definitive treatment for steroid-resistant idiopathic thrombocytopenic purpura.

C. Thrombotic thrombocytopenic purpura → Incorrect. Splenectomy is the definitive treatment for relapsing or plasma exchange-resistant thrombotic thrombocytopenic purpura.

D. Hereditary spherocytosis → Incorrect. Hereditary spherocytosis (HS) is a genetic condition that leads to spherically shaped RBCs and hemolytic anemia. Splenectomy is the definitive treatment for HS.

Diseases of the Nervous System and Special Senses

Kaitlyn Barkley, Hao-Hua Wu, Leo Wang, Drake Lebrun, Rebecca Gao, and Chuang-Kuo Wu

Introduction

Like the other chapters in this book, the key to success on the following topics is understanding the medical management of surgical diseases. In fact, although this chapter may seem like it is testing Neurosurgery, it is actually testing Neurology topics. You can refer to Gunner Goggles Neurology for more information, although the details in this chapter should be sufficient for the Surgery shelf exam. For more information, and for resources to help you succeed on your Neurosurgery clerkship, utilize the Gunner Column and Gunner Goggles app.

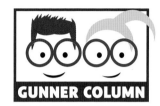

There are a few medical terms that you need to understand in order to excel:

1. **Miosis**: Very small pupil size. On the shelf exam, this is usually due to opiate use, but is also associated with an excess of parasympathetic input and, thus, can been seen with cholinergics. Additionally, miosis is seen in Horner syndrome because the sympathetic fibers are impaired.
2. **Mydriasis**: Very large pupil size. On the shelf, this can be associated with brain herniation or drug use.
3. **Aniosocoria**: Unequal pupil where at least one pupil has miosis or mydriasis. Associated with brain herniation, Horner syndrome, and other unilateral neurological disease.
4. **Palsy**: Paralysis, usually refers to impairment of extraoccular muscles. Recall that CN IV controls the superior oblique and CN VI controls the lateral rectus. CN III controls other extraoccular muscles
5. **Plegia**: Total paralysis. Used with the prefix of either quadri- or para- to mean paralysis in every limb or the lower limbs, respectively.
6. **Paresis**: Partial paralysis. Used with the prefix of either quadri- or para- to mean paralysis in every limb or the lower limbs, respectively.
7. **Anesthesia**: Lack of sensation.
8. **Paresthesia**: Abnormal sensation, "pins and needles."

9. **Fasiculations**: Twitching of a muscle indicative of denervation and lower motor neuron disease.
10. **Spasiticity**: Tightness in muscles usually associated with paralysis and upper motor neuron disease.

When trying to pick the best answer to any NBME question, your first consideration should always be the ABCs: airway, breathing, and circulation. If the patient is stable, answer choices such as "obtain a history," "perform a physical exam," or "give intravenous (IV) fluids" are probably correct. From there, try to pick the least invasive diagnostic tool or treatment. For example, if you suspect a patient has a brain tumor, get a magnetic resonance imaging (MRI) before trying to resect the tumor.

Infectious, Immunologic, and Inflammatory Disorders

Bacterial Meningitis

Buzz Words:
- **Meningitis**: nuchal rigidity + photophobia + headache + fever + college students/military recruits
- **Waterhouse-Friderichsen**: Adrenal insufficiency + petechiae + meningococcemia

Clinical Presentation: Headache, fever, meningismus progressing to altered mental status. *Neisseria meningitidis* is common in college students and military recruits, and is associated with a petechial rash (Fig. 5.1) and Waterhouse-Friderichson syndrome. *Listeria* is associated with seizures and focal (usually hindbrain) neurological deficits.

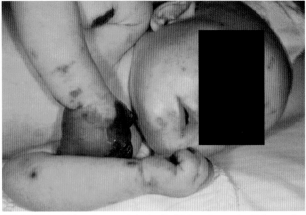

FIG. 5.1 Petechial rash associated with *Neisseria meningitidis* resulting in gangrene of the hand. (From Centers for Disease Control and Prevention, http://phil.cdc.gov/. Provided by Mr. Gust.)

- Brudzinski sign: spontaneous flexion of the hips in response to flexion of the neck
- Kernig sign: inability to extend knee with hip flexed

Prophylaxis (PPx):
- Vaccines for *N. meningitides, Streptococcus pneumonia,* and *Haemophilus influenza*
- In known *N. meningitides* exposure give rifampin, ceftriaxone, or ciprofloxacin

Mechanism of Disease (MoD): Bacteria infects the arachnoid mater causing an inflammatory response. Responsible bugs: *Actinomyces, H. influenza, Listeria,* tuberculosis, *N. meningitidis, Staphylococcus aureus/epidermidis, Streptococcus agalactiae, S. pneumoniae*

Diagnostic Steps (Dx):
1. If the presenting symptom is seizure or focal neurological sign, get a head computed tomography (CT) first.
2. Lumbar puncture to test for RBC, WBC, protein, and glucose. Refer to Table 5.1 for the expected results from different types of meningitis.

Treatment and Management Steps (Tx/Mgmt):
1. Antibiotics (until culture results are in, broad spectrum is preferred including MRSA coverage). In questions about the "next best step", it is difficult to decide if antibiotics should be started before a lumbar puncture is performed. If the patient is very sick (coma, signs of shock) then start broad spectrum antibiotics. If the patient is stable, obtain the lumbar puncture before starting antibiotics.
2. *N. meningitidis* is a public health concern, meaning that patients cannot refuse treatment for themselves or their child.

TABLE 5.1 Lumbar Puncture Results by Etiology

	RBC	WBC	Protein	Glucose
Bacterial meningitis	WNL	↑↑ (neutrophils)	↑↑	↓↓
Viral meningitis	WNL	↑ (lymphocytes)	↑↑	WNL/↓
Fungal meningitis	WNL	↑↑	↑↑	WNL/↓
HSV encephalitis	WNL/↑	↑	↑	↓
Subarachnoid hemorrhage	↑ + xanthochromia	WNL	WNL	WNL
Guillan-Barré syndrome	WNL	WNL	↑↑↑	WNL

HSV, Herpes simplex virus; *RBC,* red blood cells; *WNL,* within normal limits.

Viral Meningitis

Buzz Words: Meningismus + stable vital signs + lymphocyte predominant leukocytosis on lumbar puncture

Clinical Presentation: Similar to bacterial meningitis but less "toxic," meaning vital signs are relatively stable and the patient does not have altered mental status.

PPx: Avoid exposure (e.g., insect repellant, safe sex), vaccines (VZV, MMR)

MoD: Same as bacterial meningitis. Responsible bugs: **adenovirus**, arboviruses, echovirus, and coxsackie A & B viruses, polioviruses, **herpes simplex virus** (HSV), varicella zoster, human immunodeficiency virus (HIV), lymphocytic choriomeningitis virus, measles virus, mumps virus, St. Louis encephalitis virus, California encephalitis virus, Western equine encephalitis virus.

Dx: Lumbar puncture. Refer to Table 5.1 for results.

Tx/Mgmt:

1. Supportive care, symptomatic relief
2. Acyclovir for HSV meningitis

Other Types of Meningitis

Buzz Words: Meningismus + HIV or bull's eye rash

Clinical Presentation: Same as other types of meningitis but with a history of immunodeficiency or recent spinal injections, lumbar puncture, or neurological surgery. Lyme (*Borrelia burgdorferi*) meningitis is associated with tick exposure and bull's eye rash.

PPx: Avoid exposure, treatment, and prophylaxis for patients with HIV. See Table 5.2 for prophylaxis of opportunistic infections in HIV.

MoD: Same as bacterial meningitis:

- Fungi: *Blastomycosis dermatitidis, Cryptococcus neoformans/gattii*
- Spirochetes: *B. burgdorferi; Leptospira; Treponema pallidum* (neurosyphilis)
- Protozoans/Helminths: *Acanthamoeba, Naegleria fowleri, Strongyloides*

Dx: Lumbar puncture, refer to Table 5.1

Tx/Mgmt: Dependent on which microbe is identified. Generally: fungi respond to –azoles, spirochetes should be treated with doxycycline (*Borrelia*) or penicillin (*Treponema*), and protozoans respond to –azoles.

Herpes Simplex Virus Encephalitis

Buzz Words: Fever + signal seen on bilateral medial temporal lobes on MRI + focal neurological deficit

TABLE 5.2 Prophylaxis of Opportunistic Infections in Patients With Human Immunodeficiency Virus

CD4 Count	Management (Microbe: Antibiotic)
<200	PCP: TMP-SMX
<100	*Toxoplasma*: TMP-SMX
<50	MAC: azithromycin or clarithromycin

Other Condition	Management (Microbe: Antibiotic)
TB exposure	TB: INH+B$_6$
Histoplasma exposure plus CD4 <150	*Histoplasma*: Itraconazole

TB, Tuberculosis.

Clinical Presentation: Altered mental status, fever, ±signs of meningitis. The main distinguishing feature from meningitis is the lack of focal neurological signs in the latter.

Note: There are other causes of encephalitis, but this is the only one specifically mentioned by NBME.

PPx: Avoid HSV exposure.

MoD: Like any HSV reactivation, an event triggers the virus to begin to replicate. The virus itself does not destroy brain tissue but the immunologic response does. Subsequent swelling can be rapidly fatal.

Dx:
1. Lumbar puncture, see Table 5.1
2. Diagnosis is confirmed via cerebrospinal fluid (CSF) polymerase chain reaction (PCR) for HSV DNA

Tx/Mgmt: Fatal if untreated. Start acyclovir for any clinically suspected cases of HSV encephalitis. Do not wait for lumbar puncture, labs, or imaging.

Neoplasms

Meningioma

Buzz Words: NF2 or MEN1 + dural wing on MRI or calcifications on CT + slow growing

Clinical Presentation: Neurological symptoms depend on location. Most meningiomas are incidental findings. If symptomatic, patients often present with symptoms of mass effect including deficits of the underlying cortex or hydrocephalus.

MoD: Associated with genetic syndromes including NF2 and MEN1 and with radiation exposure. Hormones also play a role, as there is a female predominance during reproductive years.

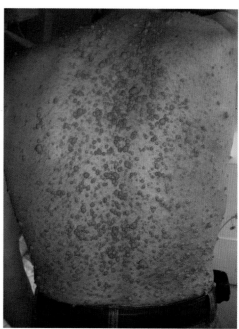

FIG. 5.2 Neurofibromas. (From Wikimedia Commons. https://commons.wikimedia.org/wiki/File:Neurofibroma02.jpg. Created by Klaus D. Peter, Gummersbach, Germany. Used under Creative Commons Attribution 3.0 Germany license: https://creativecommons.org/licenses/by/3.0/de/deed.en.)

Dx:
1. Can be seen on a CT (hyperdense due to calcifications) and MRI (will show dural wing)
2. Definitive diagnosis via biopsy

Tx/Mgmt:
1. Watch and wait
2. Surgical resection if symptomatic and amenable location

Neurofibromatosis Type 1 (von Recklinghausen Disease)

Buzz Words: Neurofibroma + optic glioma + café au lait spot + Lisch nodule + axillary and inguinal freckling

Clinical Presentation: Skin abnormalities and neurofibromas (Fig. 5.2) appear very early. Patients typically have multiple tumors early in childhood and the tumors may become malignant in adulthood.

MoD: Autosomal dominant mutation on chromosome 17 leading to defective neurofibromin, which is a GTPase-activating protein (GAP), which is involved in the mTOR pathway.

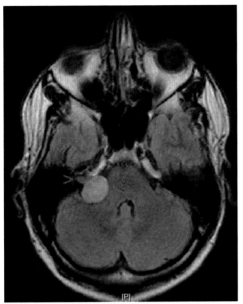

FIG. 5.3 Acoustic neuroma. (From Wikimedia Commons. https://commons.wikimedia.org/wiki/File:Akustikusneurinom_Mrt.jpg. In the public domain.)

Dx: Clinically based on symptoms or via DNA testing.

Tx/Mgmt: Treat symptomatic tumors and screen for new tumors.

Neurofibromatosis Type 2

Buzz Words: Bilateral acoustic neuromas/vestibular schwannomas (Fig. 5.3) → NF2

Clinical Presentation: Ninety-five percent will have vestibular schwannomas by the fourth decade of life. Other neural and glial tumors are common as well as cutaneous manifestations similar to NF1.

Note: Acoustic neuroma is a misnomer for a vestibular schwannoma. The true histology of these tumors is that of Schwann cells (not neurons) and often they arise from the vestibular nerve (not the cochlear nerve).

MoD: Autosomal dominant mutation on chromosome 22 leading to defective Merlin protein.

Dx: CT to detect schwannoma and neuromas. Requires presence of bilateral acoustic neuromas or a first-degree relative with NF2, and a neural or glial tumor, or two neural or glial tumors.

Tx/Mgmt: Treat symptomatic tumors and screen for new tumors

Glioblastoma Multiforme

Buzz Words: Butterfly glioma crossing corpus collosum + grade IV glioma (Fig. 5.4)

Clinical Presentation: Classically presents with gradual onset of focal neurological signs with signs of elevated intracranial pressure including headache with nausea and vomiting that is worse in the morning.

MoD: De novo or progression of lower grade glioma to a grade IV glioma, or glioblastoma multiforme (GBM). Genes to know: PTEN.

Dx:
1. CT imaging which will show a butterfly (bilateral, across the corpus callosum) mass
2. Confirmed by biopsy

Tx/Mgmt: Surgery, radiation, chemotherapy. Poor prognosis.

Astrocytoma

Buzz Words: Seizures + cystic appearance on imaging and gross exam + posterior fossa (e.g., cerebellum) + GFAP positive + children → pilocytic astrocytoma

Clinical Presentation: Two common types: Pilocytic, diffuse:
- **Pilocytic:** Slow-growing tumor usually found in the cerebellum or third ventricle in children. Those in the cerebellum may cause problems with coordination, whereas those in the third ventricle often cause

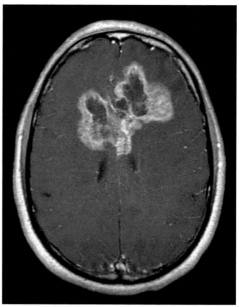

FIG. 5.4 Butterfly glioblastoma multiforme. (From Radiopaedia. https://radiopaedia.org/articles/glioblastoma.)

hydrocephalus (discussed later in this chapter). There is an association between pilocytic astrocytomas and the NF1 gene, so these patients may have other signs and symptoms related to NF1.

- **Diffuse:** Slow-growing tumors usually found in the cerebral cortex in young adults (third to fourth decade). Symptoms depend on location but seizures are common.

MoD: Series of inherited or genetic changes leading to uncontrolled cell growth. Genes to know: NF1, p53.

Dx: Suggested by imaging; confirmed by biopsy.

Tx/Mgmt: Surgical resection

Medulloblastoma

Buzz Words: Cerebellar location + drop metastases to spinal cord + ataxia + children

Clinical Presentation: Medulloblastoma is the most common malignant brain tumor of childhood. It presents with similar symptoms to pilocytic astrocytoma because it is found in the posterior fossa. Children typically have morning headache with nausea and vomiting as well as ataxia.

MoD: Series of inherited or genetic changes leading to uncontrolled cell growth. Genes to know: PTCH1, APC.

Dx: Suggested by imaging; confirmed by biopsy.

Tx/Mgmt: Surgical resection

Primary Central Nervous System Lymphoma

Buzz Words: HIV positive + solitary ring-enhancing mass

Clinical Presentation: Typically presents in a patient with immunodeficiency (such as HIV) as a focal neurological deficit related to the location of the mass. Rarely, these tumors can be leptomeningeal or spinal. May be associated with Epstein-Barr virus (EBV) or recent gastrointestinal (GI) illness.

PPx: Avoid HIV exposure.

MoD: Series of inherited or genetic changes leading to uncontrolled cell growth. It is believed that the cells arise from lymph nodes (likely B cells), which are essentially eradicated by the peripheral immune system. If a malignant cell is able to invade the central nervous system (CNS), it is able to evade the immune system and proliferate. In men, the testes should be checked since the disease can be found in both locations.

Dx:
1. Suggested by imaging and CSF studies (cytology can show lymphoma cells)
2. Confirmed by biopsy

Tx/Mgmt:
1. It is very sensitive to chemotherapy and radiation (methotrexate and whole brain radiation).
2. For immediate treatment of symptoms, steroids are helpful.

Note: rituximab is not approved for CNS lymphoma.

Metastatic Tumors (e.g., Breast, Lung, Pancreatic, Testicular, Melanoma)

Buzz Words: Mass in the gray-white junction + history of cancer

Clinical Presentation: Elderly patient with PMHx of cancer with new mass (or multiple masses) in the gray-white junction. Symptoms depend on location of the mass.

PPx: Prevention of primary cancer

MoD: Hematogenous spread of malignancy favors metastasis to the brain since the brain receives a large portion of the cardiac output.

Dx: Suggested by imaging; confirmed by biopsy

Tx/Mgmt: Typically resection, chemotherapy, or radiation

Cerebrovascular Disease

Arteriovenous Malformations

Buzz Words: Severe headache + seizure + hemorrhage w/o history of trauma + clump of vessels seen on neuroimaging

Clinical Presentation: Symptomatic arteriovenous malformations (AVMs) are typically identified when the cause intracranial hemorrhage. The hemorrhage is often intraparenchymal but may be subarachnoid (see below). Symptoms of the hemorrhage depend on location and severity. Nonruptured AVMs may also cause seizures.

MoD: Poorly understood: AVMs are a tangle of arteries and veins without capillaries. The surrounding tissue is typically gliotic, which means it lacks normal neurons. Associated with: Osler-Weber-Rendu syndrome (hereditary hemorrhagic telangiectasia).

Dx:
1. Suggested on CT or MRI
2. Angiography (CTA, MRA or DSA) can confirm. The AVM veins fill much more quickly than regular veins since the capillaries are bypassed. This results in the characteristic early venous filling.

Tx/Mgmt:
1. Surgery if accessible
2. Stereotactic radiosurgery (i.e., Gamma Knife)
3. Endovascular occlusion

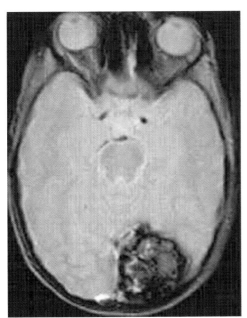

FIG. 5.5 Cavernoma "popcorn" appearance. (From Cortés Vela JJ, Concepción Aramendía L, Ballenilla Marco F, Gallego León Jl, González-Spínola San Gil J: Cerebral cavernous malformations: spectrum of neuroradiological findings. *Radiologia* 54(5):401–409, 2012.)

Cavernoma (Cavernous Malformation)

Buzz Words: Popcorn mass + hemorrhage + hemorrhage worse on radiology than clinical picture

Clinical Presentation: These vascular malformations are very similar to AVMs, although they are less common. They, too, are found in patients with intraparenchymal hemorrhage. Unlike AVMs, they are associated with developmental venous anomalies. Cavernomas usually bleed within themselves so they result in fewer neurological deficits.

MoD: Tangle of immature vessels that is well marginated. When these vessels bleed, they typically bleed into themselves without damaging surrounding tissue.

Dx: T1 and T2 MRI show a "popcorn" lesion (Fig. 5.5).

Tx/Mgmt: Surgery if accessible. Stereotactic radiosurgery is not recommended.

Transient Ischemic Attack

Buzz Words: Stroke symptoms + <24 hours + no lesions on MRI

Clinical Presentation: Focal, localizable neurological deficit that lasts less than 24 hours. See Table 5.3 for summary of stroke syndromes by vessel.

Amaurosis fugax is a transient ischemic attack (TIA) of the ophthalmic artery that is typically caused by carotid

TABLE 5.3 Clinical Stroke Syndromes

	Vessel	Syndrome
Anterior circulation	Ophthalmic	Loss of vision in one eye
	ACA	Contralateral sensory and motor impairment (legs), abulia, dyspraxia, psych changes, primitive reflexes, urinary incontinence
	MCA (dominant)	Contralateral sensory and motor impairment (arms), aphasia, eye toward infarct, homonymous hemianopsia
	MCA (nondominant)	Contralateral sensory and motor impairment (arms), neglect, eye toward infarct, homonymous hemianopsia
Posterior circulation	PCA	Homonymous hemianopsia, alexia without agraphia
	PICA	Wallenberg syndrome (lateral medullary syndrome): Pain and temperature impairment to ipsilateral face and contralateral body, CNX involvement (hoarse, dysarthria), ipsilateral Horner syndrome, hiccups, lack of sleep respiration
	AICA	Lateral pontine syndrome (AICA syndrome): Vomiting, nystagmus, dysarthria, ipsilateral facial paralysis and numbness, contralateral loss of pain and temperature
	ASA	Medial medullary syndrome: Contra body paralysis and sensation loss, tongue toward lesion
	Lacunar	Pure motor hemiparesis—posterior limb of internal capsule → arm, face, and leg equally weak without sensory sx Pure sensory stroke—VPL nucleus of thalamus Ataxic- hemiparesis—anterior limb of internal capsule Dysarthria, clumsy hand—basis pons Note: hemorrhagic strokes are often in the same vessels as lacunar strokes. The symptoms can be similar but computed tomography scans can distinguish the two.

atherosclerosis embolization. Patients describe a vertical curtain coming down over the eye, which improves gradually over the next few minutes.

PPx: Treat risk factors. Statins for atherosclerosis. Anticoagulants for atrial fibrillation and hypercoaguable states. Immunosupressants for vasculitis.

MoD: May be intrinsic or extrinsic. Classically caused by carotid atherosclerosis or embolization of atrial thrombus in atrial fibrillation.

Dx:
1. Non-con head CT
2. Brain MRI
3. Carotid duplex or CT angiogram of head/neck
4. Cardiac echo (look for thrombus in left atrium, especially in patients with Afib)

Typically damage not immediately visualized on imaging but may see on diffusion weighted imaging (DWI) sequence MRI.

Tx/Mgmt: Depends on suspected cause but generally include: aspirin, clopidogrel, antihypertensives, and statins. Also, a work-up of carotid artery disease is needed.

Ischemic Stroke

Buzz Words: Hyperlipidemia or atrial fibrillation + focal neurological symptoms

Clinical Presentation: Depends on location of stroke. See Table 5.3 for a summary of stroke syndromes.

PPx: Risk factor modifications—statins, antihypertensives, diabetes control, antiplatelet agents

MoD:
- **Thrombotic:** Cerebral vessel becomes gradually occluded by plaque or blood clot.
- **Embolic:** Material from heart (atrial thrombus or endocarditis) or elsewhere (DVT if PFO is present) travels to brain and causes acute ischemia.

Dx:
1. Non-con CT (changes seen depends on time since onset)
2. MRI (can help determine if the tissue is salvageable)
3. Carotid duplex
4. Echocardiogram

Tx/Mgmt:
1. ABCs
2. tPA if eligible: young with recent (<4.5 hours) stroke onset and without blood on head CT. Criteria may vary by institution but those rules should be enough for the NBME Exam.

3. Interventional thrombectomy if 6–8 hours
4. Warfarin
5. Anti-platelet agents
6. Secondary prevention of modifiable risk factors (e.g., hypertension [HTN])

Subarachnoid Hemorrhage

Buzz Words: Worst headache of life/thunderclap headache + aneurysm

Clinical Presentation: Variable: The Hunt Hess grading scale makes the following distinction based on clinical symptoms:

- Grade 1—Headache ± nuchal rigidity (30% mortality)
- Grade 2—Severe headache +severe nuchal rigidity ± cranial nerve deficit (40% mortality)
- Grade 3—Lethargy, confusion, focal neurological deficits (50% mortality)
- Grade 4—Stuporous, severe focal deficits (80% mortality)
- Grade 5—Comatose (90% mortality)

PPx: Treatment of aneurysms via coils, clips, or stents

MoD: Aneurysms are typically located prior to the vessels penetrating the pia. When they rupture, the blood accumulates in the subarachnoid space. The blood can irritate the arteries leading to vasospasm and severe ischemia. Rupture of berry aneurysm is common on the shelf.

Dx:

1. CT head
2. Lumbar puncture if CT is negative but high clinical suspicion (Fig. 5.6)

Tx/Mgmt:

1. ABCs
2. Discontinue antiplatelet and anticoagulant drugs
3. Aneurysms should be treated with coils, clips or stents. NBME will not expect you to know which particular method should be used.
4. Blood pressure control
5. Nimodipine for vasospasm several days to weeks later

Cerebral Aneurysm

Buzz Words: Ehlers-Danlos + polycystic kidney disease + Moyamoya

Clinical Presentation: The discussion below is for unruptured aneurysms. Ruptured aneurysms usually cause subarachnoid hemorrhage, which was discussed

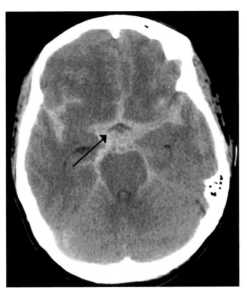

FIG. 5.6 Subarachnoid hemorrhage showing blood in the basal cisterns. (From Wikimedia Commons. https://commons.wikimedia.org/wiki/File:SubarachnoidP.png. Created by James Heilman, MD. Used under Creative Commons Attribution-Share Alike 3.0 Unported license: https://creativecommons.org/licenses/by-sa/3.0/deed.en.)

previously. Aneurysms are typically asymptomatic, but may present with headache prior to rupture. There is a slight female predominance.

PPx: Avoid risk factors (HTN, cigarette smoking)

MoD: Intrinsic or acquired weakness in vessel wall results in aneurysm formation. Typically found at branch points with the anterior communicating artery branch points being the most common. Certain diseases, such as Ehlers-Danlos, polycystic kidney disease and Moya Moya, put patients at increased risk for aneurysms.

Dx: Angiography (CTA, MRA, or DSA)

Tx/Mgmt: Generally, aneurysms greater than 7 mm are at high risk for rupture and should be treated with coils, clips, or stents.

Carotid Artery Disease

Buzz Words: Hyperlipidemia + TIA symptoms + carotid ultrasound abnormalities

Clinical Presentation: The carotid artery supplies the anterior circulation of the brain and is connected by the posterior communicating arteries to the posterior circulation,

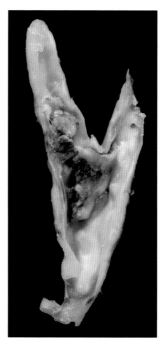

FIG. 5.7 Carotid endarterectomy specimen removed from the lumens of the common, internal, and external carotid arteries. (From Wikimedia Commons. https://commons.wikimedia.org/wiki/File:Carotid_Plaque.jpg. Created by Ed Uthman, MD. Used under Creative Commons Attribution 2.0 Generic license: https://creative-commons.org/licenses/by/2.0/deed.en.)

which is supplied via the vertebral arteries. Disease in the anterior circulation affects the anterior and middle cerebral arteries. Prior to the branching of the cerebral arteries, the ophthalmic artery and superior hypophyseal artery branch from the carotid. Carotid artery atherosclerosis may present as amaurosis fugax, which is a TIA of the ophthalmic artery.

PPx: Statins, lifestyle modification

MoD: Elevated blood cholesterol is deposited in the carotid artery.

Dx:

1. Carotid duplex (ultrasound)
2. Angiography (CTA, MRA)

Tx/Mgmt:

1. Statins
2. Antiplatelet agents (aspirin, clopidogrel)
3. Carotid endarterectomy (Fig. 5.7)
4. For greater than 80% stenosis, endovascular stenting is also an option

Vertebral Artery Disease

Buzz Words:
- **Vertebral artery dissection:** Motor vehicle collision (MVC) or chiropractor visit + vertigo + imbalance + hemianopsia

Clinical Presentation: Vertebral artery problems can be traumatic or otherwise. Trauma may occur in a MVC or by a chiropractor leading to vertebral artery dissection. Vertebral artery disease can also be caused by the same processes that leads to carotid artery disease. Symptoms can result from and distal effects on the posterior circulation. Table 5.3 summarizes stroke syndromes.

PPx: Statins, lifestyle modification

MoD: Variable

Dx: Angiography (CTA, MRA, DSA)

Tx/Mgmt: Depends on etiology. Cannot be accessed for open plaque removal so endovascular treatment is used.

Subclavian Steal Syndrome

Buzz Words: Claudication of arm (coldness, tingling, muscle pain) + visual symptoms + equilibrium problems (posterior neurologic signs) + symptoms during arm exercise

Clinical Presentation: May be related to arm or posterior fossa ischemia. In the arm: pain, fatigue, coolness, paresthesias, atrophy. Cerebral symptoms include: dizziness, vertigo, ataxia, vision changes, and hearing loss.

MoD: Reversal of flow in the vertebral artery in response to stenosis in the subclavian or innominate artery. May be due to compression at the thoracic outlet, Takayasu arteritis, or aortic coarctation.

Bloodflow in Subclavian Steal Syndrome

Dx:
1. Ultrasound
2. MRA/CTA

Tx/Mgmt:
1. Control hypertension, hyperlipidemia, diabetes, smoking cessation, lifestyle modification
2. Surgical options are available (bypass surgery)

Vascular Dementia

Buzz Words: Stepwise decline/presence of symptoms + history of stroke + elderly

Clinical Presentation: Stepwise dementia is associated with neurological deficits in an elderly patient.

PPx: Stroke prevention: statins, hypertension management, diabetes management, lifestyle modification, antiplatelets, or anticoagulants if indicated.

MoD: Small vessel strokes gradually damage the brain, leading to dementia.

Dx:
1. CT
2. Can see strokes on MRI

Tx/Mgmt:
1. Cholinesterase inhibitors
2. Prevent future strokes and ensure safety at home. If a patient has dementia to a point that it is not safe for him or her to live independently, he or she should move in with family or move to a nursing home. You may be asked ethical questions about this. Keep the safety of the patient in mind.

Hypertensive Encephalopathy

Buzz Words: Hypertension + papilledema + neurological symptoms without acute stroke

Clinical Presentation: Headache, nausea, and vomiting. Typically accompanied by visual changes. Can eventually progress to seizure, coma, and death. The blood pressure is usually more than 200/100.

PPx: Good management of chronic HTN

MoD: Elevated blood pressure causes hydrostatic pressure on the cerebral vessels leading to cerebral edema. This is considered a failure of autoregulation.

Dx: Clinical diagnosis based on ruling out other causes. Can see edema on T2 MRI, but this is not required for the diagnosis.

Tx/Mgmt: Antihypertensives (e.g., calcium channel blockers, beta blockers, and nitroprusside) to slowly reduce blood pressure. Too rapid of reduction can cause stroke.

Posterior Reversible Encephalopathy Syndrome

Buzz Words: Hypertension + preeclampsia/eclampsia or renal disease + posterior circulation symptoms

Clinical Presentation: Headache, seizure, visual disturbances (Anton syndrome common)

MoD: A few mechanisms have been suggested. A failure of autoregulation and endothelial dysfunction have been suggested. Conditions like hypertension, preeclampsia, and renal disease all put patients at risk. Immunosuppressive therapy is also a risk factor.

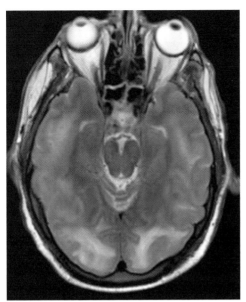

FIG. 5.8 Posterior reversible encephalopathy syndrome (PRES). (From Chawla R, Smith D, Marik PE: Near fatal posterior reversible encephalopathy syndrome complicating chronic liver failure and treated by induced hypothermia and dialysis: a case report. *J Med Case Rep* 26;3:6623, 2009.)

Dx: Can be seen on CT, but MRI is preferred (Fig. 5.8). Imaging may show symmetric white matter edema in the posterior cerebrum with or without cerebellum and brainstem involvement.

Tx/Mgmt:
1. Treat hypertension or preeclampsia if present
2. If on a cytotoxic immunosuppressive drug, the offending agent should be discontinued
3. Treat seizures with phenytoin

Venous Sinus Thrombosis

Buzz Words: Hypercoaguable state (factor V Leiden, antithrombin deficiency, protein S or C deficiency, cancer, oral contraceptive pill use, pregnancy) + dehydration (vomiting, post-exercise, post-alcohol binge)

Clinical Presentation: The classic patient is a young woman with an inherited hypercoaguable disorder (e.g., factor V Leiden) who is taking oral contraceptives and is dehydrated, usually from vomiting. Other risk factors include pregnancy and malignancy. Patients present with headache or seizures and may have focal neurological signs.

PPx: Avoid risk factors and treat genetic hypercoaguability.

MoD: Obstruction of a dural sinus leads to increased pressure in the capillary beds resulting in cerebral dysfunction and stroke. Can also result in impaired CSF drainage and hydrocephalus.

Dx:
1. MRI/MRV
2. If dx is confirmed, patient should be checked for a heritable hypercoaguable state.

Tx/Mgmt:
1. Anticoagulation with heparin and potentially warfarin if a hypercoaguable state is identified.
2. Thromboylitics like tPA can be used if symptoms are severe and no contraindications (e.g., active bleeding) are present.

Spinal Disorders

Cauda Equina Syndrome

Buzz Words: Paraplegia + urinary incontinence + fecal incontinence + saddle parasthesias

Clinical Presentation: Acute or gradual onset of back pain with pain radiating down one or both legs with decreased strength and reflexes. Urinary and fecal incontinence are also common.

See Table 5.4 and Fig. 5.9 for a comparison of the spinal disorders.

PPx: Depends on cause

MoD: The cauda equina (Latin: horse's tail) describes the 18 nerve roots in the spinal canal distal to the conus medullaris. When two or more of these roots are compressed, cauda equina syndrome results. The compression may be bony, infectious, malignant, or vascular.

Dx: Clinical diagnosis, MRI is best for visualizing the spinal canal.

Tx/Mgmt:
1. Neurosurgical emergency. Immediate decompression is required.
2. If a result of known diffuse metastatic disease, palliative care should be consulted.

Spinal Artery Occlusion

Buzz Words: Weakness + decreased pain and sensory loss (clear-cut sensory level of impairment, such as below T10 level) + preserved vibration/proprioception + in s/o surgery (particularly abdominal aortic aneurysmal repair) → ASA syndrome

TABLE 5.4 Clinical Spinal Syndromes

Problem	Syndrome
Radiculopathy (root problem)	Etiology: If the compression is cause by a disc, the disc is from the superior level (C3–C4 disc causes C4 radiculopathy). Compression may also be due to a bone spur, fluid collection (hematoma or abscess), or tumor.
C4	Motor: Deltoids (shoulder abduction) Sensory: Neck
C5	Motor: Biceps (elbow flexion) Sensory: Clavicle
C6	Motor: Wrist extensors (wrist extension) Sensory: Thumb
C7	Motor: Triceps (elbow extension) Sensory: Middle finger
C8	Motor: Hand grip (finger flexion) Sensory: Little finger
T1	Motor: Interossei (finger abduction) Sensory: Armpit
L2	Motor: Iliopsoas (hip flexion) Sensory: Difficult to localize
L3	Motor: Thigh adductors Sensory: Difficult to localize
L4	Motor: Quadriceps (knee extension) Sensory: Great toe
L5	Motor: Tibialis anterior (ankle dorsiflexion) Sensory: Dorsum of foot
S1	Motor: Soleus (ankle plantar flexion) Sensory: Plantar surface of foot
Cauda equina syndrome (L2-Co1)	Cauda equina syndrome can occur at any level after the conus medullaris, which is usually at L1–L2. The syndrome will involve the roots still present at that level. If there is compression at the L5 level, the L2–L4 roots will be spared but the L5, S1–S4, and coccygeal roots will be involved. Motor: Leg and foot movement, rectal tone (bowel and bladder incontinence) Sensory: Leg, foot, and anus
Myelopathy (cord problem)	—
Dorsal	Etiology: compression, B12 deficiency, syphilis Symptoms: Impaired fine touch and proprioception → ataxia and unnoticed foot injuries
Anterior	Etiology: compression, anterior spinal artery infarction Symptoms: Weakness and impaired pain and temperature sensation with intact fine touch and proprioception
Central	Etiology: Following extension injury in setting of degenerative changes. Or seen with syringomyelia, which is associated with Chiari 1 malformation. Symptoms: Motor and sensory impairment of upper extremity with normal lower extremity
Hemisected (Brown-Sequard syndrome)	Etiology: Following a knife assault Symptoms: Ipsilateral weakness below the level, contralateral pain and temperature starting two levels below the damage

Note: This table is an oversimplification. There is significant overlap in the muscles involved since the brachial plexus and lumbar plexus incorporate multiple roots.

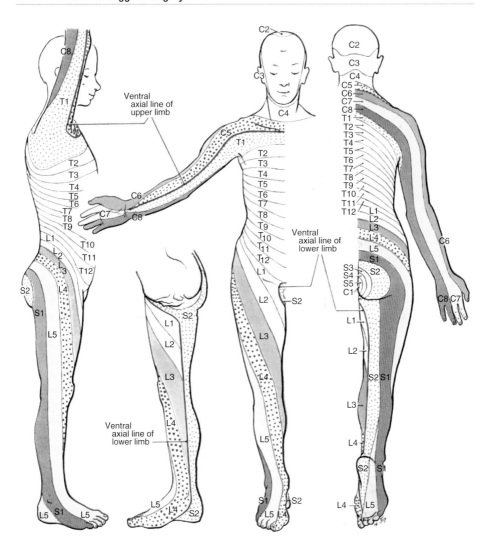

FIG. 5.9 Dermatomes. (From Wikimedia Commons. https://commons.wikimedia.org/wiki/File:Grant_1962_663.png. In the public domain.)

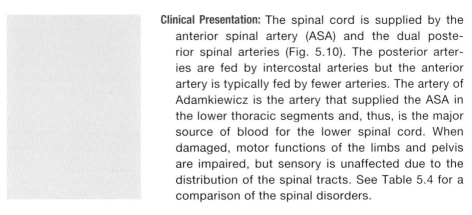

Clinical Presentation: The spinal cord is supplied by the anterior spinal artery (ASA) and the dual posterior spinal arteries (Fig. 5.10). The posterior arteries are fed by intercostal arteries but the anterior artery is typically fed by fewer arteries. The artery of Adamkiewicz is the artery that supplied the ASA in the lower thoracic segments and, thus, is the major source of blood for the lower spinal cord. When damaged, motor functions of the limbs and pelvis are impaired, but sensory is unaffected due to the distribution of the spinal tracts. See Table 5.4 for a comparison of the spinal disorders.

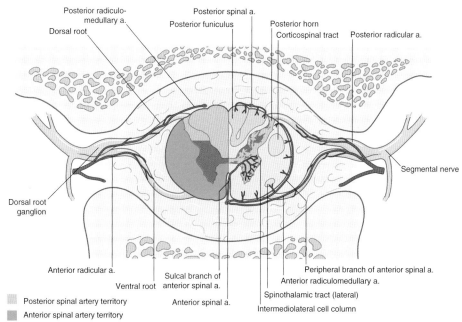

Posterior radiculo-
medullary a.
Dorsal root
Posterior spinal a.
Posterior funiculus
Posterior horn
Corticospinal tract
Posterior radicular a.

Segmental nerve

Dorsal root
ganglion

Anterior radicular a.
Ventral root
Sulcal branch of
anterior spinal a.
Anterior spinal a.
Peripheral branch of anterior spinal a.
Anterior radiculomedullary a.
Spinothalamic tract (lateral)
Intermediolateral cell column

Posterior spinal artery territory
Anterior spinal artery territory

FIG. 5.10 Blood supply of spinal cord. (Goodin DS: Neurologic complications of aortic disease and surgery. In: Aminoff MJ, Josephson SA: *Aminoff's Neurology and General Medicine*, ed 5, Philadelphia, 2014, Elsevier, fig 2.4.)

MoD: Traumatic or due to cholesterol or hypercoaguable state. Classically, damage to the spinal arteries is seen following aortic dissection or aorta surgery.

Dx:
1. Clinical diagnosis
2. MRI can show infarct in distribution of affected vessel
3. CTA may show occlusion of vessel if large

Tx/Mgmt: Endovascular management

Spinal Cord Compression

Clinical Presentation: See Table 5.4 for a comparison of the spinal disorders.

MoD: Highly variable: Can be due to bone (osteophytes), bulging discs, epidural abscess or hematoma, malignancy, nonmalignant tumors.

Dx:
1. CT is best for bony visualization
2. MRI is superior for assessing damage to the cord. If a patient cannot undergo an MRI, a CT myelogram can be used.

Tx/Mgmt: In general, compression causing neurological symptoms should be fixed with an operation. Asymptomatic compression or compression causing only pain could be fixed with an operation, depending on the patient.

Spinal Cord Transection

Buzz Words: Posterior stab wound + ipsilateral loss of position/vibration + contralateral loss of pain/temp + contralateral weakness → Brown-Sequard syndrome

Clinical Presentation: The transection that is most often tested is hemisection, also known as Brown-Sequard syndrome. Brown-Sequard syndrome presents with ipsilateral loss of motor function and contralateral loss of pain and temperature starting two dermatomes below the level of the transection.

Complete transection of the cord is often caused by high-speed MVC where the bones dislocate at the facet joints. The cervical spine is particularly susceptible to these injuries. Complete transection will result in paraplegia or quadriplegia. See Table 5.4 for a comparison of the spinal disorders.

MoD: Damage to the white matter causes failure of signaling. For Brown-Sequard, the sensory tracts take about two levels to cross to the contralateral side. This is why the sensory changes are two levels below the level of transection.

Dx:
1. Clinical diagnosis confirmed with MRI

Tx/Mgmt: Treatment is currently ineffective. New therapies are being researched but will not be tested by NBME.

Paraplegia and Quadriplegia

Buzz Words: Paralysis + numbness + incontinence

Clinical Presentation: Acutely, damage to the spinal cord will present as flaccid paralysis and numbness. These symptoms may improve as the swelling decreases and axons regenerate. Often they are permanent. Table 5.4 can be used to predict the muscles impaired with damage at each level. Fig. 5.9 also shows the dermatomes, which can be used to determine the level of injury (see Fig. 5.9). Cervical spine injuries also have effects on the neurons that supply the sympathetic chain. When impaired, there is no sympathetic drive and patients become hypotensive and bradycardic. Damage to the low-thoracic spinal cord or cauda equina can also result in autonomic dysregulation leading to incontinence and priapism.

PPx: Depends on cause

MoD: Damage to the cord severs or severely damages the axons resulting in failure of communication across the segment. Axons are capable of regenerating if the cell body is intact but this process is generally ineffective and the deficits are permanent.

Dx: Clinical diagnosis is confirmed with MRI.

MNEMONIC
MISC2 (**M**otor **I**spilateral, **S**ensory **C**ontralateral **2**) levels below

Tx/Mgmt:
1. Treat symptoms.
2. Patients with acute cervical spine injury often require intubation, fluid resuscitation, and pressors.
3. As discussed previously, the NBME will not test you on agents that may help patients regain function following spinal cord injury.

Spinal Stenosis

Buzz Words: Shopping cart sign (relief of back when leaning forward) + back pain exacerbated with extension, relieved with flexion

Clinical Presentation: In the cervical and thoracic spine, stenosis will lead to myelopathy. Patients will have a positive Hoffman sign and are hyperreflexic. In the lumbar spine, the most common presentation is neurogenic claudication. Patients describe unilateral or bilateral leg pain that is worse with activity but immediately relieved by sitting down. In contrast, vascular claudication does not improve for several minutes since reperfusion is necessary. Additionally, patients will say the pain is better when going uphill. In contrast, vascular claudication is much worse when going uphill because that increases oxygen demand. Patients will also say the pain is better when hunched over a shopping cart. Notice the theme here: the pain improves when the back is flexed. See Table 5.4 for a comparison of the spinal disorders.

PPx: Weight loss, exercise

MoD: Typically due to degenerative arthritis, which is worse in patients who are obese. Other causes include compression by tumor, postoperative fibrosis, and inherited skeletal disorders. A developmental disorder called Klippel-Feil syndrome is characterized by congenital fusion of cervical vertebrae. The spine is meant to be a mobile joint. Fusing the vertebrae may result in adjacent-level fibrosis and stenosis.

Dx:
1. CT is best for bony visualization.
2. MRI is superior for assessing damage to the cord. (If a patient cannot undergo an MRI, a CT myelogram can be used.)

Tx/Mgmt:
1. Asymptomatic compression or compression causing only pain could be fixed with an operation depending on the patient.
2. Stenosis causing neurological symptoms should be surgically fixed.

Cranial and Peripheral Nerve Disorders

Bell's Palsy

Buzz Words: Unilateral facial nerve paralysis + forehead involved + HSV or Lyme disease

Clinical Presentation: Unilateral facial paralysis with forehead involvement as evidenced by sagging eyebrow. In a stroke, the forehead is spared. There is also decreased tearing, hyperacusis (due to paralysis of the stapedius muscle) and loss of taste to the anterior two-thirds of the tongue.

MoD: An infectious agent (like HSV or *B. burgdorferi*) causes inflammation to and around the facial nerve, causing impaired functioning.

Dx:

1. Clinical diagnosis
2. HSV can be diagnosed with CSF PCR
3. Lyme disease should be considered and worked up in at risk individuals (recent hiking or camping trip in the Northeast United States).

Tx/Mgmt:

1. The most important part of management is eye care. Although the eyelid is droopy, the eye often cannot blink and has decreased tear production.
2. Antivirals and steroids can be used if HSV is suspected. For Lyme disease, doxycycline or cephalosporins can be used.

Internuclear Ophthalmoplegia

Buzz Words: MS + lesion in the MLF or PPRF + disconjugate gaze

Clinical Presentation: Weakness of adduction on contralateral gaze with nystagmus in unaffected eye (Fig. 5.11).

MoD: It is usually due to multiple sclerosis (MS) causing demyelination in the oculomotor centers. Specifically, paramedian pontine reticular formation (PPRF) signals to the abducens nucleus, which innervates the ipsilateral lateral rectus and also communicates through the medial longitudinal fasciculus (MLF) to the contralateral occulomotor nucleus, which innervates the contralateral medial rectus. MS or other damage to the MLF impairs this communication and the contralateral eye fails to adduct.

Dx: Clinical diagnosis: MRI can be used to diagnose MS.

Tx/Mgmt: Depends on cause

99 AR

Eye movements video of IOP

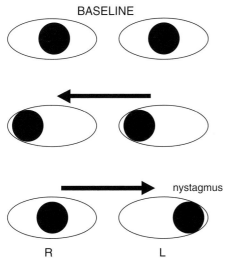

BASELINE

nystagmus

R   L

FIG. 5.11 Right internuclear ophthalmoplegia. (From Wikimedia Commons. https://commons.wikimedia.org/wiki/File:Internuclear_ophthalmoplegia.jpg. Created by Samir. Used under Creative Commons Attribution-Share Alike 3.0 Unported license: https://creativecommons.org/licenses/by-sa/3.0/deed.en.)

Nystagmus

Buzz Words: Vertigo + PCP drug abuse + Chiari malformation

Clinical Presentation: Nystagmus is any rhythmic oscillation of the eyes. There are a variety of types and associated etiologies.

MoD: Innumerable causes exist. The most likely cause is vertigo. Other causes include drugs (e.g., PCP, alcohol), lesions of the cerebellum or cranial nerve nuclei, Chiari malformation, Noonan syndrome.

Dx:
1. Clinical diagnosis
2. Caloric reflex test can be used to elicit nystagmus and the absence of nystagmus indicates a deficit in the vestibular system.
3. The Dix-Hallpike test may elicit nystagmus and suggest BPPV.
4. CT or MRI if central vertigo is suspected.

Tx/Mgmt: Treat the cause

Vestibular Neuritis, Labyrinthitis

Buzz Words: Vertigo + viral syndrome + hearing loss

Clinical Presentation: Vertigo, nystagmus, nausea, vomiting, and gait impairment. When there is unilateral hearing loss in addition to the aforementioned symptoms, the condition is called labyrinthitis.

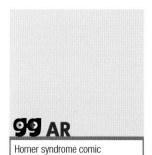
Horner syndrome comic

MoD: Viral or post-viral inflammation of the vestibular branch of the vestibulocochlear nerve

Dx: Clinical: Rule out stroke if story is suspicious.

Tx/Mgmt: Antivirals and steroids can be helpful.

Horner Syndrome

Buzz Words: Anisocoria + miosis + anhidrosis + ptosis + sympathetic chain lesion

Clinical Presentation: Patients present with the classic triad of miosis, ptosis, and anhidrosis.

Note: Ptosis alone can occur in the absence of a true Horner syndrome. Often on NBME questions, ptosis is associated with myasthenia gravis, but the differential is very broad.

MoD: The sympathetic fibers in the occuolomotor nerve cause mydriasis, proptosis, and lacrimation. When impaired, Horner syndrome results. The ptosis is only partial due to impairment of Muller's muscle, which is a minor contributor to lid elevation. The neuronal pathway begins in the brain and travels down to the spinal cord and back up to the eye via the cervical sympathetic chain and through the cavernous sinus. There are a variety of causes for Horner syndrome, including tumors, strokes, spinal cord injury, and sympathetic chain injury.

Dx: Clinical diagnosis

Tx/Mgmt: Eye care

Carpal/Cubital/Tarsal/Peroneal Tunnel Syndrome

See Table 5.5.

Mononeuritis

Buzz Words: Vasculitis + diabetes

Clinical Presentation: Symptoms depend on which nerve is involved. See Tables 5.5 and 5.6 for common peripheral nerve syndromes.

PPx: Diabetes management, good nutrition (B_{12} consumption)

MoD: Damage to nerve is usually due to metabolic disturbance, such as prolonged hyperglycemia or uremia. Also occurs in MGUS, alcoholism and B_{12} deficiency. Damage is usually permanent.

Dx: Clinical or via electromyography (EMG). May need imaging of spine and brain to rule out central cause.

Tx/Mgmt:
1. Supportive
2. Nerve pain can be treated with gabapentin.
3. Weakness should be managed with splints when possible.

TABLE 5.5 Tunnel Syndromes

Tunnel	Carpal	Cubital	Peroneal	Tarsal
Buzz Words	Median nerve, typing	Ulnar nerve	Fibular head	Tibial nerve
Clinical Presentation	Burning pain and weakness in the thumb and first two digits	Burning pain and weakness in fourth and fifth digits	Foot drop with sensory loss	Pain in the ankle, foot, and toes
PPx	Avoid compression (e.g., excessive typing)	Avoid compression (e.g., bench press)	Avoid compression (e.g., crossing legs)	Avoid compression (e.g., poor running mechanics)
MoD	Median nerve entrapment in the carpal tunnel usually due to tightening of the flexor retinaculum	Compression of ulnar nerve at medial epicondyle	Compression of peroneal nerve at the fibular head; usually from lateral leg injury or sitting with legs crossed	Compression of the tibial nerve through the tarsal tunnel
Dx	Clinical via positive Phalen or Tinel sign; EMG can confirm	Clinical but EMG can confirm	Clinical but EMG can confirm	Clinical but EMG can confirm
Tx/Mgmt	NSAIDs, splinting, surgical decompression	NSAIDs, surgical decompression	NSAIDs, surgical decompression	NSAIDs, surgical decompression

EMG, Electromyography; *NSAIDs*, nonsteroidal anti-inflammatory drugs.

TABLE 5.6 Peripheral Nerve Mononeuritis (Other Than Those Covered in Table 5.5)

Nerve	Symptoms
Long thoracic	Serratus anterior weakness → winged scapula
Axillary	Deltoid weakness → impaired arm abduction
Radial	Extensor carpi radialis weakness → wrist drop
Femoral	Iliopsoas weakness → impaired hip flexion
Obturator	Adductor weakness → impaired leg adduction
Sciatic (tibial and peroneal)	Hamstrings and lower leg weakness, pain in buttock and down leg
Lateral femoral cutaneous	Meralgia paresthetica → lateral thigh numbness

Guillain-Barré Syndrome

Buzz Words: Ascending paralysis + albuminocytologic dissociation on LP

Clinical Presentation: Symmetric paralysis that begins in the feet and ascends through the spinal cord segments. Sensory changes can be present but are typically mild. Can eventually involve the respiratory muscles, autonomic nerves, and facial muscles.

MoD: Not clear: Suspected that an infection triggers immune activation and demyelination. *Campylobacter jejuni* is commonly implicated so patients may have a recent history of diarrhea.

Dx:

1. Clinical diagnosis
2. Lumbar puncture shows normal cell counts with elevated protein, aka albuminocytologic dissociation). Antibodies that can be found in the CSF include those to GM1, GD1a, and GD1b.
3. EMG shows demyelinating polyradiculopathy lending to the name AIDP (acute inflammatory demyelinating polyradiculopathy).

Tx/Mgmt:

1. Supportive care (consider ABCs if breathing and blood pressure are impaired)
2. intravenous immunoglobulin (IVIG)

Miller Fisher Syndrome

Buzz Words: Descending paralysis + albuminocytologic dissociation on LP

Clinical Presentation: This is a variant of Guillian-Barré syndrome where the cranial nerves are affected first. The presenting symptoms are usually ophthalmoplegia and ataxia, which can descend to upper and lower extremity weakness. Miller Fisher should be considered in the differential for myasthenia gravis where the primary symptom is extraoccular weakness.

MoD: Not clear: Same theory as Guillian-Barré but is not associated with any particular predisposing infection.

Dx: CSF and EMG findings are similar to Guillian-Barré syndrome. The primary antibody found in the CSF is to GQ1b.

Tx/Mgmt:

1. Supportive care (consider ABCs if breathing and blood pressure are impaired)
2. IVIG

Charcot-Marie-Tooth Disease

Buzz Words: Hammer toes + high foot arch + polyneuropathy + family history of similar

Clinical Presentation: There are numerous types of Charcot-Marie-Tooth (CMT) disease with different presenting symptoms. They are all motor and sensory polyneuropathies. Note: Polyneuropathy can occur in other genetic diseases and in severe diabetes. These findings are not synonymous with CMT, just with neuropathy.

gg AR

Charcot Marie Tooth signs and symptoms

MoD: Many genes are responsible for causing CMT. Most of the genes code for components of peripheral myelin.

Dx: Clinical diagnosis that can be confirmed with genetic testing.

Tx/Mgmt:

1. Supportive, foot care to prevent infection from unnoticed wounds, braces
2. Surgical intervention

Herpes Zoster and Postherpetic Neuralgia

Buzz Words: Dewdrops on rose petal on the skin + neuralgia + painful lesions + dermatomal distribution

Clinical Presentation: Zoster reactivation presents initially with a burning pain in a dermatomal distribution. Vesicles erupt days later. The vesicles are often described as dewdrops on rose petals.

PPx: In immunocompromised individuals, there is a role for antivirals especially in patients with history of ocular zoster.

MoD: Following initial herpes zoster virus infection, the virus migrates up the sensory axons where it lays dormant in the dorsal root ganglia. An unknown event triggers viral reactivation, which results in inflammation of the sensory nerve. Dermatomal lesions and pain result.

Dx: Clinical diagnosis: Can PCR for varicella-zoster virus (VZV) DNA from lesion.

Tx/Mgmt:

1. Acyclovir can shorten the course and should be used for any trigeminal lesions since there is risk of damage to the eye.
2. Gabapentin and pregabalin prescribed for neuralgias.

Pain Disorders

Complex Regional Pain Syndrome (aka Reflex Sympathetic Dystrophy and Causalgia)

Clinical Presentation: These are different subtypes with associated clinical findings. In general this is a pain syndrome that occurs following surgery or trauma. The pain is accompanied by sensory changes, autonomic changes, weakness, and atrophy. The autonomic changes include pallor or rubor, piloerection, sweating, and edema.

PPx: Vitamin C (controversial)

MoD: Unknown: Cytokines and neural hypersensitivity have been implicated.

Dx: Clinical diagnosis

Tx/Mgmt: Numerous pain management options are available, including nonsteroidal anti-inflammatory drugs (NSAIDs), steroids, antidepressants, calcitonin, bisphosphonates, topical anesthetics, and injections. Severe cases may require epidural anesthesia if CPRS of lower extremity.

Fibromyalgia

Clinical Presentation: Chronic widespread musculoskeletal pain, fatigue, and psychiatric disturbance are present.

PPx: Exercise

MoD: Not well understood

Dx: Previously diagnosed based on having pain at 11/18 of tender points, which had been defined when the disease initially recognized. This has fallen out of favor and a clinical diagnosis is now favored.

Tx/Mgmt:
1. Exercise regimen
2. Tricyclic antidepressants, cyclobenzaprine, and other antidepressants

Phantom Limb Pain

Buzz Words: Perceived pain in the absence of limb + amputation

Clinical Presentation: Aching or electric-type pain is felt following amputation. Important to know for the shelf because it is a frequently seen postoperative complaint.

PPx: Epidural anesthesia prior to amputation

MoD: Poorly understood

Dx: Diagnosis of exclusion

Tx/Mgmt: Gabapentin may help

Thalamic Pain Syndrome (Dejerine-Roussy Syndrome)

Buzz Words: Lacunar stroke of thalamus + allodynia

Clinical Presentation: Severe burning pain (allodynia) occurs on one side of the body.

PPx: Stroke prevention (hypertension, hyperlipidemia, and diabetes management; smoking cessation, diet and exercise)

MoD: Lacunar stroke affecting the posteroventral thalamus unilaterally resulting in a disequilibrium of pain signals, which are misinterpreted by the cortex as severe burning pain.

Dx: Clinical diagnosis

Tx/Mgmt: Often refractory to treatment with gabapentin and antidepressants. Opioids may be required, and deep brain stimulation (DBS) may be effective.

Trigeminal Neuralgia

Buzz Words: Pain unilateral in face + many episodes per day + superior cerebellar artery (SCA) near the trigeminal nerve on MRI

Clinical Presentation: Unilateral sharp pain in the distribution of the trigeminal nerve occurring in brief paroxysms.

MoD: Compression of the trigeminal nerve typically by the SCA

Dx: Clinical diagnosis: Imaging should be done to rule out tumor or other intracranial pathology. May see compression by the SCA on imaging.

Tx/Mgmt: Carbamazepine (commonly tested on shelf)

QUICK TIPS
Trigeminal neuralgia → Tx with carbamazepine

Movement Disorders

Essential Tremor

Buzz Words: Tremor + worse with precise movement

Clinical Presentation: Tremor that occurs during movement (intention tremor). Usually involves one or both hands and can be associated with a head bob.

MoD: Heritable, but the exact cause is not known

Dx: Clinical diagnosis

Tx/Mgmt:
1. Beta blockers: Can also try primidone, gabapentin, topiramate, and botox injections.
2. Refractory cases can be treated with DBS.

QUICK TIPS
Essential tremor = worse with movement; tremor in Parkinson's = worse at rest

99 AR
Essential Tremor

Huntington Disease

Buzz Words: Chorea+ small caudate on MRI + dementia that runs in family + older relative who died in mid-adults + CAG repeat

Clinical Presentation: Progressive onset of choreiform movements, psychiatric and cognitive disturbances occur. This is one of the most high-yield diseases on the shelf because of its multidisciplinary nature.

PPx: Genetic counseling to prevent transmission to offspring

MoD: Autosomal dominant CAG repeat in the HTT gene on chromosome four resulting in translation of excess glutamine amino acids in the protein. The glutamine amino acids cause abnormal folding of the protein, which then clumps together in cells. This occurs most prominently in the caudate and putamen.

Dx:
1. Family history with progressive symptoms is sufficient
2. MRI to r/o structural etiology
3. Genetic testing can be done for the benefit of offspring

99 AR
Chorea

99 AR
hypomimia = masked facies

99 AR
Parkinson's disease

99 AR
Types of Seizures

Tx/Mgmt: Symptoms management: Chorea responds to tetrabenzine and neuroleptics. Psychiatric symptoms should be treated with antipsychotics and antidepressants.

Parkinson Disease, Including Parkinson Dementia

Buzz Words:
- **Parkinson:** Bradykinesia + rigidity + hypomimia + resting tremor
- **Lewy body dementia:** Lilliputian (benign) hallucinations + Parkinson's symptoms

Clinical Presentation: Initial symptom is variable but as the disease progresses, the entire constitution of symptoms presents. Patients have bradykinesia, hypomimia, hypophonia, resting "pill rolling" tremor, postural instability, autonomic dysregulation, and rigidity including cogwheel rigidity on exam. Nonmotor symptoms are also common, including mood disorder, psychosis, sleep disturbance, and dementia.

PPx: None

MoD: Selective loss of dopaminergic neurons in the substantia nigra result in increased inhibition of the thalamus and decreased excitation from the motor cortex.

Dx:
1. Clinical diagnosis
2. MRI/CT to r/o Parkinsonian mimics such as normal pressure hydrocephalus

Tx/Mgmt:
1. Carbidopa/levodopa
2. Dopamine agonists, MAOIs, and anticholinergics
3. Deep Brain Stimulation

Paroxysmal Disorders

Headache

See Table 5.7.

Seizure

See Table 5.8.

Traumatic and Mechanical Disorders and Disorders of Increased Intracranial Pressure

Epidural Hematoma

Buzz Words: Lenticular shape on non-con CT + lucid interval + middle meningeal artery

TABLE 5.7 Headaches

Headache	Buzz Words	Presentation	PPx	MoD	Dx	Tx
Migraine	Aura	Unilateral headache lasting 4–72 h with proceeding aura	Beta blockers, calcium channel blockers, topiramate, tricyclic antidepressants	Poorly understood	All diagnosed clinically	NSAIDs, triptans
Tension	Band-like	Steady band-like pain	Tricyclic antidepressants			NSAIDs
Cluster	Horner's	Repetitive stabbing pain behind eye lasting 15–90 min; may have Horner syndrome as well	None			Oxygen
Mixed	—	Variable	Any of the above			NSAIDs
Medication withdrawal	Opiates, NSAIDs	Pain following prolonged (>3 days) use of NSAIDs	Avoid NSAID and other headache medication overuse			Medication discontinuation
Caffeine withdrawal	Caffeine, coffee	Pain following prolonged (months) use of caffeine	Avoid caffeine overuse			Caffeine (can be found in over-the-counter headache medications)

Note: Headache disorders are discussed more extensively in the *Gunner Goggles Neurology* book. This information should suffice for the Surgery exam. *NSAIDs*, Nonsteroidal anti-inflammatory drugs.

TABLE 5.8 Seizures

Seizure Type	Presentation	PPx	MoD	Dx	Tx
Simple partial	Focal muscle jerking	Phenytoin, Carbamazepine, Valproic acid, Gabapentin, phenobarbital, Topiramate, Lamotrigine, Levetiracetam, Tiagabine	Focus of abnormal tissue causes discharge of electrical activity that spreads over cortex	EEG	Benzos
Complex partial	Focal muscle jerking with impairment in consciousness				
Tonic clonic	Generalized muscle stiffening and jerking				Benzos, phytoin
Absence	Brief impairment in consciousness often with lip smacking or other automatisms	Ethosuximide	Poorly understood		None

Note: Seizure disorders are discussed more extensively in the *Gunner Goggles Neurology* book. This information should suffice for the Surgery exam.
Dx, Diagnostic steps; *EEG,* electroencephalogram; *PPx,* prophylaxis; *MoD,* mechanism of disease; *Tx,* treatment.

Clinical Presentation: An epidural hematoma is often associated with a "lucid interval" after the trauma followed by progressive deterioration.

MoD: Classically, it is due to trauma on the pterion leading to damage of the middle meningeal artery. An epidural hematoma is lenticular in shape (biconcave).

Dx: Head CT

Tx/Mgmt: Surgery if GCS <8, volume >30 mL, or pupillary asymmetry

Subdural Hematoma

Buzz Words: Crescent shape on non-con CT + alcohol + elderly + bridging veins

Clinical Presentation: Subdural hematomas often cause weakness that may only be noticeable as a pronator drift in the contralateral arm.

PPx: Avoid trauma

MoD: Classically, it is due to deceleration injury with damage to the bridging veins. The bridging veins are most stretched in the elderly and alcoholics because their brains have shrunken. A subdural hematoma is crescent shaped.

Dx: Head CT

Tx/Mgmt: Surgery if greater than 10 mm thick or greater than 5 mm shift or GCS <8

Spinal Epidural Hematoma

Buzz Words: Hypertension + spinal cord symptoms + trauma

Clinical Presentation: Myelopathy or radiculopathy depending on level of lesion. See Table 5.4 for possible symptoms. Often these patients present following lumbar puncture or post-traumatic event. Epidural abscess is associated with endocarditis and has similar imaging, so history is important.

PPx: In a patient with thrombocytopenia or coagulopathy, administration of platelets or anticoagulant reversal should be considered prior to lumbar puncture.

MoD: Venous or arterial bleeding resulting in epidural collection

Dx: MRI

Tx/Mgmt: Prompt decompression via aspiration or spine surgery

Intraparenchymal Hemorrhage

Buzz Words: Hypertension + focal neurological symptoms

Clinical Presentation: Depends on location: See Table 5.3 for summary of symptoms by vessel.

PPx: Avoid trauma, hypertension management

MoD: Damage to a small vessel within the brain causes hemorrhage in this location. If atraumatic, hypertensive hemorrhage often occurs as a result of hypertensive damage to small vessels. These are typically the same vessels that result in lacunar strokes.

Dx: Head CT

Tx/Mgmt:
1. Reduce intracranial pressure to slow bleeding.
2. Surgery if hemorrhage is in the posterior fossa.

Pseudotumor Cerebri (Idiopathic Intracranial Hypertension)

Buzz Words: Obese woman + papilledema+ blindness + vitamin A + doxycycline

Clinical Presentation: Classically, patient is a young adult obese female who is taking isotretinoin (vitamin A derivative) and doxycycline for acne who presents with headache and visual field changes. Examination will reveal papilledema (Fig. 5.12) and sometimes extraocular muscles palsy.

MoD: Unknown: Theories include venous hypertension and elevated intraabdominal pressures.

Dx: Clinical symptoms + elevated opening pressure on lumbar puncture. Certain findings on MRI are associated with the disease but are not diagnostic.

Tx/Mgmt: Treatment is primarily to prevent blindness.
1. Diuretics (loop diuretics and carbonic anhydrase inhibitors)

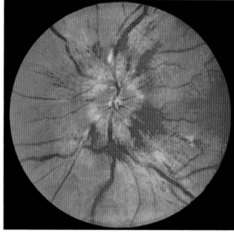

FIG. 5.12 Papilledema. (From Wikimedia Commons. https://commons.wikimedia.org/wiki/File:Papilledema.jpg. Created by Jonathan Trobe, M.D., University of Michigan Kellogg Eye Center. Used under Creative Commons Attribution 3.0 Unported license: https://creativecommons.org/licenses/by/3.0/deed.en.)

AR

Posterior fossa decompression

2. Corticosteroids and migraine medications for headache
3. Surgical treatments (shunting and optic nerve fenestration)

Torticollis/Cervical Dystonia

Buzz Words: Antipsychotics + neck stuck in one position
Clinical Presentation: Neck is twisted to one side. Can be constant or paroxysmal. Tenderness to palpation of SCM.
PPx: Torticollis due to antipsychotic use can be prevented with trihexyphenidyl.
MoD: Can be congenital or acquired: Acquired torticollis may be due to antipsychotics, spinal cord compression (via tumor, blood, abscess, or bone), retropharyngeal abscess, or simply muscle inflammation.
Dx: Clinical diagnosis
Tx/Mgmt: Trihexyphenidyl can prevent the spasm. Botox can be used for persistent torticollis.

Normal Pressure Hydrocephalus

AR

Wet, wild, and wacky comic

Buzz Words: Wet (urinary incontinence) + wacky (dementia) + wobbly (ataxia)
Clinical Presentation: The mnemonic "wet, wacky, wobbly" can be used to describe these patients. They have urinary incontinence (wet), impaired cognition (wacky), and gait dysfunction (wobbly).

MoD: Thought to be due to initial elevated pressure hydro-cephalus followed by a period of pressure normalization.

Dx:
1. Confirmed on imaging (CT or MRI)
2. Lumbar puncture

Tx/Mgmt: Shunting via external ventricular drain (EVD) or ventriculo-peritoneal shunt (VPS) can be used but may not be effective.

Traumatic Brain Injury (Concussion)/ Post-concussion Syndrome (Dementia Pugilistica)

Buzz Words: Head trauma + seeing stars

Clinical Presentation:
- **Concussion:** Confusion following head trauma. Speech, memory, and attention can all be affected. Seizures may also result.
- **Post-concussion syndrome:** Headache and dizziness with impaired cognition and psychiatric symptoms are possible.
- **Dementia pugilistica:** It follows numerous concussions characterized by memory impairment. Boxers, wrestlers, and football players are at greatest risk.

PPx: Trauma prevention: use of helmets, seatbelts, etc.

MoD: Trauma causes disruption of neuronal networks

Dx:
1. Clinical diagnosis
2. Neuroimaging is usually normal but should be done to rule out any intracranial hemorrhage.

Tx/Mgmt:
1. Observation for deterioration (which would occur if intracranial hemorrhage is present)
2. Avoid recurrent concussion

Congenital Disorders

Friedreich Ataxia

Buzz Words:
- 22 years old (onset during teenage) + gait ataxia + frequent falling + dysarthria + hypertrophic cardiomyopathy + diabetes + hammer toes + pes cavus + scoliosis
- Ataxia + cardiomyopathy + loss of position/vibration + pain/temp intact

Clinical Presentation: Neurological dysfunction with cardiomyopathy and diabetes occurs. The neurologic dysfunction is characterized by ataxia, weakness, and sensory dysfunction. Children may present with scoliosis and clumsiness. Most common cause of death is cardiomyopathy, then respiratory causes. Pes cavus can also be CMT so be sure to keep both diseases in your differential.

MoD: Loss of function of frataxin gene on chromosome 9 due to GAA trinucleotide repeat. Frataxin is a mitochondrial protein involved in iron metabolism. The mutation results in increased oxidative stress to the cells, resulting in cell dysfunction and death. Neurological dysfunction is due to damage of the posterior columns.

Dx:
1. Clinical exam
2. Genetic testing
3. Echo to look for HCM

Tx/Mgmt:
1. Physical therapy
2. Endocrine and cardiology follow up

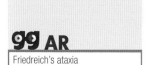

99 AR
Friedreich's ataxia

Neural Tube Defects (e.g., Spina Bifida, Holoprosencephaly, Anencephaly)

Buzz Words: Folate deficiency + elevated AFP → spina bifida

Clinical Presentation: Can be identified prenatally or postnatally: Prenatally, mothers may have elevated AFP. Postnatally, the defect can be visible or associated with a tuft of hair that signifies underlying defect (Fig. 5.13).

PPx: Maternal folate supplementation: 400 μg for pregnant women; 4000 μg for pregnant women with history of neural tube defect in previous pregnancy.

MoD: Failure or embryogenesis at the time of the neural tube closure.

Dx: Clinical diagnosis

Tx/Mgmt: Conservative versus surgical management depends on severity. Holoprosencephaly and anencephaly are managed with palliative care.

Microcephaly

Buzz Words: Neural tube defect + TORCH or fetal alcohol syndrome + small head

Clinical Presentation: Small head circumference

PPx: Avoid intrauterine infections via vaccination; take folate to prevent neural tube defects.

MoD: Can be isolated or associated with certain syndromes. Can be seen with neural tube defects, TORCH infections, and fetal alcohol syndrome.

Dx: Head circumference

Tx/Mgmt: Work-up for specific syndrome depending on other symptoms present.

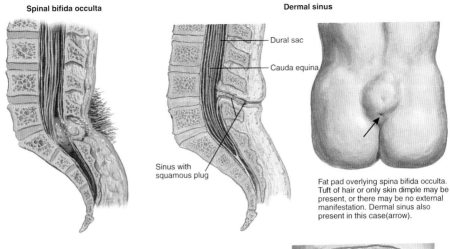

Spinal bifida occulta

Dermal sinus

Dural sac

Cauda equina

Sinus with squamous plug

Fat pad overlying spina bifida occulta. Tuft of hair or only skin dimple may be present, or there may be no external manifestation. Dermal sinus also present in this case(arrow).

Types of spina bifida aperta with protrusion of spinal contents

Meningocele

Meningomyelocele

Arnold-Chiari syndrome decompression

FIG. 5.13 Neural tube defects. (Copyright 2017 Elsevier Inc. All rights reserved. www.netterimages.com.)

Sturge-Weber Syndrome

Buzz Words: Port-wine stain + CNS angiomas

Clinical Presentation: Usually diagnosed due to appearance of port-wine stain on face (Fig. 5.14) and CNS angiomas. Children will also have eye involvement, intellectual impairment, and seizures.

MoD: Nonheritable genetic disorder caused by mutation in the GNAQ gene, which is involved in cellular signaling.

Dx: Clinical diagnosis

Tx/Mgmt: Treat symptoms: Skin lesions can be reduced with laser treatments. Seizures should be managed with antiepileptics.

Tuberous Sclerosis

Buzz Words: Hamartomas + ash leaf spots+ shagreen patches + giant cell tumors

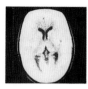

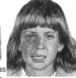

Sturge–Weber Disease

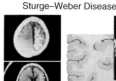

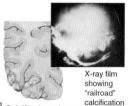

CT scan. Showing one of many calcified lesions in periventricular area

Multiple small tumors in kidney

Rhabdomyomas of heart muscle

Facial nevus

CT scan. Showing calcifications and atrophy in temporoparietal area

Calcific deposits and hypervascularity. In leptomeninges and gray matter of brain

X-ray film showing "railroad" calcification

FIG. 5.14 Sturge-Weber syndrome findings. (Copyright 2017 Elsevier Inc. All rights reserved. www. netterimages.com.)

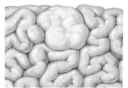

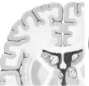

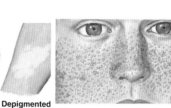

Tuber of cerebral cortex. Consisting of many astrocytes, scanty nerve cells, some abnormal sites

Multiple small tumors. Caudate nucleus and thalamus projecting into ventricles

Tuber of ocular fundus

Depigmented skin area

Adenoma sebaceum. Over both cheeks and bridge of nose

FIG. 5.15 Tuberous sclerosis findings. (Copyright 2017 Elsevier Inc. All rights reserved. www.netterimages. com.)

Clinical Presentation: Presents in infancy or early childhood with benign tumors and cognitive deficits. The tumors associated with tuberous sclerosis are CNS hamartomas, subependymal giant cell tumors, cardiac rhabdomyosarcomas, and renal angiomyolipomas (Fig. 5.15). Additional findings include: seizures, white matter heterotopia, cognitive delay, autism spectrum disorder, and infiltrating lung disease.

MoD: TSC gene is a tumor suppressor. It is inherited.

Dx: Clinical, but can confirm with genetic testing.

Tx/Mgmt: Tumor surveillance and symptom management

von Hippel-Lindau Disease

Buzz Words: CNS hemangioblastomas + renal cell carcinoma + pheochromocytoma

Clinical Presentation: Highly variable depending on tumor that develops first. Tumors include: CNS hemangioblastomas, renal cell carcinoma, pheochromocytoma, pancreatic carcinoma, pancreatic neuroendocrine tumors, tumors of the middle ear, tumors of the broad ligament.

MoD: von Hippel-Lindau (VHL) gene is located on chromosome 25 and follows the "two hit" model of carcinogenesis. A germline mutation is often transmitted to a child. If the second chromosome 25 develops a mutation or the VHL gene is hypermethylated, a tumor may result. VHL functions as a tumor suppressor gene.

Dx: Clinical diagnosis is based on finding greater than 1 VHL-related tumor. Genetic testing can confirm.

Tx/Mgmt: Annual tumor surveillance: Tumors should be resected when possible.

Congenital Hydrocephalus

Buzz Words: Prematurity + neural tube defects + aqueductal stenosis

Clinical Presentation: In newborns with patent fontanelles, hydrocephalus presents with increasing head circumference (macrocephaly).

PPx: Depends on etiology

MoD: Numerous: The best way to think about hydrocephalus is by the cause. The cause may be decreased circulation of CSF (outflow obstruction), decreased absorption of CSF by arachoind granulations, or overproduction of CSF by choroid plexus.

Dx: Brain imaging can confirm in patient with macrocephaly.

Tx/Mgmt:
1. Determine cause
2. EVD or VPS are usually necessary
3. Ventriculostomy and serial lumbar punctures may be used.

Chiari 1 Malformation

Buzz Words: Headaches+ cervical spine syrinx + scoliosis

Clinical Presentation: Usually found in teenage years. May be asymptomatic or present with occipital headache, syringomyelia, scoliosis, myelopathy, and cranial nerve dysfunction.

MoD: Greater than 5 mm herniation of the cerebellar tonsils through the foramen magnum. The herniation will result in a syrinx, which may present as scoliosis.

Dx: Sagittal MRI

Tx/Mgmt: Surgical decompression

Chiari 2 Malformation (Arnold-Chiari Syndrome)

Buzz Words: Myelomeningocele + VACTERL, or Noonan syndrome, or NF1

Clinical Presentation: Typically found prenatally in association with other defects. If not, child will present with progressive hydrocephalus.

MoD: Dysgenesis of the brainstem results in sagging of the cerebellar tonsils.

Dx: Sagittal MRI

Tx/Mgmt: Surgical decompression

GUNNER PRACTICE

1. A 25-year-old male presents to the emergency department with complaints of headache and fever for the past 2 days. The headache is diffuse and radiates down his posterior neck. He works as a mechanic and lives with two male roommates. His vital signs are temperature 101.3°F, pulse 108/min, blood pressure 118/75, and respirations of 16/min. He is alert and oriented to person, place, and time. Cranial nerves II–XII are normal with 5/5 strength in all extremities, and sensation is intact. A lumbar puncture is performed and the results are shown below:

Opening pressure	19 cm H_2O (10–12 cm H_2O)
Color	clear
Nucleated cells	150/μL (0–5/μL)
Neutrophils	22%
Erythrocytes	9/μL
Protein	90 mg/dL
Glucose	60 mg/dL
Gram stain and culture pending	—

What is the appropriate management of this patient?
A. IV normal saline
B. Vancomycin and ceftriaxone
C. Vancomycin, ampicillin, and meropenam
D. Dexamethasone and doxycycline
E. Insertion of EVD
F. Decompressive hemicraniectomy

2. A 45-year-old female presents to her family doctor after her husband noticed her smile is asymmetric. She lives in Vermont and is an avid hiker. On exam, her doctor notes that her left face is weak, including the forehead. Which of the following is the most likely cause?
A. Cortical brain tumor
B. Ischemic stroke
C. Facial nerve trauma
D. Spirochete infection

3. A 64-year-old male is brought to the trauma bay by emergency medical services (EMS) following a car accident. He is moaning and not opening his eyes. He flexes his arms in response to pain. He has obvious bilateral femur fractures and respirations are 38/minute with pulse oximetry 84% and blood pressure of 62/45. A FAST (focused assessment with sonography

for trauma) scan does not reveal any bleeding. What is the next best step?

A. Rapid sequence intubation
B. Intravenous epinephrine
C. Intramuscular epinephrine
D. Place c-spine collar and CT cervical spine
E. Reduction and fixation of femurs

ANSWERS: What Would Gunner Jess/Jim Do?

1. WWGJD? A 25-year-old male presents to the emergency department with complaints of **headache and fever for the past 2 days.** The headache is diffuse and radiates down his **posterior neck.** He works as a mechanic and lives with two male roommates. His vital signs are temperature **101.3°F,** pulse 108/min, blood pressure 118/75 and respirations of 16/min. He is alert and oriented to person, place, and time. Cranial nerves II-XII are normal with 5/5 strength in all extremities, and sensation is intact. **[Normal physical exam].** A **lumbar puncture** is performed and the results are shown below:

Opening pressure	19 cm H_2O (10–12 nmL)
Color	Clear
Nucleated cells	150/µL (0–5 nmL) **[High]**
Neutrophils	22% **[Virus]**
Erythrocytes	9/µL
Protein	90 mg/dL
Glucose	60 mg/dL
Gram stain and culture	—
pending	

What is the appropriate management of this patient?
Answer: A, Intravenous normal saline.

    Explanation: The patient has viral meningitis. We can rule out bacterial meningitis because the CSF is lymphocyte predominant (low % neutrophils). This rules out choices B, C, and D. (B would be treatment for suspected bacterial meningitis; C is for meningitis in the setting of immunodeficiency or ventriculoperitoneal shunt; and D is for Lyme meningitis.) E and F are extreme answers. Surgical intervention is usually only indicated in a patient with poor physical exam and these are never used for treatment of viral meningitis. In general, if IV fluids is an answer and the patient is stable, it is the correct answer.

2. WWGJD? A 45-year-old female presents to her family doctor after her husband noticed her **smile is asymmetric.** She lives in **Vermont** and is an avid **hiker. [She has tick exposure].** On exam, her doctor notes that her left face is weak including the forehead.
Answer: D, spirochete infection.

    Explanation: Lyme disease is a common cause of Bell's palsy. A cortical brain tumor or stroke could cause weakness of the face if it was in the motor strip, but other symptoms would be expected. Also, central facial weakness usually spares the forehead. For this reason, A and B can be ruled out. Facial nerve trauma would cause a peripheral facial weakness, which would involve the forehead on the ipsilateral side only. However, the question gives no history of trauma so this answer is not a strong as D.

3. WWGJD? A 64-year-old male is brought to the trauma bay by EMS following a car accident. He is moaning and not opening his eyes. He flexes his arms in response to pain. He has obvious bilateral femur fractures and respirations are 38/min with pulse oximetry 84% and blood pressure of 62/45. FAST scan does not reveal any bleeding. What is the next best step?

Answer: A, rapid sequence intubation.

Explanation: The patient is not breathing effectively and needs to be intubated. In trauma always consider ABC (airway, breathing, and circulation). His airway and breathing are at risk so intubation is required first. The patient is also hypotensive, so following intubation he will require IV fluids and maybe even pressors like epinephrine. But answer A should be done prior to B or C. The patient probably has a cervical spine injury and should be placed in a cervical collar (answer D) and he should undergo a CT scan, but not before intubation. Cervical spine injury can disrupt the sympathetic chain causing hypotension with an abnormal FAST exam. Arguably, the FAST exam should not have been done prior to intubation, which may have been distracting. Do not assume that because a trauma has progressed to a FAST exam that the ABCs have been managed. Lastly, the femurs should be reduced and fixated (answer E) but that can be done once the patient is hemodynamically stable.

Cardiovascular Disorders

Hao-Hua Wu, Junqian Zhang, Leo Wang, Drake Lebrun, Rebecca Gao, and Sean Harbison

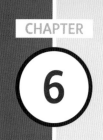

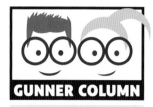

GUNNER COLUMN

Introduction

The heart is one of the most dynamic organs in the human body. It provides driving force in the circulatory system and has the ability to adapt to a wide range of hemodynamic conditions. Dysfunction of the cardiovascular system can occur in many acute and chronic contexts and has both local and systemic manifestations. The heart itself can be afflicted by disease including ischemia, valvular dysfunction, infection, and arrhythmias to name a few. In addition, the vascular system may also have pathology, some of which may be independent of cardiac disease.

From 10 to 15 questions on the Surgery shelf will be from content covered in this chapter. Organization of this chapter is based on pathology within the cardiovascular system: (1) The Heart and Great Vessels, (2) Ischemic Heart Disease, (3) Arrhythmias, (4) Heart Failure, (5) Valvular Heart Disease, (6) Pericardial Disease, (7) Endocarditis and Myocarditis, (8) Cardiac Trauma, (9) Congenital Cardiac Malformations, (10) Cardiac Neoplasms, (11) Hypertension and Hypotension, (12) Vascular Disease, (13) Dyslipidemia, (14) Medication Side Effects Involving the Heart, and (15) Gunner Practice.

The NBME Surgery shelf assesses both factual knowledge as well as the application of principles in the context of the cardiovascular system. First, ensure a solid foundation of knowledge with regard to etiologies, risk factors, diagnostic criteria, and treatment for specific cardiac pathologies. Second, associate Buzz Words with specific diseases. Finally, and most importantly, conceptualize the cardiovascular system (pump + pipes analogy works well) and work through different scenarios on how you would expect the heart (heart rate, stroke volume) and vasculature (systemic vascular resistance, mixed venous oxygen saturation) to respond to changing conditions in the circulatory system.

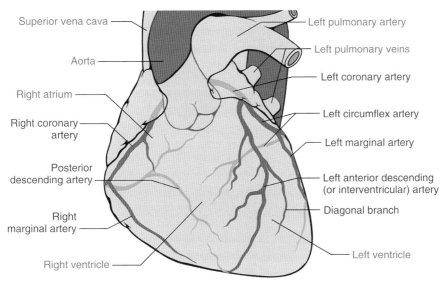

FIG. 6.1 Coronary circulation. (From Wikimedia Commons. https://commons.wikimedia.org/wiki/File:Coronary_arteries.svg. Created by Patrick J. Lynch. Used under Creative Commons Attribution-Share Alike 3.0 Unported license: https://creativecommons.org/licenses/by-sa/3.0/deed.en.)

The Heart and Great Vessels

Like any great surgery student, know your anatomy. Know the coronary circulation (Fig. 6.1) well and be able to correlate arteries with areas of ischemia.

- Left anterior descending artery (LAD) supplies the left ventricle (LV).
- Right coronary artery (RCA) supplies the right ventricle (RV) and both the sinoatrial (SA) and atrioventricular (AV) nodes.
- The majority of individuals have a right-dominant circulation: this means that the posterior descending artery (PDA) comes off of the RCA (and not the left circumflex artery).

Ischemic Heart Disease

Stable Angina

Buzz Words: Sub-sternal chest pressure or pain on EXERTION that goes away with rest

Clinical Presentation: Sub-sternal chest pressure or pain that may radiate to the arm, shoulder, neck, or jaw. Other features may include diaphoresis and shortness of breath. Note that women and the elderly may have atypical symptoms, including epigastric pain. No elevation in cardiac enzymes (troponin, creatine kinase).

Prophylaxis (PPx): Control risk factors including atherosclerosis, hyperlipidemia, and DM

Mechanism of Disease (MoD): Chronic atherosclerotic disease of coronary vessels prevents adequate delivery of blood to the myocardium during periods of high oxygen demand.

Diagnostic Steps (Dx):

1. Baseline electrocardiogram (EKG)
2. Exercise EKG (aka stress test):
   - Exercise EKG is only indicated if baseline EKG is normal
   - For patients with abnormal baseline EKG or who cannot tolerate exercise → pharmacologic stress (with coronary vasodilators—dipyridamole, regadenoson) echocardiography
3. Cardiac enzymes—no elevation in troponin or creatine kinase
4. Coronary angiogram:
   - Indicated in patients with abnormal noninvasive testing (i.e., EKG or echocardiogram)

Treatment and Management Steps (Tx/Mgmt):

- Treat modifiable risk factors—obesity, diabetes mellitus, cholesterol
- Sublingual nitroglycerin for acute exacerbations
- β-Blockers, calcium channel blockers (CCBs), or long-acting nitrates (isosorbide mononitrate) for chronic stable angina

Unstable Angina

Buzz Words: Sub-sternal chest pressure or pain with exertion that occurs AT rest

Clinical Presentation: Sub-sternal chest pressure or pain that may radiate to the arm, shoulder, neck, or jaw that is not necessarily related to exertion. Other features may include diaphoresis and shortness of breath. No elevation in cardiac enzymes (troponin, creatine kinase).

PPx: Control risk factors including atherosclerosis, hyperlipidemia, and DM

MoD: Atherosclerotic plaque instability that leads to temporary partial occlusion of coronary artery with subsequent resolution. Note that the distinction between stable and unstable angina is based on clinical findings and not necessarily related to the degree of coronary occlusion.

Dx:

(1) EKG (transient ST-segment depression or T wave inversion during acute symptoms), (2) cardiac enzymes (NO elevation in troponin or creatine kinase)

Tx/Mgmt:
- Sublingual nitroglycerin for acute symptoms
- Aspirin, β-blockers, heparin
- Coronary angiography ± angioplasty or CABG

Non-ST-Elevation Myocardial Infarction

Buzz Words: ST-depressions in the setting of anginal chest pain ± radiation to the arm and jaw

Clinical Presentation: Non-ST-elevation myocardial infarction (non-STEMI): Typical anginal chest pain (crushing substernal chest pressure is classic) ± radiation to jaw, shoulder, or arm ± diaphoresis, nausea, or vomiting.

PPx: Control risk factors including atherosclerosis, hyperlipidemia, and DM

MoD: Acute plaque rupture within coronary circulation with partial occlusion or transient total occlusion that leads to partial-thickness myocardial infarction

Dx:
(1) EKG (ST-depressions or T wave inversions in contiguous leads), (2) cardiac enzymes (elevation of troponin and creatine kinase)

Tx/Mgmt:
- OH BATMAN—oxygen, heparin, β-blockers, aspirin, thrombolysis, morphine, angiotensin converting enzyme (ACE) inhibitors, nitroglycerine:
  - Give aspirin and typically heparin prior to coronary catheterization
- Secondary prevention of future acute coronary syndrome with: aspirin, β-blocker, ACE inhibitors or angiotensin receptor blockers (ARBs), statin, spironolactone:
  - Avoid β-blockers in patients with bradycardia, decompensated heart failure with low ejection fraction, heart block, asthma, and COPD
  - ARBs can be used in patients who are allergic to ACE inhibitors

ST-Elevation Myocardial Infarction

Buzz Words: ST-elevation in contiguous leads in the setting of typical anginal chest pain (crushing substernal chest pressure is classic) ± radiation to jaw, shoulder, or arm ± diaphoresis, nausea, or vomiting

Clinical Presentation: Typical anginal chest pain (crushing substernal chest pressure is classic) ± radiation to jaw, shoulder, or arm ± diaphoresis, nausea, or vomiting. Note that women and the elderly may have atypical symptoms including epigastric pain.

NSTEMI and unstable angina

MNEMONIC
OH BATMAN for the treatment of NSTEMI (oxygen, heparin, β-blockers, aspirin, thrombolysis, morphine, ACE inhibitors, nitroglycerine)

FOR THE WARDS
Unlike Medicine, you do NOT need to interpret EKGs for the Surgery shelf.

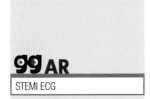

PPx: Control risk factors including atherosclerosis, hyper-lipidemia, and DM

MoD: Acute plaque rupture within coronary circulation with complete occlusion leading to full-thickness myocardial infarction

Dx:

1. EKG (ST-elevations >1 mm in contiguous leads).
2. Cardiac enzymes (elevation of troponin and creatine kinase):
   - Troponin is more sensitive but stays elevated for up to 2 weeks after MI → use CK-MB if suspicious for repeat-MI

Tx/Mgmt:

- **OH BATMAN**—oxygen, heparin, β-blockers, aspirin, thrombolysis, morphine, ACE inhibitors, nitroglycerine:
  - Give aspirin and typically heparin prior to coronary catheterization
- Coronary catheterization (door-to-balloon time <90 minutes is ideal).
- Secondary prevention of future acute coronary syndrome is with: aspirin, β-blocker, ACE inhibitors or ARBs, statin, spironolactone.
- Avoid β-blockers in patients with bradycardia, decompensated heart failure with low ejection fraction, heart block, asthma, and COPD.
- ARBs can be used in patients who are allergic to ACE inhibitors.
- Ventricular arrhythmias are common after MI and are the most common cause of cardiac failure and death in the immediate post-MI period.
- Ventricular free-wall rupture, septal rupture, and papillary muscle rupture most commonly occur during the first 7–10 days after MI:
  - Posteromedial papillary muscle is most prone to rupture due to single blood supply from the RCA.
- Ventricular aneurysms tend to occur months after MI.

Printzmetal Angina (Variant Angina)

Buzz Words: Young, female smokers with anginal chest pain + nighttime

Clinical Presentation: Young and middle-aged female smokers who present with typical chest pain, especially at night. Associated with migraines and Raynaud phenomenon (i.e., other vasospasm-related disorders); can also occur secondary to cocaine use.

MoD: Coronary artery vasospasm leading to tissue ischemia/infarction

Dx:

(1) EKG (typically normal but may show ST-segment abnormalities during episodes of vasospasm), (2) coronary angiography with provocation testing with ergonovine or acetylcholine is the gold standard.

Tx/Mgmt:
- CCBs or nitrates
- β-blockers are contraindicated as they can lead to exacerbation of vasospasm (i.e., unopposed α-adrenergic stimulation)

Arrhythmias

Atrial Arrhythmia

Atrial Fibrillation

Buzz Words: Irregularly irregular rhythm + absence of P-waves

Clinical Presentation: Can be paroxysmal or chronic: Patients can be asymptomatic or have symptoms ranging from palpitations, chest discomfort, lightheadedness, and syncope to hemodynamic instability. This is the most high-yield arrhythmia on the Surgery shelf:
- Atrial fibrillation with rapid ventricular response indicates rapid conduction through the AV node and ↑ventricular rate.
- Long-standing tachycardia can lead to dilated cardiomyopathy.

MoD: Ectopic atrial conduction originating from around the pulmonary veins. Causes of atrial fibrillation include but are not limited to: structural heart disease, valvular heart disease (mitral regurgitation [MR], mitral stenosis), asthma and COPD, hyperthyroidism, hypertension, obstructive sleep apnea, and alcohol consumption.

Dx:

(1) EKG (absence of P-waves and irregularly irregular rhythm), (2) Holter monitor for paroxysmal atrial fibrillation

Tx/Mgmt:
- Hemodynamically unstable → synchronized cardioversion
- Hemodynamically stable:
  - Onset less than 48 hours:
    - Rate control—**β-blockers** (metoprolol), non-dihydropyridine CCBs (verapamil, diltiazem)

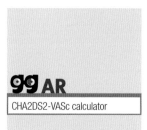

- Onset greater than 48 hours:
  - Use CHA$_2$DS$_2$-VASc:
    - Score of 0 in males or 1 in females → no anticoagulation needed
    - Score of 1 in males → consider anticoagulation
    - Score ≥2 → anticoagulate
  - Consider rate control, rhythm control (class I and III antiarrhythmics), synchronized cardioversion, or catheter ablation of the electrical pathways near the pulmonary veins

Atrial Flutter

Buzz Words: Sawtooth waves on EKG

Clinical Presentation: Patients can be asymptomatic or have symptoms ranging from palpitations, chest discomfort, lightheadedness, and syncope to hemodynamic instability.

MoD: Ectopic atrial conduction originating from around the **tricuspid annulus.** Causes of atrial flutter include but are not limited to: structural heart disease, valvular heart disease (MR, mitral stenosis), asthma and COPD, hyperthyroidism, hypertension, and obstructive sleep apnea.

Dx: EKG showing sawtooth pattern between 250 and 300 bpm with no discernable P-waves

Tx/Mgmt:

- Hemodynamically unstable → synchronized cardioversion
- Hemodynamically stable:
  - β-Blockers, CCBs + anticoagulation for at least 4 weeks
  - Anticoagulation for at least 4 weeks then cardioversion
  - Ablation

Multifocal Atrial Tachycardia

Buzz Words: Irregularly irregular supraventricular tachycardia (VT) with at least three different P-wave morphologies

Clinical Presentation: Patients can be asymptomatic or have symptoms ranging from palpitations, chest discomfort, lightheadedness, and syncope to hemodynamic instability. Particularly common in older people with COPD.

MoD: Multiple atrial foci (≥3) of electrical activity

Dx:
- Tachycardia with at least three different P-wave morphologies
- Irregularly irregular rhythm
- Vagal maneuvers and adenosine can break re-entrant supraventricular tachycardias but are not as useful for multifocal atrial tachycardia (MAT)

Tx/Mgmt:
(1) Treatment of underlying cause, (2) β-blockers and CCBs can be used for rate control

Re-Entrant Tachycardia

Buzz Words: Narrow-complex tachycardia

Clinical Presentation: Asymptomatic or palpitations, chest pain, SOB, lightheadedness, syncope.

MoD: Rapid electrical conduction with re-entrant conduction through an accessory pathway between the atria and ventricles (most commonly seen in Wolf-Parkinson-White syndrome [WPW]) or within the AV node itself (AV nodal re-entrant tachycardia)

Dx:
(1) AV re-entry → see section on WPW syndrome, (2) AV nodal re-entry → EKG with narrow complex tachycardia and retrograde P-waves

Tx/Mgmt: AV nodal re-entry → vagal maneuvers; medications that slow conduction through the AV node: adenosine, CCBs, β-blockers

Ventricular Arrhythmia

Ventricular Tachycardia

Buzz Words: Wide-complex monomorphic tachycardia

Clinical Presentation: Patient may have palpitations, lightheadedness, SOB, syncope that can lead to cardiac arrest.

MoD: Ectopic pacemaker in the ventricles or re-entrant circuit around area of infarcted myocardium → monomorphic VT. **Torsades de pointes** is a polymorphic VT that is associated with prolonged QT interval. Common causes of torsades de pointes include: hypokalemia, hypomagnesemia, drugs (fluoroquinolones, erythromycin, typical antipsychotics). Treat with magnesium sulfate (**high yield!**).

Dx: EKG with wide-complex tachycardia

Tx/Mgmt:
- Hemodynamically unstable → cardioversion:
  - Pulseless VT → defibrillation
- Hemodynamically stable:
  - Procainamide, sotalol, amiodarone

99 AR

Re-entrant tachycardia

99 AR

Ventricular tachycardia

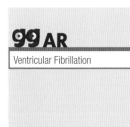

Ventricular Fibrillation

Ventricular Fibrillation

Buzz Words: Low-amplitude undulating EKG without QRS complexes

Clinical Presentation: Patient may present in cardiac arrest leading to hypotension, syncope, and/or sudden death.

MoD: Uncoordinated electrical activity in the ventricles leading to systolic dysfunction and collapse of the systemic circulation

Dx: EKG showing fine or coarse fibrillating line

Tx/Mgmt:

Defibrillation ± epinephrine, amiodarone

Pulseless electrical activity = cardiac rhythm on EKG that is expected to produce a pulse but does not. Treat with cardiopulmonary resuscitation (CPR) + epinephrine → defibrillation if reverts to pulseless VT or ventricular fibrillation (VF).

Asystole = absence of cardiac electrical activity (flat line on EKG). Treat with CPR + epinephrine → defibrillation if reverts to pulseless VT or VF.

Conduction Blocks and Bundle Branch Blocks

Intro to heart blocks

These are frequently tested on Medicine but less tested on Surgery since you won't be expected to interpret an EKG. However, the question stem may contain Buzz Words about conduction blocks that prompt you to recognize the disease without the corresponding EKG. However, left and right bundle branch block are very difficult to identify with Buzz Words alone, are rarely tested, and thus not covered.

First Degree Heart Block

Buzz Words: Prolonged PR interval ≥0.2 seconds + regular rhythm

Clinical Presentation: Prolonged PR interval ≥0.2 seconds, asymptomatic

MoD: Delay of conduction in the AV node

Dx: EKG—PR prolongation ≥0.2 seconds

Tx/Mgmt: None

Second Degree Heart Block (Mobitz Type I [Wenckebach])

Buzz Words: Prolonging of the PR interval followed by a dropped beat; grouped beating + abnormal rhythm

Clinical Presentation: Progressive prolonging of **PR interval** ending with a dropped beat → compare the PR intervals of the beats just before and just after the dropped beat. QRS interval is normal.

MoD: Delay of conduction at the level of the AV node

Dx: EKG—progressive prolonging of the PR interval followed by a drop beat

Tx/Mgmt: Benign, no treatment needed

QUICK TIPS
Compare the PR interval of the last beat before the dropped beat with the first beat following the dropped beat.

Mobitz Type II

Buzz Words: Constant PR interval followed by a dropped beat; grouped beating

Clinical Presentation: **PR interval is constant** prior to dropped beat. QRS interval is typically **prolonged.**

MoD: Delay of conduction in the bundle of His

Dx: EKG—constant PR interval before and after a dropped beat with prolongation of the QRS complex ≥0.12 seconds

Tx/Mgmt: Typically requires pacemaker insertion to prevent complete heart block

Third-Degree (Complete) Heart Block

Buzz Words: Complete dissociation of the electrical activity between the atria and the ventricles

Clinical Presentation: Complete dissociation of the atria and ventricles. Spontaneous atrial and ventricular pacemakers are firing independently → no association between P-waves and QRS complexes.

MoD: Damage to the AV node (most commonly by ischemia) leads to loss of conduction of atrial signals into the ventricles.

Dx: EKG showing dissociation between P-waves and QRS complexes (typically ≥0.1 second). The duration between successive P-waves is constant. The duration between successive QRS complexes is also constant.

Tx/Mgmt: **Pacemaker insertion**

QUICK TIPS
Look for buried P-waves presenting as weird blips in QRS or T-waves

Long-QT Syndromes

Be familiar with two long-QT syndromes with eponyms that are useful for ruling out answer choices:

- **Romano-Ward syndrome** = autosomal dominant long-QT syndrome
- **Jervell and Lange-Nielsen syndrome** = autosomal recessive long-QT syndrome + sensorineural hearing loss

Sick Sinus Syndrome

Buzz Words: Impaired conduction from the sinus node that may cause periods of tachycardia and periods of conduction block/bradycardia

AR

Tachy-brady syndrome. Note the transition from tachycardia to bradycardia.

Clinical Presentation: May be asymptomatic or present with palpitations, chest pain, lightheadedness, and syncope. **Tachy-Brady syndrome** = subset of sick sinus syndrome with periods of tachycardia and bradycardia is often associated with ischemic or valvular heart disease.

MoD: Scarring, degeneration, or damage to the conduction system that impairs conduction from the sinus node

Dx:

(1) EKG—showing periods of arrhythmia (sinus block, sinus bradycardia, atrial fibrillation, etc.) during acute events. (2) Holter monitor is often necessary as conduction blocks may be transient.

Tx/Mgmt:

- Patients with bradyarrhythmias require pacemaker
- Patients with isolated tachyarrhythmias may be managed medically with β-blockers and CCBs

Wolf–Parkinson–White Syndrome

Buzz Words: Up-sloping first segment of QRS (**delta wave**), prolonged QRS, decreased PR-interval

Clinical Presentation: Typically asymptomatic when not in re-entrant rhythm. Palpitations, lightheadedness, syncope are possible for re-entrant tachycardia.

MoD: Presence of an accessory conduction tract between the atria and ventricles (Bundle of Kent) that allows for bypass of the AV node. Re-entrant rhythm can occur with retrograde conduction from the ventricles through the accessory tract and back into the atria.

Dx:

1. EKG:
   - Decreased PR-interval
   - Characteristic up-sloping first segment of QRS (delta wave)
   - Prolonged QRS

Tx/Mgmt: Procainamide or amiodarone for tachyarrhythmias associated with WPW

Heart Failure

Congestive Heart Failure

Systolic Dysfunction (Heart Failure With Reduced Ejection Fraction/HFrEF)

Buzz Words: Orthopnea, reduced ejection fraction (EF ≤ 55%), pulmonary edema

Clinical Presentation:
- Left-sided heart failure (HF)—SOB, pulmonary edema (rales, crackles), orthopnea, paroxysmal nocturnal dyspnea, decreased perfusion (cyanosis, acute kidney injury [AKI], hepatic injury, etc.)
- Right-sided HF—edema, ascites, ↑JVP (jugular venous pulse), liver enlargement (nutmeg liver), hepatojugular reflux, decreased perfusion (cyanosis, AKI, hepatic injury, etc.)

PPx: Control of risk factors—hypertension (HTN), EtOH, atherosclerosis/coronary artery disease (CAD) risk factors

MoD: Variable but all lead to impaired ventricular contraction (↓ejection fraction)

Dx:
(1) EKG (left ventricular hypertrophy [LVH]/right ventricular hypertrophy [RVH] → high amplitude QRS complex), (2) echocardiogram showing reduced ejection fraction, (3) elevated levels of pro-brain natriuretic peptide (pro-BNP)

Tx/Mgmt:
- Acute HF—diuretics (furosemide), noninvasive positive pressure ventilation
- Chronic HF:
  - Survival benefit: ACE inhibitors, ARBs, β-blockers, spironolactone
  - Symptom management without survival benefit: diuretics, digoxin, hydralazine

Diastolic Dysfunction (Heart Failure With Preserved Ejection Fraction/HFpEF)

Buzz Words: Preserved ejection fraction (EF ≥ 55%)

Clinical Presentation: Similar to systolic heart failure as described above

MoD: Impaired relaxation (diastolic dysfunction) of the ventricles → increased left ventricular end-diastolic pressure → back-up of pressure through the left heart, pulmonary circulation, and right heart

Dx:
(1) EKG, (2) echocardiography showing preserved ejection fraction, (3) elevated levels of pro-brain natriuretic peptide (pro-BNP)

Tx/Mgmt:
- Current treatments do not improve survival
- β-Blockers, ACEIs, and diuretics for symptom management

QUICK TIPS

Nutmeg liver is caused by venous congestion of hepatic vessels (dark areas) and areas of uninvolved tissue.

99 AR

2013 ACCF/AHA guidelines for treatment of heart failure

QUICK TIPS

The only β-blockers shown to improve survival are metoprolol tartrate, carvedilol, and bisoprolol.

QUICK TIPS

Hydralazine can be of benefit in African-Americans with NYHA class III–IV heart failure.

High-Output Cardiac Failure

Buzz Words: Increased ejection fraction + hyper-dynamic circulation + bounding pulses with widened pulse pressure

Clinical Presentation:
- SOB, dyspnea, pulmonary edema, peripheral edema in the setting of **increased EF** (hyper-dynamic circulation)
- Tachycardia w/ a bounding pulse with widened pulse pressure

MoD:
- **Anemia**—blood is unable to provide enough oxygen for tissues → requires faster circulation
- **Arterio-venous fistulas** (e.g., hereditary hemorrhagic telangiectasia, knife wound in the thigh causing a shunt)—shunting of blood from the arterial to venous system simulates anemia (tissues are not getting enough oxygen) so the heart must pump faster to deliver more blood
- **Paget disease of the bone**—increased vascularization of metabolically active bone
- **Sepsis**—dilation of peripheral vasculature
- **Thyrotoxicosis**
- **Wet beriberi** (vitamin B1 deficiency)

Dx:
(1) EKG, (2) echocardiography—evidence of increased ejection fraction and hyperdynamic circulation, (3) pro-BNP levels can be used for evidence of ventricular strain

Tx/Mgmt:
Treatment of underlying etiology:
- **Anemia**—blood transfusions or iron supplementation depending on the cause of anemia
- **AV-fistulas**—surgical repair
- **Paget disease of the bone**—bisphosphonates, calcitonin
- **Thyrotoxicosis**—depends on the cause (radioactive iodine for Graves, surgical resection for hot thyroid nodule)
- **Wet beriberi**—replete vitamin B1 (thiamine)

Valvular Heart Disease

Aortic Valve Disease

Valvular heart disease is frequently tested on the shelf. Know the characteristics of heart murmurs and you will ace this topic.

Aortic Stenosis

Buzz Words: Pulsus parvus et tardus (weak and late-arriving pulse) + crescendo-decrescendo murmur at the right upper sternal border that radiates to carotids

Clinical Presentation:

- SAD—syncope, angina, dyspnea
- *Pulsus parvus et tardus*—weak and late arriving carotid pulse
- Early systolic ejection murmur radiating to carotids—crescendo-decrescendo murmur best heard at the right upper sternal border
- Soft aortic component of the second heart sound

Aortic stenosis murmur

MoD: Narrowing of aortic valve increases afterload → LV strain, weak pulses, inadequate delivery of blood. Typically occurs in older individuals → most commonly due to senile **sclerocalcific changes** of the aortic valve. Aortic stenosis (AS) in younger individuals is often caused by **bicuspid**/unicuspid **aortic valves** or **rheumatic fever** (developing nations).

Dx: Echocardiography to visualize valve, measure flow, pressure gradient, and valve area

Tx/Mgmt:

Aortic valve replacement is indicated in:

- Patients with symptomatic disease
- Patients with severe AS (pressure gradient ≥40 mm Hg) with left ventricular ejection fraction (LVEF) ≤40% or undergoing other cardiac surgery

Aortic Regurgitation

Buzz Words: Water hammer pulse, decrescendo murmur at the right upper sternal border

Clinical Presentation:

- Dyspnea on exertion, orthopnea, chest pain
- Early diastolic murmur—decrescendo murmur best heard at the right upper sternal border

Aortic stenosis murmur

- Increased pulse pressure (difference between systolic and diastolic blood pressures) → bounding pulses
- Austin Flint murmur = rumbling mid-diastolic murmur heard in severe aortic regurgitation (AR)

MoD: Most often caused by **dilation of the aortic root**—can occur with bicuspid aortic valve, collagen vascular diseases (Marfan syndrome, Ehlers-Danlos syndrome), rheumatic fever, ankylosing spondylitis, or idiopathic. Loss of adequate valve coaptation leads to backflow of blood into the LV after ventricular systole.

Dx: Echocardiography to visualize valve and measure flow

Tx/Mgmt:
- **Aortic valve replacement** is the treatment of choice:
  - Indications include symptomatic disease or with EF ≤ 50%
- ACEIs, ARBs, CCBs may be useful in patients with AR and HTN to reduce afterload on the strained LV.

Mitral Valve Disease

Mitral Stenosis

Buzz Words: Opening snap with a mid-diastolic, low-pitched, rumbling murmur

Clinical Presentation:
- Mid-diastolic, low-pitched, rumbling murmur with opening snap
- Dyspnea on exertion, orthopnea, chest pain
- Secondary atrial fibrillation

PPx: Prevention of rheumatic heart disease

MoD:
- Thickened, fibrotic, calcified mitral valve → reduced diastolic flow through the mitral valve → ↑left atrial pressures → back up of pressure into the pulmonary circulation
- Chronic increase in left atrial pressures leads to dilatation → disruption of electrical conduction system → atrial fibrillation

Dx:
(1) EKG; (2) echocardiography—visualize valve, measure flow, pressure gradient, and valve area

Tx/Mgmt:
- For patients with mild mitral stenosis:
  - Dietary sodium restriction
  - Careful titration of β-blockers while avoiding medications that reduce afterload (to prevent hypotension)
  - Rheumatic fever PPx with penicillin or azithromycin
  - Monitor for sequelae of mitral stenosis → atrial fibrillation (anticoagulated as necessary)
- **Mitral valve replacement** or balloon valvuloplasty for refractory disease or recurrent embolization due to atrial fibrillation

Mitral Valve Prolapse

Buzz Words: Mid-systolic click followed by a systolic decrescendo murmur

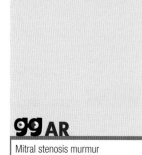

99 AR

Mitral stenosis murmur

QUICK TIPS

Treatment of group A streptococcal pharyngitis is with penicillin or azithromycin.

Clinical Presentation:
- Mid-systolic click followed by decrescendo murmur (systolic):
  - Murmur increases in duration with Valsalva or decreasing preload
- Risk factors include: collagen vascular disorders (Marfan syndrome, Ehlers-Danlos syndrome), polycystic kidney disease, Graves disease

MoD: Myxomatous valve degeneration

Dx: Echocardiography showing variable prolapse of the mitral valve leaflets into the left atrium (LA) during ventricular systole

Tx/Mgmt:
- Most patients require no treatment
- Those with symptomatic mitral valve prolapse (MVP) can be treated with β-blockers
- No antibiotic PPx for dental procedures in otherwise healthy patients with MVP

Mitral Regurgitation

Buzz Words: Mid-systolic, blowing murmur that radiates to the axilla

Clinical Presentation:
- Signs of congestive heart failure—SOB, orthopnea, paroxysmal nocturnal dyspnea
- Atrial fibrillation due to LA dilation → *P mitrale* = broad P-wave with two peaks
- Initially see increased ejection fraction → decrease in EF suggests systolic heart failure

MoD: Mitral valve prolapse is the most common predisposing factor. Other causes include ischemic heart disease, rheumatic fever, and connective tissue disease. Posterior MI can lead to ischemia of the postero-medial papillary muscle → acute MR.

Dx: Echocardiography—measure degree of regurgitation

Tx/Mgmt:
- Medical management is aimed at decreasing afterload with ACEIs or hydralazine to increase the forward ejection fraction while minimizing the regurgitant fraction
- Surgical repair for ↓EF, severe pulmonary hypertension, or new onset atrial fibrillation

Tricuspid Valve Disease

Tricuspid Stenosis

Buzz Words: Mid-diastolic murmur that is best heard over the left sternal border

99 AR

Mitral prolapse and regurgitation

QUICK TIPS

For posterior MI, look for inverse changes (ST-depressions) in the anterior precordial leads V_1 and V_2.

Clinical Presentation:
- Mid-diastolic murmur that is best heard over the left sternal border, which may increase with inspiration
- Right-heart dysfunction with backup of pressure into the venous system:
  - May result in hepatic congestion and peripheral edema
  - Jugular venous pressure is increased

MoD: Almost always caused by rheumatic heart disease

Dx: Echocardiography

Tx/Mgmt:
- Medical management with diuretics and salt restriction to decrease preload on right heart
- Balloon valvuloplasty or surgical replacement for refractory symptomatic disease

Tricuspid Regurgitation

Buzz Words: Blowing systolic murmur best heard at the lower left sternal border that increases with inspiration, large C-V waves on jugular venous tracings

Clinical Presentation:
- Right-sided heart failure—ascites, peripheral edema
- Pan-systolic murmur that increases with inspiration
- Large C-V waves in the jugular venous pulse

MoD: Dilation of the tricuspid annulus—most commonly 2/2 RV dilation; rheumatic heart disease, myxomatous degeneration

Dx: Echocardiography

Tx/Mgmt:
- For patients with left-sided heart failure leading to tricuspid regurgitation:
  - Diuretics and ACE inhibitors
- Tricuspid valve replacement for symptomatic patients or those with RV dysfunction

Pulmonic Valve Disease

Pulmonic Stenosis

Buzz Words: Systolic ejection murmur at the right upper sternal border, right-sided S_4, loud S_2

Clinical Presentation:
- Asymptomatic or dyspnea on exertion/signs of right-sided heart failure
- Systolic ejection murmur at the right upper sternal border
- Loud S_2
- RVH → may present with right-sided S_4

gg AR

Tricuspid regurgitation murmur

MoD:
- **Congenital**: Tetralogy of Fallot, Noonan syndrome, congenital rubella syndrome, Williams syndrome, Alagile syndrome
- **Acquired**: carcinoid syndrome

Dx: Echocardiography showing reduced flow through the pulmonic valve

Tx/Mgmt: Balloon valvotomy

Pulmonic Regurgitation

Buzz Words: Diastolic murmur best heard at the right upper sternal border

Clinical Presentation:
- Patients are typically asymptomatic prior to right ventricular dysfunction
- Dyspnea on exertion, lightheadedness, syncope, peripheral edema, hepatic congestion
- Graham-Steell murmur = early, diastolic murmur heard best at the left sternal edge with the patient in full inspiration

MoD: Etiologies include: iatrogenic, endocarditis, rheumatic heart disease, carcinoid disease, congenital (tetralogy of Fallot)

Dx: Echocardiography showing retrograde flow through the pulmonic valve

Tx/Mgmt:
- Mild pulmonic regurgitation typically does not require treatment as the right-sided heart can adapt to the low pressure volume overload
- Surgical valve repair in cases of RV strain or failure

Pericardial Disease

Pericardial Effusion

Buzz Words: Water bottle heart, enlarged cardiac silhouette, low-voltage on EKG with electrical alternans, pulsus paradoxus (Figs. 6.2 and 6.3).

Clinical Presentation:
- Variable depending on rate of formation and volume of effusion:
  - Large volumes can accumulate with long-standing, slow effusions
  - Rapid effusions cause cardiac dysfunction almost immediately
- Cardiac tamponade = effusion that results in equalization of intracardiac pressures → bulging of

Heart murmurs

QUICK TIPS

EKG for pericardial effusion showing electrical alternans may be seen on the Surgery shelf; however, you can make the diagnosis WITHOUT knowing how to interpret the EKG.

interventricular septum into the LV → ↓stroke volume → cardiogenic shock:

- Pulsus paraxodus = drop of >10 mm Hg in systolic blood pressure (BP) with inspiration

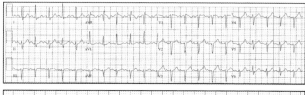
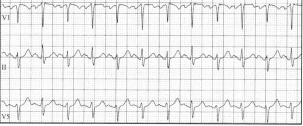

FIG. 6.2 Electrical alternans. Note the alternating amplitudes of the QRS complex as the heart swings in a pericardial effusion. (From Wikimedia Commons. https://commons.wikimedia.org/wiki/File:Electrical_Alternans.JPG. Created by James Heilman, MD. Used under Creative Commons Attribution-Share Alike 3.0 Unported license: https://creativecommons.org/licenses/by-sa/3.0/deed.en.)

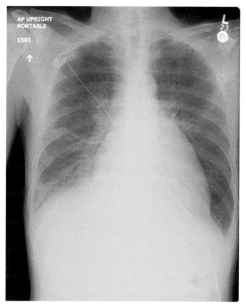

FIG. 6.3 Pericardial effusion. Note the enlarged cardiac silhouette. (From Wikimedia Commons. https://commons.wikimedia.org/wiki/File:Water_bottle.png. Used under Creative Commons Attribution-Share Alike 3.0 Unported license: https://creativecommons.org/licenses/by-sa/3.0/deed.en.)

MoD: Post-myocardial infarction or cardiac surgery, auto-immune disease, acute pericarditis, malignancy, uremia, blunt cardiac trauma.

Dx:

1. CXR—enlarged cardiac silhouette (water bottle heart)
2. EKG:
   - Low voltage—low amplitude QRS
   - Electrical alternans—alternating amplitude of QRS with each beat (heart is moving in sac of fluid so the major axis of EKG changes with each beat)
3. Echocardiography
4. Diagnostic and therapeutic pericardiocentesis—if the etiology of the effusion is not known

Tx/Mgmt:

- Asymptomatic, small effusions can be monitored if the patient is hemodynamically stable
- Hemodynamically unstable patients (i.e., tamponade) require pericardiocentesis:
  - Patients with large effusions typically require eventual treatment, even if they are asymptomatic

Pericarditis

Acute

Buzz Words: Friction rub + diffuse ST-elevations with PR-depressions + improvement with sitting up and leaning forward

Clinical Presentation:

- Sharp chest pain that is classically improved while sitting up and leaning forward
- **Diffuse ST-elevations** and **PR-depressions** in all leads except aVR on EKG
- Pericardial **friction rub** on auscultation

MoD: Inflammation of the pericardium 2/2 **infection, uremia**, autoimmune (Dressler syndrome), or post-MI/pericardiotomy syndrome

Dx: Clinical Presentation + EKG changes

Tx/Mgmt:

- Nonsteroidal anti-inflammatory drugs (NSAIDs) ± colchicine > steroids
- Treatment of underlying cause in uremia or autoimmune disease

Constrictive

Buzz Words: Pericardial calcification

99 AR

Pericarditis EKG

QUICK TIPS

Note that patients with uremic pericarditis (usually with BUN ≥60 mg/dL) often do not have classic EKG changes.

Clinical Presentation:
- Hypotension, syncope
- Kussmaul sign = ↑ in JVD with inspiration
- Pericardial calcification
- Pericardial knock (early diastolic sound) on auscultation

MoD: Calcification and fibrosis of the pericardium leading to diastolic dysfunction and impaired filling:
- Developed countries—viral (coxsackievirus, echo-virus adenovirus), radiation, cardiac surgery
- Undeveloped countries—tuberculosis (TB)

Dx: Echocardiography showing calcifications and elevated diastolic pressures

Tx/Mgmt: Pericardiotomy

Endocarditis and Myocarditis

Endocarditis

Infectious

Buzz Words: Splinter hemorrhage, Roth spots, Janeway lesions, Osler nodes

Clinical Presentation:
- One of the highest yield disease processes on the Surgery shelf. Can also appear on Medicine, Pediatrics, Ob/Gyn shelf exams.
- Fever, malaise
- Splinter hemorrhage (Fig. 6.4), Roth spots (retinal hemorrhage with pale center), Janeway lesions (painless microabscess/embolus) (Fig. 6.5), Osler nodes (Osler = Ouch!; painful nodules in fingers—immune complex)
- Embolic disease—stroke, arterial occlusion, seeding of bacteria causing local infection

MoD:
- Native valve—*Staphylococcus aureus*
- Damaged valves—*Staphylococcus epidermidis, S. aureus*
- Dental procedures—Viridans group streptococci (*Streptococcus mutans, Streptococcus mitis, Streptococcus sanguinis*)
- Intravenous drug user (IVDU)—*S. aureus, Candida, Pseudomonas*
- Genitourinary (GU) procedures—*Enterococci*
- Colon cancer—*Streptococcus gallolyticus* (*Streptococcus bovis*), *Clostridium septicum*
- Culture negative infectious endocarditis—HACEK organisms (although some are now able to be cultured), *Coxiella, Bartonella, Chlamydia*

99 AR
Duke criteria for endocarditis

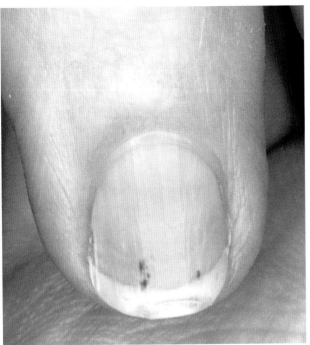

FIG. 6.4 Splinter hemorrhages. (From Wikimedia Commons. https://commons.wikimedia.org/wiki/File:Splinter_hemorrhage.jpg. In the public domain.)

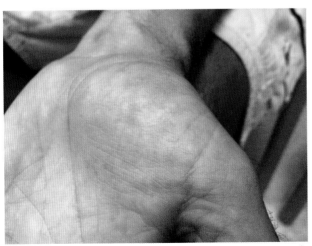

FIG. 6.5 Janeway lesions. These are painless lesions, most commonly seen on the acral extremities, which are caused by bacterial emboli. (From Wikimedia Commons. https://commons.wikimedia.org/wiki/File:Janeway_lesion.JPG. Used under Creative Commons Attribution-Share Alike 4.0 International license: https://creativecommons.org/licenses/by-sa/4.0/deed.en.)

Dx:

(1) Large-volume blood cultures, (2) echocardiography

Tx/Mgmt: Antibiotics ± surgical debridement/valve replacement

Noninfectious (Marantic Endocarditis)

Buzz Words: Sterile vegetations on cardiac valves associated with malignancy and autoimmune disease

Clinical Presentation:

- Sterile deposits on cardiac valves → can flick off and cause thrombotic disease
- Libman-Sacks endocarditis is associated with systemic lupus erythematosus and presents with deposits on both the atrial and ventricular surfaces of cardiac valves:
  - Most commonly causes valve dysfunction > embolic disease

Dx: Echocardiography

Tx/Mgmt:

- Anticoagulation
- Treatment of underlying disease
- Surgical valve repair/replacement

Myocarditis

Buzz Words: Acute-onset heart failure in a young or middle-aged, otherwise healthy individual

Clinical Presentation:

- May have viral prodrome—upper respiratory tract infection (URI) symptoms, myalgias, fever
- Cardiac manifestations are variable:
  - Asymptomatic, chest pain, palpitations, arrhythmias, sudden cardiac death
  - Signs of heart failure—SOB, orthopnea, paroxysmal nocturnal dyspnea

MoD:

- Viral infection is the most common cause: Coxsackie B, adenovirus, hepatitis C virus (HCV), cytomegalovirus (CMV), Epstein-Barr virus (EBV), echovirus, parvovirus B19, influenza:
  - Initial viral infection and subsequent immune response cause damage to cardiac myocytes
- Bacterial, fungal, and parasitic causes are also possible but are less common
- Noninfectious etiologies include: giant cell myocarditis (rapidly progressive), alcohol, hypereosinophilic syndrome (Loeffler syndrome), sarcoidosis, thyrotoxicosis

Dx:
(1) Endomyocardial biopsy is the gold standard but is not always required, (2) echocardiography or other cardiac imaging to assess cardiac function

Tx/Mgmt:
(1) Treat symptoms of heart failure—diuretics, ACEI, oxygen, ± β-blockers; (2) avoid NSAIDs, EtOH, and heavy exercise to prevent further cardiac stress

Cardiac Trauma

Cardiac trauma is very high yield on the Surgery shelf due to the need for surgical intervention.

Myocardial Contusion

Buzz Words: Associated with sternal fracture, presents with new-onset bundle branch block and ST-segment abnormalities

Clinical Presentation:
- New onset bundle branch block or arrhythmia (may be delayed up to 72 hours)
- RV is the most commonly affected as it is the most anterior
- Often associated with sternal fracture

MoD: Blunt chest trauma

Dx:
(1) EKG—new-onset bundle branch block and/or ST-segment abnormalities, (2) echocardiography—wall-motion abnormalities, (3) cardiac enzymes—troponin and creatine kinase are typically elevated

Tx/Mgmt: Supportive care

Myocardial Free Wall Rupture

Buzz Words: Sudden-onset pulseless electrical activity (PEA) arrest 3–7 days after MI

Clinical Presentation:
- Rapid onset cardiovascular collapse and death unless tamponade occurs:
  - PEA arrest is common
- Hypotension, tachycardia, ↑JVP, signs of cardiogenic shock

MoD: Typically occurs 3–7 days after MI or occasionally after myocardial trauma. Risk factors include: female gender, first ischemic event (i.e., scar tissue is tougher and less prone to rupture), low body mass index (BMI), and no myocardial hypertrophy.

Dx: Typically by Clinical Presentation (hypotension, PEA arrest) or at autopsy

Tx/Mgmt: Immediate surgical repair

Traumatic Aortic Rupture

Buzz Words: Acceleration-deceleration injury causing a tear at the attachment of the ligamentum arteriosum

Clinical Presentation:

- May be difficult to diagnose clinically because of other trauma that typically co-presents
- Some patients may have differential blood pressures between upper and lower extremities
- Most commonly occurs just proximal to the attachment site of the ligamentum arteriosum (immobile part of the aorta):
  - Rupture occurs in the descending aorta, near the branch point of the left subclavian artery

MoD: Acceleration-deceleration forces cause shearing of the aorta at places where the aorta is relatively immobile (i.e., tethered by the ligamentum arteriosum).

Dx:

- Chest x-ray (CXR) may show widened mediastinum
- Computed tomography (CT) angiogram if patient stable

Tx/Mgmt:

- Blood pressure control with labetalol or nitroprusside to prevent complete tear
- Immediate surgical or endovascular repair

Congenital Cardiac Malformations

Ventricular Septal Defect

Buzz Words: Harsh, holosystolic blowing murmur along the left lower sternal border with palpable thrill

Clinical Presentation:

- Small ventricular septal defects (VSDs) are typically asymptomatic and may close spontaneously.
- Large VSDs allow passage of significant volume of blood from the LV to the RV → ↑RV pressures, ↑pulmonary blood flow:
  - Over time the flow may reverse as pressures in the pulmonary and right heart increase (Eisenmenger syndrome) → late-onset cyanosis.

MoD: Communication between the LV and RV allows for blood flow from the high-pressure left-heart system into the low-pressure right heart.

AR

Eisenmenger syndrome

QUICK TIPS

Small VSDs typically have louder murmurs due to increased turbulence.

Dx:
(1) Harsh, holosystolic blowing murmur along the left lower sternal border ± palpable thrill, (2) echocardiography

Tx/Mgmt:
- No treatment for small VSDs
- Surgical or catheter-based closures can be considered for symptomatic, large VSDs

Atrial Septal Defect

Buzz Words: Fixed splitting of S_2 + paradoxical embolization

Clinical Presentation:
- Typically asymptomatic into early adulthood. May eventually present with dyspnea on exertion, palpitations, and easy fatigueability → Eisenmenger syndrome occurs late.
- Paradoxical emboli—venous emboli bypasses the lungs to cause obstruction in the arterial system.
- **Patent foramen ovale** = incomplete closure of the foramen ovale occurs (fetal connection between the LA and right atrium [RA]).

MoD: Incomplete closure of the inter-atrial septum—most commonly due to ostium secundum defect. Associated diseases include: Down syndrome, Ebstein anomaly, fetal alcohol syndrome.

Dx:
(1) Echocardiography, (2) Doppler bubble study—inject air into the right atrium and look for bubbles in the left atrium

Tx/Mgmt: Percutaneous or surgical closure for symptomatic or large atrial septal defects (ASDs)

Patent Foramen Ovale

Buzz Words: Incomplete closure of the foramen ovale from fetal circulation, paradoxical embolization

Clinical Presentation: Typically asymptomatic: May lead to paradoxical emboli—venous emboli that bypasses the lungs to cause obstruction in the arterial system.

MoD: Incomplete closure of the foramen ovale (between the LA and RA) from fetal circulation

Dx:
(1) Echocardiography, (2) Doppler bubble study—inject air into the right atrium and look for bubbles in the left atrium

Tx/Mgmt: No treatment for asymptomatic disease; percutaneous/catheter closure if needed

Patient ductus arteriosis

Patent Ductus Arteriosus

Buzz Words: Continuous machine-like murmur, widened pulse pressure and bounding pulse

Clinical Presentation:
- Affected infants are initially asymptomatic but may have increased work of breathing if the patent ductus arteriosus (PDA) is large.
- Increased blood flow from the aorta into the pulmonary artery → widened pulse pressure / bounding pulse:
  - **Late cyanosis** in lower extremities > upper extremities due to increased pressure in the pulmonary circulation
    - Continuous, machine-like murmur best heard at the right upper sternal border
    - May be associated with transposition of the great vessels → give **prostaglandin E2** to keep the PDA open
  - Need to keep the ductus arteriosus open in order to have mixing of blood from the otherwise separate pulmonary and systemic circulations in transposition of the great vessels.

MoD: Connection between the aorta and pulmonary trunk that persists after the immediate neonatal period. Blood flows from high pressure systemic circulation (aorta) into the low pressure pulmonary circulation. Associated with: congenital rubella syndrome, preterm birth, and chromosomal abnormalities (Down syndrome).

Dx: Echocardiography

Tx/Mgmt:
- NSAIDs (**indomethacin**) can be used to close PDA in the neonatal period
- Surgical repair for later diagnosed lesions

Tetralogy of Fallot

Buzz Words: Boot-shaped heart + pulmonic stenosis + tet spells + overriding aorta +DiGeorge syndrome (Figs. 6.6 and 6.7)

Clinical Presentation:
- Major anomalies in tetralogy of Fallot (ToF):
  - Pulmonic stenosis—the most important factor in the degree of the cyanosis
- VSD:
  - RVH
  - Overriding aorta

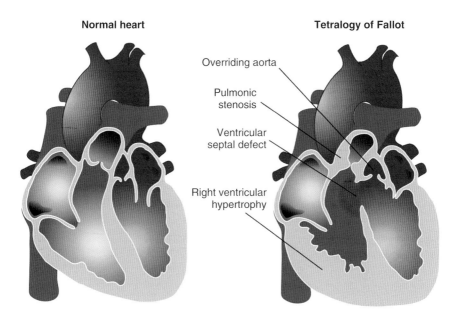

Normal heart

Tetralogy of Fallot

Overriding aorta

Pulmonic stenosis

Ventricular septal defect

Right ventricular hypertrophy

FIG. 6.6 Tetralogy of Fallot. (From Wikimedia Commons. https://commons.wikimedia.org/wiki/File:Tetralogy_of_Fallot.svg. Created by Mariana Ruiz. In the public domain.)

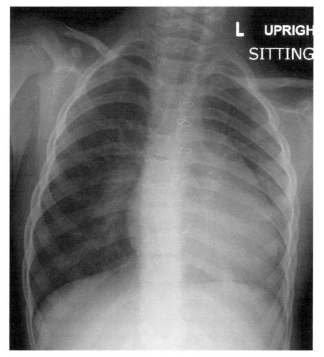

FIG. 6.7 Boot-shaped heart. Note the boot-shaped protrusion caused by right ventricular hypertrophy seen in tetralogy of Fallot. (From Wikimedia Commons. https://commons.wikimedia.org/wiki/File:HeartTOP.jpg. Created by James Heilman, MD. Used under Creative Commons Attribution-Share Alike 3.0 Unported license: https://creativecommons.org/licenses/by-sa/3.0/deed.en.)

- Tet spells = acute onset cyanotic spells in which affected children will often squat (↑systemic vascular resistance [SVR] leads to ↑pulmonary blood flow)
- Most common cyanotic heart disease after the neonatal period
- Single S_2 (pulmonic stenosis)

MoD: Pulmonic stenosis reduces blood flow to lungs → cyanosis; associated with DiGeorge syndrome (aka 22q11.2 deletion syndrome)

Dx:
(1) CXR with boot-shaped heart, (2) echocardiography

Tx/Mgmt:
(1) Surgical correction, (2) β-blockers, morphine, intranasal fentanyl for tet spells

Transposition of the Great Vessels

Buzz Words: Egg-on-a-string heart (narrow mediastinum) + single S_2 + cyanosis within the first 24 hours of life (Fig. 6.8)

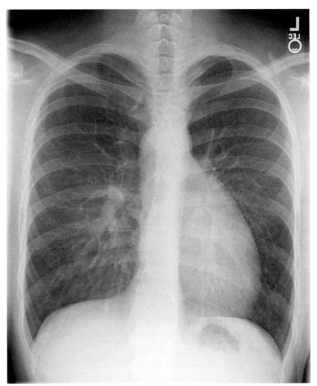

FIG. 6.8 Transposition of great vessels; looks like egg on its side. (From Wikimedia Commons. https://commons.wikimedia.org/wiki/File:Transposition-of-great-vessels.jpg. Used under Creative Commons Attribution-Share Alike 3.0 Unported license: https://creativecommons.org/licenses/by-sa/3.0/deed.en.)

Clinical Presentation:
- Cyanosis within the first 24 hours of life
- Single S_2
- ASD, VSD, or PDA will be present

MoD: Caused by failure of spiralization of the aorticopulmonary septum; may be associated with maternal diabetes mellitus

Dx:
(1) Echocardiography, (2) CXR with egg-on-a-string heart

Tx/Mgmt:
- Prostaglandin E2 to keep PDA open
- Surgical repair

Total Anomalous Pulmonary Venous Return

Buzz Words: Young baby with cyanosis, right ventricular hypertrophy

Clinical Presentation: RVH, right axis deviation in a cyanotic baby

MoD: Pulmonary veins empty into the RA instead of the LA

Dx: CXR with snowman sign/figure-of-8 sign

Tx/Mgmt: Surgical repair (Fig. 6.9)

Truncus Arteriosus

Buzz Words: Common arterial trunk for the aorta and the pulmonary artery

Clinical Presentation: Baby with dyspnea, pulmonary congestion, and edema

MoD: Failure of septum formation in the common arterial trunk → increased flow through the pulmonary circulation; associated with DiGeorge syndrome

Dx: Echocardiography

Tx/Mgmt: Surgical repair

Tricuspid Atresia

Buzz Words: Complete absence of the tricuspid valve with hypoplasia of the RV

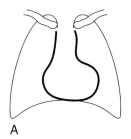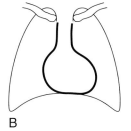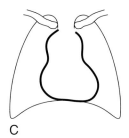

A   B   C

FIG. 6.9 (A) Tetralogy of Fallot. (B) Transposition of the great vessels. (C) Total anomalous pulmonary venous return.

Clinical Presentation:

- Progressive cyanosis
- Left axis deviation with LVH

MoD: Complete absence of the tricuspid valve with RV hypoplasia → LV must function as the sole ventricle for pumping blood through the pulmonary and systemic circulations.

Dx: Echocardiography

Tx/Mgmt: Surgical repair

Cardiac Neoplasms

Atrial Myxoma

Buzz Words: Ball valve-type obstruction, tumor plop, most common primary cardiac tumor in adults

Clinical Presentation:

- Shortness of breath, palpitations, dizziness, paroxysmal nocturnal dyspnea, fever
- Tumor emboli can cause arterial obstruction

MoD:

- Most common primary cardiac tumor rhabdomyosarcoma is the most common in children):
  - Metastatic disease is much more common—lung, breast, esophagus, melanoma, lymphoma/leukemia
- Most commonly located in the left atrium

Dx:

1. Echocardiography
2. Tumor plop heard on auscultation (mid-diastolic rumble that is similar to mitral stenosis)

Tx/Mgmt: Surgical removal is the treatment of choice.

Hypertension and Hypotension

Hypotension

Orthostatic Hypotension

Buzz Words: Syncope, decrease in systolic BP of ≥20 mm Hg or diastolic BP of ≥10 mm Hg when moving from supine to sitting to standing position

Clinical Presentation: Dizziness, lightheadedness, syncope, temporary decrease in vision or hearing

MoD: Intravascular volume depletion, autonomic dysfunction (diabetes mellitus, multiple system atrophy), medication side effect (tricyclic antidepressants, α1-antagonists (doxazosin, prazosin, tamsulosin, terazosin)

Dx: Orthostatic vital signs–decrease in systolic BP of ≥20 mm Hg or diastolic BP of ≥10 mm Hg taken 3 minutes after moving from supine to sitting to standing position

Tx/Mgmt:
- Increase fluid intake
- Medications to increase blood pressure: midodrine (α1-agonist), dopamine antagonists, tyramine, indomethacin

Carotid Sinus Hypersensitivity

Buzz Words: Bradycardia, hypotension, or syncope with constriction of the neck (e.g., when wearing a tight-fitting collared shirt)

Clinical Presentation: Patients present with bradycardia and hypotension with light contact with the carotid area of the neck (e.g., when shaving or with a tight-fitting shirt collar)

MoD: Hypersensitivity of the carotid baroreceptor leads to increased vagal tone with light external compression of the carotid area.

Dx:
1. Carotid sinus massage can reproduce symptoms.
2. Rule out other common causes of syncope:
   - Orthostatic syncope—orthostatic vital signs
   - Vasovagal—tilt-table test
   - Cardiogenic—EKG, echocardiogram

Tx/Mgmt:
1. Patient should not be allowed to drive until treatment.
2. Maintain adequate hydration and increase electrolyte intake.
3. Pacemaker insertion can be considered for patients with recurrent episodes associated with bradycardia.

Hypertension

Buzz Words: Blood pressure ≥140/90 mm Hg

Clinical Presentation: Insidious and asymptomatic until secondary effects become evident. There is increased risk for cardiovascular disease, renal disease, and stroke.

MoD: May be primary (idiopathic/essential) or secondary to other pathology. Causes of secondary hypertension include:
- Chronic renal failure
- Renal artery stenosis—classically in older males with a history of atherosclerotic disease
- Fibromuscular dysplasia—classically in younger women
- Hyperaldosteronism—via increased sodium absorption in the distal convoluted tubule

- Hyper- or hypothyroidism—via hyperdynamic circulation (hyperthyroidism) or vasoconstriction (hypothyroidism)
- Obstructive sleep apnea
- Others—scleroderma, pheochromocytoma

Dx: Blood pressure ≥140/90 mm Hg on two separate occasions; Dx of renal artery stenosis and fibromuscular dysplasia through CT angiogram

Tx/Mgmt:

1. Lifestyle modification—weight loss, reduce dietary sodium
2. Medication:
   - In patients with chronic kidney disease (CKD) → start with ACE inhibitor or ARB
   - In patients without CKD:
     - If African-American → HCTZ or CCB
     - Otherwise → HCTZ or ACE inhibitor or ARB or CCB

Hypertensive Urgency

Buzz Words: Systolic BP ≥ 180 mm Hg or diastolic BP ≥ 110 mm Hg without evidence of end-organ dysfunction

Clinical Presentation: Systolic BP ≥ 180 mm Hg or diastolic BP ≥ 110 mm Hg without evidence of end-organ dysfunction

MoD: Possible etiologies include: medication noncompliance, cocaine, monoamine oxidase inhibitor (MAOI) with tyramine ingestion (from cured meats, wine, and cheese), pheochromocytoma

Dx:

1. Systolic BP ≥ 180 mm Hg or diastolic BP ≥ 110 mm Hg without evidence of end-organ dysfunction
2. Neurologic exam, funduscopic exam, EKG, urinalysis

Tx/Mgmt: Gradual lowering of blood pressure with oral agents—HCTZ, CCBs

Hypertensive Emergency

Buzz Words: Systolic BP ≥ 180 mm Hg or diastolic BP ≥ 120 mm Hg in the setting of end-organ dysfunction

Clinical Presentation: Systolic BP ≥ 180 mm Hg or diastolic BP ≥ 120 mm Hg occurs in the setting of end-organ dysfunction (i.e., headache, vision changes, oliguria, chest pain, SOB, etc.). Complications include: stroke, encephalopathy, subarachnoid hemorrhage, MI, renal damage, aortic dissection, pulmonary edema.

MoD: Pressure-related damage to small blood vessels leading to end-organ dysfunction

Dx: Systolic BP ≥ 180 mm Hg or diastolic BP ≥ 120 mm Hg in the setting of end-organ dysfunction

Tx/Mgmt:

1. Rapid control of blood pressure with IV antihypertensive agents including – labetalol, sodium nitroprusside, fenoldopam (dopamine-1-receptor agonist), or clevidipine (CCB)
2. In neurologic emergencies → aim to lower the mean arterial pressure by 25% over 8 hours:
   - Labetalol and nifedipine are the preferred medications for neurologic pathology associated with hypertensive emergency.

Vascular Disease

Arterial Disease

Peripheral Artery Disease

Buzz Words: Cool, pale extremities with weak or absent pulses; loss of hair, shiny skin

Clinical Presentation: Cool, pale extremities, weak/absent pulses, loss of hair, atrophy, necrosis, gangrene; intermittent limb claudication (pain with activity)

PPx: Management of risk factors—abstain from **smoking**, control of DM, HLD, and HTN

MoD: Destruction or chronic occlusive disease of peripheral vessels occurs → ↓ perfusion of extremities. Smoking damages the vascular endothelium and promotes atherosclerotic changes.

Dx:

1. Ankle brachial index (ABI) ≤ 0.9
2. Duplex ultrasound and Doppler studies

Tx/Mgmt:

1. Smoking cessation, management of comorbid conditions:
   a. Cessation of smoking prevents further accelerated vascular disease but does not necessarily significantly improve existing vascular pathology.
2. Supervised exercise program
3. Medications—**cilostazol** (anti-platelet + vasodilator), **pentoxyfylline**
4. Surgical intervention—angioplasty, stenting, bypass, thrombolysis

Thromboangiitis Obliterans (Buerger Disease)

Buzz Words: Corkscrew arteries on imaging, tobacco-associated vascular inflammation leading to thrombosis

> **QUICK TIPS**
> Claudication is to the limb and angina is to the heart.

> **QUICK TIPS**
> Patients with calcification of the peripheral vasculature may have falsely elevated ABI.

Clinical Presentation: Inflammation of the peripheral vasculature leading to: limb claudication, decreased/absent peripheral pulses, cyanosis, hair loss and shiny skin, ulcerations and gangrene

MoD: Unknown but exposure to tobacco is a very strong risk factor

Dx:

1. Dx of thromboangiitis obliterans often necessitates exclusion of other pathology:
   - Patients are usually males between 20 and 40 years old with a history of current or recent tobacco use.
   - Distal extremity ischemia is present, as evidenced by claudication, ulceration, or gangrene.
   - Vasculitis, embolic disease, diabetes mellitus, and hypercoagulable states are excluded.
   - Arteriographic findings are consistent with arterial occlusion.

Tx/Mgmt:

1. Smoking cessation is key
2. Medical therapy:
   a. Iloprost (prostaglandin) can be used for vasodilation and improve symptoms without changing the course of disease.
   b. Thrombolytic agents have been used as an experimental treatment.
3. Hyperbaric oxygen may help with wound healing.
4. Surgical revascularization can be attempted in select patients with suitable obstruction that can be bypassed.

Embolic Disease

Buzz Words: Amaurosis fugax +livedo with blue toes + acute arterial thrombus

Clinical Presentation: Acute embolization causing end-organ dysfunction depending on the vessel that is occluded:

- Carotid plaque rupture → amaurosis fugax, Hollenhorst plaques in the retinal vasculature, transient ischemic attack, stroke
- Cholesterol embolism classically presents after vascular manipulation in patients with underlying atherosclerotic disease:
  - Livedoid skin changes with blue toes is classic.
  - Variable organ dysfunction—renal, gastrointestinal, central nervous system—occurs, depending on the location of embolus.

MoD:
- Unstable atherosclerotic plaques in the aorta, carotid, or heart can embolize.
- Vegetations from endocarditis can also embolize.

Dx:
1. Echocardiogram
2. Carotid duplex ultrasound
3. Skin biopsy showing cholesterol clefts (in cholesterol embolism)

Tx/Mgmt:
1. Anticoagulation with warfarin for patients with cardiac thrombus
2. Carotid endarterectomy for patients with carotid stenosis ≥50% and history of transient ischemic attack or stroke in the preceding 6 months
3. Statins for patients with cholesterol emboli

Compartment Syndrome

Buzz Words: Pain, pulselessness, paresthesias, paralysis, pallor, poikilothermia; compartment pressures ≥30 mm Hg

Clinical Presentation: 6Ps—**pain, pulselessness, paresthesias, paralysis, pallor, poikilothermia** (difference in temperature between affected segment and surrounding areas). Complications include permanent muscle or nerve damage → rhabdomyolysis.

MoD:
Etiologies include:
- Bleeding into a limb
- Crush injuries (tissue edema + bleeding)
- Ischemic reperfusion injury
- Tissue swelling after casting

Dx:
1. Clinical diagnosis
2. Intra-compartmental pressure ≥30 mm Hg is suggestive

Tx/Mgmt:
Emergent fasciotomy

Venous Disease

Deep Vein Thrombosis

Buzz Words: Swelling and pain of a limb with limb asymmetry, Homan sign

Clinical Presentation:
- Swelling, pain, redness of the affected limb ± engorgement of superficial veins
- **Homan sign** = pain with dorsiflexion of the foot (this test is historical and is not sensitive or specific)

QUICK TIPS
Recall the four compartments of the thigh—anterior, lateral, deep posterior, and superficial posterior

PPx: Ambulation, compression stockings, anticoagulation (heparin or enoxaparin)

MoD: Most commonly occurs in the proximal deep veins of the lower extremities (femoral veins, popliteal veins, iliac veins). Risk factors include: hypercoagulable state (factor V Leiden, malignancy, recent surgery, hormone replacement therapy), endothelial cell damage, and venous stasis.

Dx:

1. Duplex ultrasound
2. D-dimer—can be used to rule out deep vein thrombosis (DVT) if negative
3. If D-dimer equivocal → spiral CT chest

Tx/Mgmt:

1. Provoked DVT—an underlying factor can be identified to explain the DVT (e.g., concurrent malignancy, prior immobilization, recent surgery):
   a. Anticoagulation with warfarin or low-molecular weight heparin for 3 months
2. Unprovoked DVT—no underlying factor can be identified:
   a. Anticoagulation with warfarin for 3–6 months for the first episode
   b. Anticoagulation for 12 months to indefinite for the second episode
3. Inferior vena cava filter (if patient is unable to tolerate anticoagulation)

Venous Insufficiency

Buzz Words: Lower extremity edema with evidence of stasis dermatitis ± prominent varicose veins due to venous valvular insufficiency

Clinical Presentation:

- Lower extremity edema with hyperpigmentation, scaling, and shiny, indurated appearance of the skin (**stasis dermatitis**)
- Prominent varicose veins
- Lipodermatosclerosis = chronic panniculitis (inflammation of fat) with sclerosis and inverted champagne bottle appearance of the lower leg

MoD: Dysfunction or destruction of venous valves leads to backflow and pooling in the dependent veins of the body

Dx: Clinical exam

Tx/Mgmt: Compression stockings and leg elevation

Disorders of the Great Vessels

Aortic Aneurysm

Buzz Words: Widened mediastinum (thoracic aortic aneurysm), pulsatile abdominal mass (abdominal aortic aneurysm [AAA])

Clinical Presentation:

- AAA—pulsatile abdominal mass:
  - Risk factors include: atherosclerosis, smoking, and hypertension
- Thoracic aortic aneurysm—widened mediastinum on chest radiograph:
  - Risk factors include: smoking, hypertension, and atherosclerosis

MoD: Weakening of the vascular wall (through atherosclerosis or intrinsic defects in collagen and support proteins) leads to ballooning and formation of an aneurysm.

Dx:

1. Male smokers between 65 and 75 years old should be screened with a one-time abdominal ultrasound
2. Echocardiogram or CT angiogram for thoracic aortic aneurysms
3. CT angiogram can also be used for accurate assessment of abdominal aortic aneurysms.

Tx/Mgmt:

1. Modification of risk factors—statins, smoking cessation, and control of blood pressure
2. Surgical treatment is indicated for those at higher risk for rupture:
   - AAA—diameter >5.5 cm, rate of growth >1 cm/year, current smokers
   - Thoracic aortic aneurysm—aneurysms >5–6 cm

Aortic Dissection

Buzz Words: Tearing chest pain that radiates to the back (Fig. 6.10).

Clinical Presentation:

- Extremely high-yield condition because it is life-threatening.
- **Acute onset, severe, tearing chest pain that radiates to the back.**
- May be associated with hypertension or hypotension, aortic insufficiency, acute MI, or acute stroke depending on location and progression of dissection.

> **QUICK TIPS**
> Patients with connective tissue disease (Marfan syndrome, Ehlers-Danlos syndrome, Loeys-Dietz syndrome) as well as those with syphilitic aortitis are at increased risk for thoracic aortic aneurysms.

- Dissection of the subclavian artery may lead to different blood pressure readings between arms.

PPx: Blood pressure control

MoD: Tearing of the tunica intima of the aorta → blood flow between the layers of the aorta leading to dissection. Risk factors include: **hypertension**, collagen vascular disease (Marfan syndrome, Ehlers-Danlos syndrome), bicuspid aortic valve, and tertiary syphilis

Dx:

1. **Transesophageal echocardiography** is the diagnostic test of choice because of speed:
   - **Magnetic resonance imaging (MRI)** is the gold standard (more sensitive and equal specificity compared to CT angiography).
   - Aortography is not typically used anymore.

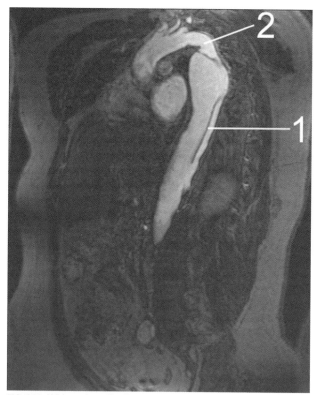

FIG. 6.10 Widened mediastinum on magnetic resonance imaging (MRI). (1) Aorta descendens; (2) aorta isthmus. (From Wikimedia Commons. https://commons.wikimedia.org/wiki/File:AoDiss_MRT. jpg. Created by Dr. Lars Grenacher. Used under Creative Commons Attribution-Share Alike 3.0 Unported license: https://creativecommons. org/licenses/by-sa/3.0/deed.en.)

2. **CT angiography** is often used in the emergent setting because of high sensitivity and speed.
3. CXR may show **widened mediastinum**.

Tx/Mgmt:
1. Blood pressure control with β-blockers (**labetalol**) or **CCBs** ± nitroprusside
2. Dissection of the ascending aorta (Stanford type A) → **surgery**
3. Dissection of the descending aorta (Stanford type B) → **medical management**

Dyslipidemia

Familial Hypercholesterolemia

Buzz Words: Early atherosclerotic disease, tendon xanthoma, increased serum cholesterol (Figs. 6.11 and 6.12)

Clinical Presentation: Early atherosclerotic disease (CAD, MI, peripheral arterial disease [PAD]), tendon xanthoma, corneal arcus, xanthelasma (yellow bumps on eyelids)

MoD: Mutation in the low-density lipoprotein (LDL) receptor or ApoB that results in ability of the liver to clear cholesterol from the blood.

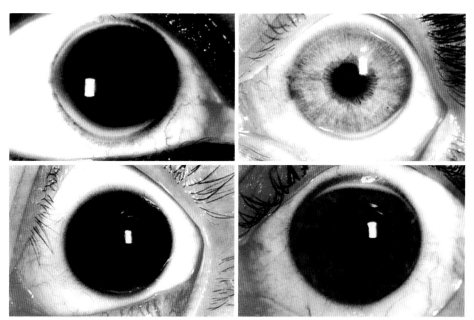

FIG. 6.11 Corneal arcus. Deposition of cholesterol in the limbic area of the pupil resulting in a white ring seen in hypercholesterolemia and in the elderly. (From Wikimedia Commons. https://commons.wikimedia.org/wiki/File:Four_representative_slides_of_corneal_arcus.jpg. Created by Loren A. Zech Jr. and Jeffery M. Hoeg. Used under Creative Commons Attribution 2.0 Generic license: https://creativecommons.org/licenses/by/2.0/deed.en.)

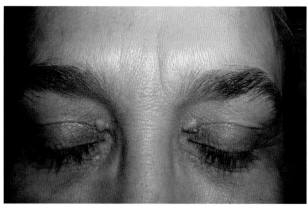

FIG. 6.12 Xanthelasma. Note the yellow-hued papules around the eyelids representing deposits of cholesterol. This may be seen in patients with hypercholesterolemia but may also be seen in normo-cholesterolemic patients. (From Wikimedia Commons. https://commons.wikimedia.org/wiki/File:Xanthelasma.jpg. Created by Klaus D. Peter, Gummersbach, Germany. Used under Creative Commons Attribution 3.0 Germany license: https://creativecommons.org/licenses/by/3.0/de/deed.en.)

Dx:

1. Total serum cholesterol:
   - 350–550 mg/dL is suggestive of heterozygous state.
   - 650–1000 mg/dL is suggestive of homozygous state.
2. Mutation analysis

Tx/Mgmt:

1. Homozygous mutants—high-dose statins + lipid apheresis, liver transplant
2. Heterozygous mutants—statins ± bile acid sequestrants (cholestyramine), niacin

Familial Hyperchylomicronemia (Lipoprotein Lipase Deficiency)

Buzz Words: Creamy layer in supernatant of blood sample, serum fasting triglycerides

Clinical Presentation: Eruptive xathomas, acute pancreatitis (due to ↑↑ triglycerides); no increased risk of atherosclerotic disease

MoD: Caused by deficiency in lipoprotein lipase

Dx:

1. Blood testing showing increased fasting triglycerides >1000 mg/dL
2. Milky, creamy plasma with increased hyperchylomicronemia

Tx/Mgmt:
1. Low-fat diet and avoidance of simple carbohydrates
2. Lipid-lowering medications—omega-3-fatty acids, gemofibrozil

Familial Hypertriglyceridemia—Increased Risk of Pancreatitis (Triglycerides >1000 mg/dL)

Buzz Words: Triglycerides greater than 1000 mg/dL
Clinical Presentation: Xanthoma, corneal arcus, xanthelasma, acute pancreatitis (due to ↑↑ triglycerides)
MoD: Mutations in the ApoA5 and lipase I genes
Dx: Fasting serum triglycerides greater than 1000 mg/dL
Tx/Mgmt:
1. Low-fat diet and avoidance of simple carbohydrates
2. Lipid-lowering medications—omega-3-fatty acids, gemofibrozil

Medication Side Effects Involving the Heart

Cardiotoxic Drugs

- **Doxorubicin**—causes dose-dependent cardiomyopathy; **dexrazoxane** can be used to mitigate cardiotoxicity
- **Traztuzumab** (Herceptin)—cardiomyopathy → CHF
- **Cocaine**—may cause coronary artery vasospasm and typical ACS chest pain, diaphoresis, HTN. Treat with **CCBs** preferred; **avoid β-blockers** as they can cause unopposed α-adrenergic activity.

QT-Prolonging Medications

- Antiemetics—ondansetron
- Antipsychotics
- Tricyclic antidepressant
- Anti-arrhythmics—amiodarone, sotalol, flecainide
- Antibiotics—macrolides, fluoroquinolones, azole antifungals

Anti-Hypertensives

- CCBs can cause reflex tachycardia and peripheral edema.

GUNNER PRACTICE

1. A 33-year-old male is brought to the emergency department by ambulance after being the victim of a witnessed stabbing. The patient was initially complaining of chest pain and difficulty breathing in the ambulance. However,

he is completely unresponsive upon arrival to the emergency room. There is a stab wound at the left sternal border between his fourth and fifth ribs. His temperature is 99.1°F, blood pressure is 77/52 mm Hg, pulse is 122/min, respiratory rate is 28/min, and SpO$_2$ is 98% on room air. Heart sounds are muffled on auscultation. Distended jugular veins are noted. Pupils are equally round and reactive to light. Lung sounds are clear to auscultation bilaterally. No other signs of trauma are noted. What is the next best step in the management of this patient?

A. Chest radiograph
B. Chest needle decompression and oxygen supplementation
C. Pericardiocentesis and volume resuscitation
D. Electrocardiogram
E. Wound debridement

2. A 16-year-old male with a history of well-controlled asthma collapses during a basketball game. He is unconscious and pulseless. A bystander initiates CPR and an ambulance is called. Despite adequate CPR, the patient is pronounced dead when the ambulance arrives. His family history is notable for an uncle who died suddenly of unknown causes at the age of 25. A review of the patient's medical records reveals a distant history of a cardiac murmur in early childhood. Which of the following would likely be seen on autopsy?

A. Mitral valve leaflet commissural fusion and an enlarged left atrium
B. Dilated right and left ventricular walls
C. Bicuspid aortic valve
D. Asymmetrically enlarged ventricular septum
E. Ruptured chorda tendinae

3. A 59-year-old African-American male presents to his primary care doctor complaining of lower extremity pain and numbness. He reports that over the past 6 months, he has started to develop cramping bilateral buttock and leg pain that is worse on the left. The pain develops during ambulation and is relieved by rest. The pain has gotten progressively worse over the past 6 months. The patient also reports that he has experienced difficulty maintaining an erection over the same time period. His history is notable for a prior myocardial infarction, hypertension, and hyperlipidemia. He is currently taking aspirin, lisinopril, atorvastatin, and propranolol. On exam, femoral pulses are decreased bilaterally and calf

atrophy is noted on the left. Which of the following will most likely be found in this patient?

A. MRI demonstrating disc herniation at the L4–L5 junction
B. Doppler ultrasound demonstrating a thrombus in the left femoral vein
C. Ankle systolic pressure less than 90% of brachial systolic pressure
D. Abdominal ultrasound revealing an abdominal aortic aneurysm below the renal arteries
E. Muscle biopsy demonstrating ragged red fibers

ANSWERS: What Would Gunner Jess/Jim Do?

1. WWGJD? A 33-year-old male is brought in to the emergency department by ambulance after being the victim of a witnessed **stabbing.** The patient was initially complaining of **chest pain and difficulty breathing** in the ambulance. However, he is **completely unresponsive upon arrival** to the emergency room. There is a **stab wound at the left sternal border between his fourth and fifth ribs.** His temperature is 99.1°F, **blood pressure is 77/52 mm Hg, pulse is 122/min, respiratory rate is 28/min,** and SpO$_2$ is 98% on room air. Heart sounds are **muffled** on auscultation. **Distended jugular veins** are noted. Pupils are equally round and reactive to light. Lung sounds are clear to auscultation bilaterally. No other signs of trauma are noted. **What is the next best step in the management of this patient?**

Answer: C, pericardiocentesis and volume resuscitation.

Explanation: This patient presents with hypotension, tachycardia, muffled heart sounds, and distended neck veins following penetrating chest trauma to the left chest. This presentation is consistent with **cardiac tamponade.** Cardiac tamponade occurs when fluid builds up in the pericardial sac and restricts adequate ventricular filling of the heart. This leads to a decrease in cardiac output and hemodynamic collapse. **Beck triad** is a classic set of physical exam findings in cardiac tamponade that includes (1) hypotension, (2) muffled heart sounds, and (3) distended jugular veins. This patient is hemodynamically unstable and requires urgent pericardiocentesis to drain the pericardial fluid collection and restore ventricular filling. This patient also will benefit from rapid volume expansion to increase preload and cardiac output.

A. Chest radiograph → Incorrect. This patient is rapidly decompensating and requires urgent intervention to restore cardiac output. Chest radiograph may reveal an enlarged heart in cases of pericardial tamponade; however, it is not appropriate in this case.

B. Chest needle decompression and oxygen supplementation → Incorrect. Needle decompression is indicated in cases of tension pneumothorax to relieve pressure in the pleural space. Tension pneumothorax can present following penetrating chest trauma and lead to unilateral absent breath sounds and hyper-resonance on percussion. Since this

patient has clear lungs and good oxygen saturation, tension pneumothorax is not the cause of his
hemodynamic instability.

D. Electrocardiogram → Incorrect. This patient is rapidly decompensating and requires urgent intervention to restore cardiac output. Electrocardiogram
may reveal **electrical alternans** — variability in the
QRS magnitudes — in cases of pericardial tamponade; however, it is not appropriate in this case.

E. Wound debridement → Incorrect. This patient is
rapidly decompensating and requires urgent intervention to restore cardiac output. Wound care is
not appropriate at this time.

2. WWGJD? A 16-year-old male with a history of well-
controlled asthma collapses during a basketball game.
He is unconscious and pulseless. A bystander initiates
CPR and an ambulance is called. Despite adequate
CPR, the patient is pronounced dead when the ambulance arrives. His family history is notable for an uncle
who died suddenly of unknown causes at the age of
25. A review of the patient's medical records reveals a
distant history of a cardiac murmur in early childhood.
Which of the following would likely be seen on autopsy?

Answer: D, asymmetrically enlarged ventricular septum.

Explanation: This previously healthy young athlete
experiences sudden cardiac death during exertion.
The most common cause of death in young healthy
athletes is **hypertrophic cardiomyopathy (HCM).**
HCM is characterized by thickened (hypertrophied)
ventricular walls and an asymmetrically enlarged
ventricular septum. Death from HCM can result from
either obstruction of the left ventricular outflow tract or
ventricular tachyarrhythmias.

A. Mitral valve leaflet commissural fusion and an
enlarged left atrium → Incorrect. Rheumatic heart
disease can lead to mitral stenosis, which is characterized by fused mitral valve leaflets and eventual
enlargement of the left atrium due to restricted
flow through the mitral valve. This may present
later in life with symptoms of left-sided heart failure
(dyspnea, orthopnea) but is not a cause of sudden
cardiac death.

B. Dilated right and left ventricular walls → Incorrect.
Dilated ventricular walls occur in dilated cardiomyopathy. Dilated cardiomyopathy presents with
progressive dyspnea, fatigue, and edema. It does
not typically cause sudden death in athletes.

C. Bicuspid aortic valve → Incorrect. Bicuspid aortic valves predispose patients to early aortic stenosis. However, it would not cause sudden death in an otherwise healthy adolescent athlete.

E. Ruptured chorda tendinae → Incorrect. Chordae tendinae rupture results in mitral valve regurgitation. It typically occurs secondary to connective tissue disorders or bacterial endocarditis and would not cause sudden death in a healthy young person.

3. **WWGJD?** A 59-year-old African-American male presents to his primary care doctor complaining of lower extremity pain and numbness. He reports that over the past 6 months, he has started to develop cramping bilateral buttock and leg pain that is worse on the left. The pain develops during ambulation and is relieved by rest. The pain has gotten progressively worse over the past 6 months. The patient also reports that he has experienced difficulty maintaining an erection over the same time period. His history is notable for a prior myocardial infarction, hypertension, and hyperlipidemia. He is currently taking aspirin, lisinopril, atorvastatin, and propranolol. On exam, femoral pulses are decreased bilaterally and calf atrophy is noted on the left. Which of the following will most likely be found in this patient?

Answer: C, Ankle systolic pressure less than 90% of brachial systolic pressure.

Explanation: This patient has exertional lower extremity pain and numbness that occurs with exertion and improves with rest. This condition is known as **claudication.** The triad of buttock claudication, decreased femoral pulses, and male impotence is most consistent with **aortoiliac disease (Leriche syndrome),** which is a form of **peripheral arterial disease (PAD).** In Leriche syndrome, the aortoiliac vessels are partially occluded leading to vascular insufficiency distal to the site of occlusion. An **ankle-brachial index** can be used in the setting of PAD to measure the difference in systolic blood pressure between the ankle and brachial arteries. In cases of PAD, the ankle systolic pressure will be less than 90% of the brachial systolic pressure.

A. MRI demonstrating disc herniation at the L4–L5 junction → Incorrect. Herniated intervertebral discs can compress the sciatic nerve and lead to radiating lower extremity pain. The pain is typically not exertional and is not associated with decreased femoral pulses or impotence.

B. Doppler ultrasound demonstrating a thrombus in the left femoral vein → Incorrect. Deep venous thrombosis can cause lower extremity pain and swelling in the affected limb. However, the pain is generally not exertional and is not associated with decreased femoral pulses, muscle atrophy, or impotence.

D. Abdominal ultrasound revealing an abdominal aortic aneurysm (AAA) distal to renal arteries → Incorrect. AAAs can be asymptomatic or present with a pulsatile abdominal mass, back pain, and/or abdominal discomfort. They can be associated with lower extremity vascular insufficiency but the triad of claudication, impotence, and decreased femoral pulses are most consistent with Leriche syndrome.

E. Muscle biopsy demonstrating fatty replacement of muscle tissue → Incorrect. Replacement of muscle tissue by fat and connective tissue occurs in muscular dystrophies. Muscular dystrophies typically arise earlier in the life and lead to proximal muscle weakening.

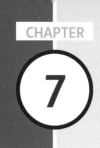
Diseases of the Respiratory System

William Plum, Drake Lebrun, Hao-Hua Wu, Leo Wang, Rebecca Gao, and Sean Harbison

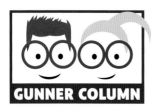

GUNNER COLUMN

Introduction

Diseases of the respiratory system are more than fair game for the Clinical Surgery shelf and comprise 8%–12% of your exam. The respiratory system includes upper and lower airways, lungs, pleura, and the diaphragm. We will introduce and cover various pathologies in these categories. However, not all topics are covered equally. Some of the higher yield topics, which we will focus on with a heavier hand in this chapter, are worth giving your time to achieve mastery. Such higher yield topics include: solitary pulmonary nodules (SPNs), malignant lung neoplasms, pulmonary embolism, acute respiratory distress syndrome (ARDS), atelectasis, and penetrating and blunt chest wounds. Focus on the different aspects of such pathology while still learning the breadth of the entire material in this chapter.

When a respiratory system question is presented, your first job as the acting clinician is to narrow down the diagnosis to either a respiratory, cardiovascular, or gastrointestinal (GI) pathology. Certain "Buzz Words" will be used for each of the different categories, which you must learn to quickly pick out from amidst the noise. After you narrow down the diagnosis to a specific organ system and pathology, you will need to decide if the patient needs a surgical or medical management. Although this is your "Surgery" shelf, a lot of the management you will be doing for your test will be medical. Remember, just because an answer choice focuses on surgical management, does not necessarily mean this is the right answer for your Surgery shelf.

Neoplasms

Benign Neoplasms
Upper Airways
Vocal Cord Polyps
Buzz Words: Hoarseness, scratchy, lump in throat, unilateral, smoker

Clinical Presentation: Hoarseness, scratchy throat, or "lump in throat" sensation in the setting of chronic irritation.

Polyps tend to be unilateral and present in the anterior one-third of the vocal fold. They are more common in males and in smokers.

Prophylaxis (PPx): Smoking cessation

Mechanism of Disease (MoD): Chronic vocal cord irritation

Diagnostic Steps (Dx):

1. Physical examination
2. Laryngoscopy

Treatment and Management Steps (Tx/Mgmt):

1. Voice rest
2. Smoking cessation
3. Surgery

Nasal Polyps

Buzz Words: Chronic rhinosinusitis, cystic fibrosis, and aspirin/non-steroidal anti-inflammatory drug (NSAID)-induced bronchospasm

Clinical Presentation: Recurrent nasal discharge/congestion with bilateral, shiny mucoid masses are present. Anosmia leads to possible change in taste.

Dx:

1. Physical exam including rhinoscopy
2. Nasal endoscopy
3. Head computed tomography (CT) or magnetic resonance imaging (MRI)
4. Allergy tests
5. Test for cystic fibrosis

Tx/Mgmt:

1. Intranasal glucocorticoids
2. Oral glucocorticoids if severe or refractory to intranasal delivery
3. Surgery, although polyps tend to return

Lungs and Pleura
Solitary Pulmonary Nodule

Buzz Words: Singular nodule/lesion, accidental finding (Fig. 7.1)

Clinical Presentation: Single, well-defined, round opacity are surrounded completely by pulmonary parenchyma, and ≤3 cm. Image: If imaging also depicts atelectasis, lymph node enlargement, or pleural effusion the lesion is not a SPN. Usually found accidently on chest x-ray. For SPN, it is more important to focus on the Dx and Mgmt rather than the cause of the nodule.

MoD:

- Benign neoplasia: hamartoma, fibroma, chondroma, or neural tumor

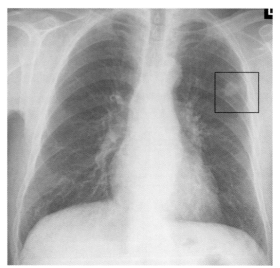

FIG. 7.1 Solitary pulmonary nodule. (From Wikimedia Commons: https://commons.wikimedia.org/wiki/File:Thorax_pa_peripheres_Bronchialcarcinom_li_OF_markiert.jpg. Created by Lange123 at the German language Wikipedia. Used under Creative Commons Attribution-Share Alike 3.0 Unported license: https://creativecommons.org/licenses/by-sa/3.0/deed.en.)

- Infectious: tuberculosis, fungal infection, abscess, nocardia, nontuberculosis mycobacteria, round pneumonia, septic embolus
- Malignant neoplasia: bronchogenic carcinoma, carcinoid/neuroendocrine, metastasis, lymphoma, teratoma, leiomyoma
- Inflammatory: granulomatosis with polyangiitis, rheumatoid nodule, sarcoidosis
- Vascular: arteriovenous malformation, hematoma, pulmonary artery aneurysm, pulmonary venous varix, pulmonary infarct
- Bronchial: bronchogenic cyst

Dx:
1. Compare with previous imaging.
2. If low risk for malignancy (Table 7.1), or 2-year radiographic stability, no further testing and follow yearly with serial chest CT scans.
3. If intermediate risk of malignancy, either fine-needle aspiration (FNA) or positron emission tomography (PET) scan is acceptable. If the results suggest malignancy, surgical resection is the next step. However, if the results are non-diagnostic, active surveillance is the correct course of action.
4. If high risk for malignancy, surgical excision of nodule is recommended.

TABLE 7.1 Cancer Risk Factors in Solitary Pulmonary Nodule

Variable	Low Cancer Risk	Intermediate Cancer Risk	High Cancer Risk
Age	<45	45–60	>60
Diameter	<0.5 cm	0.5–2 cm	>2 cm
Tobacco use	Never smoker	Current smoker <1 pack/day	Current smoker ≥1 pack/day
Smoking cessation	Quit ≥7 years prior	Quit <7 years ago	Current smoker
Margins	Smooth	—	Spiculated
Calcification pattern	Laminated, central, or diffuse	Not calcified	Stippled

Tx/Mgmt: See the criteria above:
1. Serial chest CT scans
2. CT-FNA
3. PET scan
4. Surgical excision

99 AR

Management of SPN

Bronchial Carcinoid Tumor

Buzz Words: Recurrent PNA in same pulmonary segment + indolent

Clinical Presentation: Most of these tumors arise in the proximal airways and lead to symptoms due to obstruction from the mass or bleeding from its hypervascularity. Presentation includes a cough or wheeze, chest pain, recurrent pneumonia in same pulmonary segment, or hemoptysis. Bronchial carcinoid tumors produce less serotonin than midgut carcinoid tumors. Therefore, they are less likely to present with cutaneous flushing, diarrhea, bronchospasms, and right-sided valvular heat disease. Most common metastatic site for carcinoid tumors is the liver.

MoD: Thought to arise from specialized Kulchitsky cell, a type of neuroendocrine cell.

Dx:
1. Chest CT scan
2. Bronchoscopic biopsy for central lesions
3. Transthoracic needle biopsy for peripheral lesions
4. Abdominal CT scan looking for metastatic liver lesions

Tx/Mgmt: Surgical resection

> **QUICK TIP**
> Despite being a rare tumor, bronchial carcinoid tumors are the most common primary lung neoplasm of children.

Malignant Neoplasms

Upper Airways

Lip—Squamous Cell Carcinoma

Buzz Words: Smoker + alcohol use + "persistent" papules, plaques, erosions, or ulcers

Clinical Presentation: Exophytic or ulcerative lesion is likely associated with pain. Slow-growing, local tumor with a low potential to metastasize.

PPx: Smoking cessation, alcohol cessation, adequate sun protection

MoD: Malignant proliferation of squamous keratinocytes

Dx: Physical exam, biopsy

Tx/Mgmt:
1. Mohs surgery or excision
2. Topical imiquimod and 5-fluorouracil

> Lip squamous cell carcinoma (SCC) is more commonly found on lower lip due to greater sun exposure.

Oral Cavity—Squamous Cell Carcinoma

Buzz Words: Smoker + alcoholic + "non-healing" ulcer + immunocompromised

Clinical Presentation: A persistent, non-healing ulcer or mass that is associated with pain. May also present as a bleeding sore, growth or lump, painful chewing or swallowing, sore throat, and poorly fitting dentures. More likely to occur in smokers, alcohol abusers, and the immunocompromised. The effect of smoking and alcohol is multiplicative with the increased risk of developing cancers of the oral cavity. A subset of oropharyngeal SCC is associated with human papillomavirus infection (HVP-16). Up to two-thirds of primary tongue lesions have nodal involvement. Also remember that oral leukoplakia (Fig. 7.2) is a precancerous lesion presenting as white patches or plaques.

PPx: Smoking cessation, alcohol cessation

MoD: Malignant proliferation of squamous keratinocytes; progression from untreated leukoplakia

Dx: Physical exam, biopsy, head and neck CT scan

Tx/Mgmt: Surgery and radiation: May require chemotherapy with cisplatin plus fluorouracil if more advanced.

> Smoking and alcohol are the two most common risk factors associated with head and neck SCC.

Pharynx-Squamous Cell Carcinoma

Buzz Words: Smoker + painful swallowing + cystic neck mass

Clinical Presentation: Dysphagia and odynophagia are often in the setting of smoking and alcohol abuse. May also present with snoring and obstructive sleep apnea (OSA), bleeding, or a neck mass. Human papillomavirus

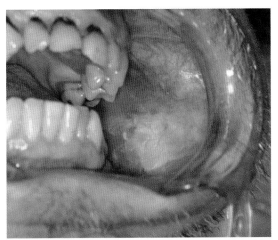

FIG. 7.2 Oral leukoplakia. (From Wikimedia Commons: https://commons.wikimedia.org/wiki/File:Leukoplakia02-04-06.jpg. Created by Michael Gaither. Used under Creative Commons Attribution-Share Alike 3.0 Unported license: https://creativecommons.org/licenses/by-sa/3.0/deed.en.)

(HPV)-associated oropharyngeal cancers (HPV-16) often present with cystic neck masses. These may often be mistaken for branchial cleft cyst carcinomas, although these are remarkably rare. If patient is presenting with a cystic neck mass, metastatic cystic SCC should be excluded.

PPx: Smoking cessation, alcohol cessation

MoD: Malignant proliferation of squamous keratinocytes

Dx:

1. Head and neck CT scan
2. Triple endoscopy if smoking and/or alcohol abuse history
3. Direct laryngoscopy if lack of smoking and/or alcohol abuse history
4. Biopsy
5. Chest CT scan to rule out metastases

Tx/Mgmt: Surgery and radiation: May require chemotherapy with cisplatin plus fluorouracil if more advanced.

> Triple endoscopy: direct laryngoscopy, bronchoscopy, and esophagoscopy

Larynx—Squamous Cell Carcinoma

Buzz Words: Smoker + alcohol use + hoarseness

Clinical Presentation: Presentation depends on location of tumor. Persistent hoarseness is the initial complaint in glottic lesions. Symptoms may progress to dysphagia, referred otalgia, persistent cough, hemoptysis, and stridor. Supraglottic lesions are more indolent and are often discovered later from airway obstruction or from palpable lymph nodes.

PPx: Smoking cessation, alcohol cessation
MoD: Malignant proliferation of squamous keratinocytes
Dx: Same as SCC pharynx
Tx/Mgmt: Same as SCC pharynx

Trachea, Lower Airways, and Pleura
Bronchus and/or Lung
Squamous Cell Carcinoma

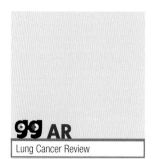

99 AR
Lung Cancer Review

99 AR
Paraneoplastic Syndromes

Buzz Words: Smoker, persistent cough, hemoptysis, hypercalcemia, superior vena cava (SVC) syndrome, Horner

Clinical Presentation: Intrathoracic symptoms of SCC include a persistent cough, hemoptysis, chest pain, dyspnea, hoarseness, and wheezing. Constitutional symptoms, especially in a smoker, such as weight loss, decreased appetite, and weakness should raise your suspicion for lung cancer. Be on the lookout for recurrent pneumonia in the same lobe, as this could be a sign of postobstructive pneumonia.

Local invasion may lead to SVC syndrome, Horner syndrome, Pancoast syndrome, phrenic nerve palsy, recurrent laryngeal nerve palsy, and malignant pleural effusion. SVC syndrome presents with facial and upper extremity edema, dilated neck and chest veins, and a feeling of facial fullness. Horner syndrome presents with unilateral facial anhidrosis, ptosis, and miosis (PAM is horny: ptosis, anhidrosis, miosis). Pancoast syndrome presents with shoulder pain that may radiate down the arm, atrophy of hand muscles, and upper extremity weakness. Phrenic nerve palsy presents with dyspnea from hemidiaphragmatic paralysis. Recurrent laryngeal nerve presents with persistent hoarseness. Malignant pleural effusion will show up on imaging and have a poor prognosis, as they are considered incurable.

Paraneoplastic syndromes seen in SCC include hypertrophic pulmonary osteoarthropathy and PTHrP secretion. Hypertrophic osteoarthropathy presents with clubbing and a symmetrical, painful arthropathy in the ankles, knees, wrists, and elbows. PTHrP secretion will lead to symptoms of hypercalcemia, such as decreased appetite, nausea, vomiting, constipation, lethargy, polyuria, polydipsia, and dehydration. Labs in such instances will depict decreased PTH and increased PTHrP. Do not forget that hypercalcemia in cancer patients may also be due to other causes, such as bony metastasis. Speaking of metastasis, frequent sites of metastasis of lung cancer include liver, adrenal glands, bones, and brain.

PPx: Smoking cessation, avoiding asbestos, and avoiding radon. Low-dose CT screening for those aged 55–77

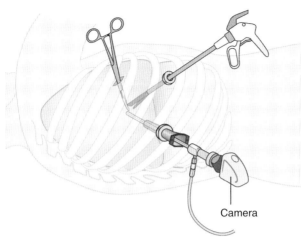

Camera

FIG. 7.3 Video-assisted thoracic surgery. (From Cancer Research UK/Wikimedia Commons: https://commons.wikimedia.org/wiki/ File:Diagram_showing_video_assisted_thoracoscopy_(VATS)_ CRUK_378.svg. Used under Creative Commons Attribution-Share Alike 4.0 International license: https://creativecommons.org/ licenses/by-sa/4.0/deed.en.)

who have no symptoms and have a 30-pack-year smoking history.

Dx:
1. Chest x-ray (obtain prior chest imaging)
2. Chest CT scan
3. Whole-body PET scan
4. Biopsy: Bronchoscopy with endobronchial ultrasound (EBUS)-directed biopsy for central primary tumors and mediastinal lymph nodes; transthoracic needle biopsy for peripheral lesions; mediastinoscopy for staging the mediastinum; video-assisted thoracic surgery (VATS; Fig. 7.3) for patients who are good surgical candidates.
5. Pulmonary function: Forced expiratory volume in 1 second (FEV1) and diffusing capacity for carbon monoxide (DLCO). Patients with preoperative values of FEV1 >2L and DLCO >80% predicted should be able to tolerate surgery including pneumonectomy.

Tx/Mgmt: Surgical resection, lobectomy. Adjuvant chemotherapy may be indicated for tumors ≥4 cm. Radiation therapy (RT) for patients with postoperative positive margins and who are not candidates for surgery.

Adenocarcinoma

Buzz Words: Persistent cough, hemoptysis, peripheral, osteoarthropathy, normal calcium level

Clinical Presentation: It is similar to SCC of the lung, see above. However, adenocarcinoma tends to be found

99 AR

Lung Cancer Staging

in more of a peripheral location, has higher incidence of hypertrophic pulmonary osteoarthropathy, and does not produce PTHrP. It is the most common primary lung malignancy in smokers and nonsmokers. Suspect adenocarcinoma when presenting symptoms are found in a nonsmoker.

PPx: Smoking cessation (although adenocarcinoma has the lowest association with smoking), avoiding asbestos, and avoiding radon; low-dose CT screening for those aged 55–77 who have no symptoms and have a 30-pack/year smoking history.

MoD: Malignant neoplastic gland formation possibly containing intracytoplasmic mucin

Dx: Same as lung SCC

Tx/Mgmt: Same as lung SCC

Large Cell Carcinoma

Buzz Words: Smoker, persistent cough, hemoptysis

Clinical Presentation: It is similar to SCC of the lung, see above. However, large cell carcinoma (LCC) tends to be found both centrally and peripherally. It is rare to encounter paraneoplastic syndromes in LCC except hypereosinophilia.

PPx: Smoking cessation, avoiding asbestos, and avoiding radon; low-dose CT screening for those age 55–77 who have no symptoms and have a 30-pack/year smoking history.

MoD: Undifferentiated epithelial neoplasm lacking both glandular and squamous cells; highly aggressive with a poor prognosis

Dx: Same as lung SCC

Tx/Mgmt: Same as lung SCC

Small Cell Carcinoma

Buzz Words: Smoker, persistent cough, hemoptysis, hyponatremia, Cushing's

Clinical Presentation: It is similar to SCC of the lung, see above. However, small cell carcinoma tends to be found more centrally and have different paraneoplastic syndromes. Paraneoplastic syndromes associated with small cell carcinoma include syndrome of inappropriate antidiuretic hormone secretion (SIADH), Cushing syndrome, and Eaton-Lambert syndrome. SIADH presents with symptoms of hyponatremia including anorexia, nausea, and vomiting. If the onset of hyponatremia is rapid, symptoms of cerebral edema, such as irritability, restlessness, confusion, and seizures may occur.

Cushing syndrome presents with muscle weakness, weight loss, hypertension, hirsutism, osteoporosis, hypokalemic, alkalosis, and hyperglycemia. Eaton-Lambert presents with symmetrical, proximal muscle weakness (that improves with use) and autonomic dysfunction, such as dry mouth and erectile dysfunction.

PPx: Smoking cessation, avoiding asbestos, and avoiding radon; low-dose CT screening for those aged 55–77 who have no symptoms and have a 30-pack/year smoking history.

MoD: Malignant, poorly differentiated small cells arising from neuroendocrine (Kulchitsky) cells; SIADH-ectopic secretion of antidiuretic hormone (ADH); Cushing syndrome-ectopic secretion of ACTH; Eaton-Lambert syndrome-antibodies against presynaptic voltage-gated calcium channel leads to decreased release of acetylcholine.

Dx: Same as lung SCC

Tx/Mgmt: Surgery and radiation ± chemotherapy for early-stage tumors that are resectable.

Pleura
Mesothelioma

Buzz Words: Asbestos, plumber, construction worker, unilateral pleural effusion

Clinical Presentation: Gradual onset of symptoms, such as chest pain, dyspnea, hoarseness, night sweats, or dysphagia occurs. Majority of cases occur in older patients. Tends to present decades after exposure to asbestos. Constitutional symptoms may also be present, such as fatigue and weight loss. Can present with a large, unilateral pleural effusion (Fig. 7.4), which will lead to unilateral dullness to percussion and decreased aeration at the lung base during a physical exam. Has very poor prognosis.

PPx: Avoiding asbestos, avoiding radiation

MoD: Malignant proliferation of mesothelial surfaces of the pleura

Dx:
1. Chest x-ray
2. Chest CT scan
3. Thoracentesis of pleural effusion
4. Pleural and mediastinal biopsy
5. PET scan for staging

Tx/Mgmt: Surgery, radiation, chemotherapy

Metastasis to Lung

Buzz Words: Multiple pulmonary nodules

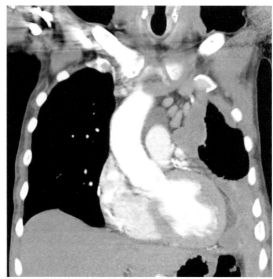

FIG. 7.4 Computed tomography scan of mesothelioma. (From Wikimedia Commons: https://commons.wikimedia.org/wiki/File:MesotheliomaCT.jpg. Created by Frank Gaillard. Used under Creative Commons Attribution-Share Alike 3.0 Unported license: https://creativecommons.org/licenses/by-sa/3.0/deed.en.)

Clinical Presentation: Symptoms include persistent cough, hemoptysis, chest pain, dyspnea, hoarseness, and wheezing. Constitutional symptoms such as weight loss, decreased appetite, and weakness may also be present. Imaging will depict multiple pulmonary nodules that are ≥1 cm in diameter and in different stages of growth. Metastatic lesions tend to be round with sharply demarcated borders and have a predilection for the bases (Fig. 7.5).

MoD: Tumors that tend to metastasize to the lungs include breast cancer, colon cancer, prostate cancer, bladder cancer, and sarcoma.

Dx:

1. CT scan
2. PET scan
3. Biopsy (see Dx section of lung SCC)

Tx/Mgmt: Treatment based on primary tumor

Metastasis to Pleura

Clinical Presentation: Gradual onset of symptoms include chest pain, dyspnea, hoarseness, night sweats, or dysphagia. Constitutional symptoms may also be present, such as fatigue and weight loss. Pleural effusion is likely to be present.

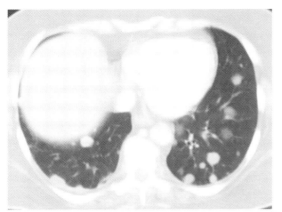

FIG. 7.5 Computed tomography scan of lung metastasis. (From Wikimedia Commons: https://commons.wikimedia.org/wiki/ File:MetsToLungs.png. Created by James Heilman, MD. Used under Creative Commons Attribution-Share Alike 4.0 International license: https://creativecommons.org/licenses/by-sa/4.0/deed.en.)

MoD: Tumors that tend to metastasize to the pleura include lung cancer, breast cancer, stomach cancer, kidney cancer, ovarian cancer, thymus cancer, and prostate cancer.

Dx: Same as Dx of mesothelioma (see above)

Tx/Mgmt: Treatment based on primary tumor

Respiratory Failure/Respiratory Arrest and Pulmonary Vascular Disorders

Acute Respiratory Distress Syndrome

Buzz Words: Dyspnea, hypoxemia refractory to oxygen, bilateral diffuse pulmonary infiltrates, "White-out" on chest x-ray

Clinical Presentation: Respiratory distress presents with dyspnea, tachypnea, hypoxemia, and diaphoresis. Chest x-ray will clearly depict bilateral alveolar infiltrates (Fig. 7.6) PaO_2/FiO_2 ≤200 mm Hg, brain natriuretic peptide (BNP) <100 pg/mL, and pulmonary capillary wedge pressure (PCWP) ≤18 mm Hg. Important to remember cardiogenic pulmonary edema presents in a similar manner and must be distinguished from ARDS (look for signs of volume overload, CHF, jugular venous distension [JVD], edema, and hepatomegaly). Complications include permanent lung injury or barotrauma from high-pressure mechanical ventilation.

MoD: ARDS is a consequence of alveolar injury producing massive alveolar damage. This injury leads to the release of pro-inflammatory cytokines, which recruit

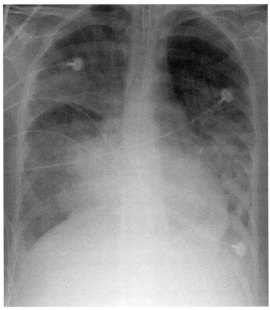

FIG. 7.6 X-ray of acute respiratory distress syndrome. (From Wikimedia Commons: https://commons.wikimedia.org/wiki/File:AARDS_X-ray_cropped.jpg. Used under Creative Commons Attribution-Share Alike 3.0 Unported license: https://creativecommons.org/licenses/by-sa/3.0/deed.en.)

neutrophils to the lungs. These neutrophils release toxic mediators that lead to damage to the capillaries and alveoli. Ultimately, the airspaces will fill with edema fluid and debris from damaged cells causing: ventilation-perfusion mismatching from physiological shunting (A-a gradient), decreased lung compliance from lung stiffness, increased dead space from obstruction and destruction of pulmonary capillary bed, and pulmonary hypertension (PH) from hypoxic vasoconstriction.

Dx:
1. Chest x-ray ("White-out")
2. Arterial blood gas, calculate PaO_2/FiO_2
3. BNP
4. Swan-Ganz catheter-PCWP

Tx/Mgmt:
1. Mechanical ventilation: high FiO_2 for appropriate oxygenation, low tidal volume (will lead to permissive hypercapnia) to protect from barotrauma, and positive end-expiratory pressure (PEEP) to open collapsed alveoli and decrease shunting.
2. Manage fluids to prevent volume overload.
3. Treat underlying condition.

Pulmonary Hypertension

Buzz Words: Loud pulmonic heart sound, fatigue, right heart failure, mPAP ≥25 mm Hg at rest or 30 mm Hg during exercise

Clinical Presentation: PH is defined by a mean pulmonary arterial pressure (mPAP) ≥25 mm Hg at rest or 30 mm Hg during exercise. Patients often present with dyspnea on exertion, fatigue, atypical chest pain, and syncope. On physical exam, patient may have a loud pulmonic component of the second heart sound. As the disease progresses and right ventricular failure occurs, signs will include JVD, hepatomegaly, ascites, and peripheral edema/anasarca.

MoD: PH occurs ultimately due to vascular remodeling and increased pulmonary vascular resistance. PH is classified as one of five groups:

- Group 1: Pulmonary arterial hypertension (PAH), which includes causes, such as sporadic idiopathic PAH, heritable PAH, drugs and toxins, systemic sclerosis, HIV, and congenital heart disease.
- Group 2: PH from left heart disease, which includes causes such as mitral and aortic valve disease, left ventricular systolic or diastolic dysfunction, or restrictive cardiomyopathy.
- Group 3: PH from lung disease, which includes causes such as COPD and interstitial lung disease.
- Group 4: PH from thromboembolic disease such as chronic thromboembolic occlusion of pulmonary vessels.
- Group 5: PH from multifactorial causes.

Classification of PH

Dx:

1. Echocardiogram
2. Electrocardiogram (ECG)
3. Chest x-ray
4. Right heart catheterization

Tx/Mgmt:

1. Fluid management with diuretics
2. Oxygen
3. Anticoagulant therapy (group 4)
4. Calcium channel blocker (CCB), such as dihydropyridine or diltiazem (group 1)
5. Prostacyclin analogs (esoprostenol [group 1])
6. Endothelin agonists (ambrisentan, bosentan, or macitentan [group 1])
7. Oral phosphodiesterase inhibitors (sildenafil [group 1])
8. Lung transplant

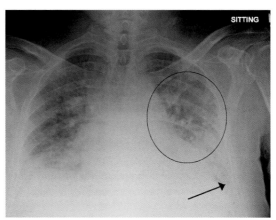

FIG. 7.7 X-ray of pulmonary edema. (From Wikimedia Commons: https://commons.wikimedia.org/wiki/File:PulmEdema.PNG. Created by James Heilman, MD. Used under Creative Commons Attribution-Share Alike 3.0 Unported license: https://creativecommons.org/licenses/by-sa/3.0/deed.en.)

Pulmonary Arteriovenous Malformations

Buzz Words: Hereditary hemorrhagic telangiectasia, hemoptysis

Clinical Presentation: It is most commonly asymptomatic and found accidently on imaging. If patient has symptoms they may include dyspnea and hemoptysis. Complications from pulmonary arteriovenous malformations (PAVM) also includes stroke, brain abscess, and PH.

MoD: Abnormal communications occur between pulmonary arteries and veins, which may lead to right-to-left shunt.

Dx:
1. Transthoracic contrast echocardiogram
2. Chest CT scan

Tx/Mgmt:
1. Yearly clinical observation and a CT every 3–5 years.
2. If symptomatic, use embolotherapy via angiographic occlusion of the feeding artery.
3. Surgery for patients who fail multiple embolization.
4. Lifelong antibiotics prophylaxis prior to dental procedures.

Non-cardiogenic Pulmonary Edema

Buzz Words: Respiratory distress, crackles (Fig. 7.7)

Clinical Presentation: Dyspnea, hypoxemia, and crackles are found on lung auscultation. It is important to rule out cardiogenic causes.

MoD: Movement of excess fluid into the alveoli. In non-cardiogenic pulmonary edema (PCWP ≤18 mm Hg), this accumulation of fluid and protein in the alveolar leads hinders diffusion capacity. Major causes include ARDS, high altitude, neurogenic pulmonary edema, opioid overdose, massive pulmonary embolism, and eclampsia.

Dx:
1. Chest x-ray
2. ABG
3. ECG/echocardiogram
4. BNP

Tx/Mgmt:
1. Oxygen
2. Manage fluids to prevent volume overload
3. Treat underlying condition

Cardiogenic Pulmonary Edema

Buzz Words: Respiratory distress, crackles, history of orthopnea and/or paroxysmal nocturnal dyspnea (PND), S3 or S4, JVD

Clinical Presentation: Dyspnea, hypoxemia, and crackles are found on lung auscultation. Patients may have tachy-cardia and hypertension. S3 or S4, JVD, and peripheral edema may also be present.

PPx: Patient compliance: adherence to medications and dietary restrictions

MoD: Most often it is the result of acute decompensated heart failure (ADHF) due to ventricular systolic or diastolic dysfunction leading to a rapid and acute increase in left ventricular filling pressures and left atrial pressure. Ultimately, this causes increased transudation of protein-poor fluid into the alveolar spaces. Causes of left ventricular systolic dysfunction include coronary heart disease, hypertension, valvular disease, and dilated cardiomyopathy. Causes of left ventricular diastolic dysfunction include hypertrophic and restrictive cardiomyopathies.

Dx:
1. Chest x-ray
2. ABG
3. ECG/echocardiogram
4. BNP

Tx/Mgmt:
1. Place patient sitting up with legs dangling from bed
2. Diuresis with daily assessment of weight
3. Supplemental oxygen and assisted ventilation
4. Nitrates
5. Morphine

QUICK TIPS

The most common mechanism of noncardiogenic pulmonary edema is an increased in capillary permeability.

Pulmonary Embolism

Buzz Words: Dyspnea, chest pain, post-op

Clinical Presentation: The most common presenting symptom is dyspnea followed by pleuritic chest pain, cough, and symptoms of DVT. Rarely, as in the case of a massive PE, do patients present with hemoptysis, shock, syncope, and/or right bundle branch block. Many patients are asymptomatic or have mild symptoms. What is important to remember are the risk factors for PE. Inherited risk factors include factor V Leiden mutation, prothrombin gene mutation, protein S or C deficiency, and antithrombin deficiency. Acquired risk factors include malignancy, surgery (especially orthopedic procedures), trauma, prior DVT/PE, pregnancy, oral contraceptives, immobilization, congestive heart failure, obesity, and nephrotic syndrome.

PPx: Mobility after surgery

MoD: Virchow triad leads to a thrombus. This thrombus, originating in another location of the body, embolizes to the pulmonary vasculature leading to three possible pathophysiologic responses: Pulmonary infarction, abnormal gas exchange, and cardiovascular compromise. Pulmonary infarction is due to small thrombi travelling distally to the segmental and subsegmental vessels. Abnormal gas exchange is due to mechanical obstruction altering the ventilation to perfusion ratio, which creates dead space. Cardiovascular compromise is caused by increased pulmonary vascular resistance, which ultimately leads to an impeded right ventricular outflow and causes right heart strain.

Dx:

1. Modified Wells Criteria determined to determine likelihood of PE
2. D-dimer to help RULE OUT PE
3. Spiral CT for likely probability of PE
4. Leg ultrasound if spiral CT is inconclusive or cannot be performed
5. V/Q scan is reserved for those with suspected PE in whom spiral CT is contraindicated (renal insufficiency), inconclusive, or negative in the face of high clinical suspicion

Tx/Mgmt:

1. Oxygen and fluids
2. Low-molecular-weight heparin or unfractionated heparin (Box 7.1)
3. Inferior vena cava (IVC) filter placement for those with contraindications to anticoagulation

---

BOX 7.1 Contraindications of Anticoagulation

Absolute Contraindications	Relative Contraindications
Active bleeding Severe bleeding diathesis Platelet <50,000/μL Recent, planned, or emergent high bleeding-risk surgery Major trauma Recent intracranial hemorrhage	Recurrent bleeding from multiple gastrointestinal telangiectasias Intracranial or spinal tumors Platelet <150,000/μL Large abdominal aortic aneurysm with concurrent severe hypertension Stable aortic dissection Recent, planned, or emergent low bleeding-risk surgery

---

4. Thrombolytic therapy, catheter-directed therapy, and/or thrombectomy for hemodynamically unstable patients.
5. Long-term anticoagulation with factor Xa inhibitors (apixaban, edoxaban, rivaroxaban), direct thrombin inhibitors (dabigatran), or warfarin.

Air Embolism

Buzz Words: Dyspnea, trauma, surgery, audible air suction during a procedure

Clinical Presentation: In cases of venous embolism, dyspnea is accompanied by substernal chest pain, lightheadedness, or dizziness. Massive air embolism can present with acute onset right-sided heart failure, syncope, shock, or cardiac arrest. Signs may include tachypnea, tachycardia, hypotension, wheezing, crackles, and elevated jugular venous pressure. Arterial embolism presents differently based on what organ is affected. The most commonly affected organ is the brain, and these patients present with an abrupt change in mental status and/or focal neurological deficits.

MoD: Most common causes include surgery, trauma, vascular interventions, and barotrauma from mechanical ventilation

Dx:
1. ABG
2. Chest x-ray
3. ECG/echocardiogram
4. Chest or head CT scan

Tx/Mgmt:
1. Position patient in left lateral decubitus or Trendelenburg for venous air embolism
2. Position patient in supine position for arterial embolism

3. Oxygen and/or ventilation
4. Fluids
5. Vasopressors
6. Hyperbaric oxygen, manual removal of air, and closed chest cardiac massage for severe cases

Fat Embolism

Buzz Words: Dyspnea, petechial rash, post op, long bone fracture

Clinical Presentation: Presents 24–72 hours after the original insult (e.g., femur fracture) with the classical triad of hypoxemia, neurological abnormalities and a petechial rash.

PPx: Early immobilization of fractures, prophylactic corticosteroids

MoD: Result of fat globules entering the bloodstream usually from bone marrow or adipose tissue

Dx: Clinical diagnosis

Tx/Mgmt: Supportive care, oxygen and fluid management

Respiratory Failure due to Enteral Feeding

Buzz Words: Dyspnea, enteral nutrition

Clinical Presentation: Respiratory distress occurs after enteral feeding. Patient will present with dyspnea and hypoxia. May also have a delayed presentation that includes cough, fever, tachypnea, or frothy sputum.

PPx: Backrest elevation, post-pyloric feeding, enteral feeding via percutaneous gastrostomy, and the use of motility agents to promote gastric emptying.

MoD: Enteral nutrition is associated with an increased incidence of aspiration. Patients who are very ill or post-op are unable to protect their airways during tube feedings. Large volumes of aspiration may lead to hypoxia or pneumonitis.

Dx: Chest x-ray

Tx/Mgmt: Supportive care, antibiotics if aspiration pneumonia is suspected–clindamycin

Disorders of the Pleura, Mediastinum, and Chest Wall

Chylothorax

Buzz Words: Milky fluid, pleural effusion, dyspnea

Clinical Presentation: Patients present with gradual signs and symptoms that are due to the mechanical effects of a pleural effusion, such as decreased exercise tolerance, dyspnea, fatigue, and a heavy feeling in the chest.

BOX 7.2 Pleural Fluid Analysis

Gross appearance:
    White blood cell count with differential
    pH
    Triglycerides
    Cholesterol
    Glucose
    Lactic dehydrogenase
    Total protein
    Cytology
    Microbiologic smear and culture

Remember that chyle in the pleural space does not create an inflammatory response; therefore, patients won't present with fever and chest pain.

MoD: Chylothorax is due to the disruption or obstruction of the thoracic duct that leads to the leakage of lymphatic fluid known as chyle into the pleural space. The etiology of chylothorax is broken down into nontraumatic and traumatic causes. Nontraumatic causes are often caused by malignancy such as lymphoma, chronic lymphocytic leukemia (CLL), and metastatic cancer. Surgical procedures near the thoracic duct account for the majority of cases of traumatic chylothorax. Esophagectomy, pulmonary resection, and heart surgery appear to carry the greatest risk of resulting in chylothorax.

Dx:
1. Chest x-ray
2. Thoracentesis
3. Analysis of pleural fluid, which can be milky, sanguineous, or serous (Box 7.2)
4. Chest CT scan

Tx/Mgmt:
1. Therapeutic pleural drainage accompanied by therapeutic thoracentesis, tube thoracostomy, or indwelling pleural catheter
2. Dietary control with high-protein, low-fat diet
3. Talc via thoracoscope for pleural sclerosing or surgical pleurodesis
4. Surgical thoracic duct ligation

Costochondritis

Buzz Words: Chest pain reproduced with palpation

Clinical Presentation: Musculoskeletal chest pain often presents as an insidious and persistent pain. It can also be sharp and localized to a specific area. Pain is often reproducible upon palpation, which is key to differentiating costochondritis from other more serious causes of chest pain. The majority of chest wall pain associated with costochondritis is positional and will be exacerbated by deep breathing and movement. Patients will often not have the typical risk factors for cardiac causes of chest pain.

MoD: Inflammation of cartilage that connects ribs to sternum; can be caused by physical strain, blow to the chest, arthritis, or joint infection.

Dx: Clinical diagnosis, EKG to rule out cardiac causes

Tx/Mgmt: Avoid strenuous activity; stretching; heat/cold packs and NSAIDs

Empyema

Buzz Words: Prolonged duration of pneumonia

Clinical Presentation: Signs and symptoms of bacterial pneumonia include cough, fever, pleuritic chest pain, dyspnea, and increased sputum production. Patients with increased duration of such signs and symptoms of pneumonia are more likely to develop empyema. On auscultation, patients may have decreased breath sounds and decreased fremitus (unlike the crackles, egophony, and increased fremitus typical of consolidation).

PPx: Early treatment of pneumonia

MoD: Bacterial infection of the pleural fluid that leads to either pus or the presence of bacterial organisms on Gram stain.

Dx:
1. Chest x-ray
2. Ultrasound
3. Chest CT scan
4. Thoracentesis/analysis of pleural fluid (see Box 7.2)

Tx/Mgmt:
1. Antibiotics
2. Pleural drainage: tube thoracostomy, VATS, open decortication, and open thoracostomy

Mediastinitis

Buzz Words: Sternal purulent discharge, bacteremia

Clinical Presentation: Patients present with fever, tachycardia, chest pain, and/or signs of sternal wound infection. Postoperative mediastinitis can be either fulminant or subacute. Bacteremia is a common occurrence in postoperative mediastinitis. Risk factors include diabetes, obesity, peripheral artery disease, tobacco use, and prolonged surgical procedure.

QUICK TIPS
Start with antibiotic that includes anaerobic coverage such as clindamycin, amoxicillin-clavulanate, piperacillin-tazobactam, or imipenem.

PPx: Smoking cessation, preoperative antibiotic prophylaxis with first- or second-generation cephalosporins in high-risk patients

MoD: Before the modern area of cardiothoracic surgery, most cases of mediastinitis were due to esophageal perforation or from the spread of odontogenic or retropharyngeal infections. However, currently, the majority of cases of mediastinitis occur as a postoperative complication of cardiothoracic procedures due to wound contamination during surgery. The most common organisms isolated from cases of mediastinitis are *Staphylococcus aureus* (MSSA and MRSA), Gram-negative bacilli, coagulase-negative staphylococci, and streptococci.

Dx:
1. Blood cultures
2. Chest CT scan
3. Subxiphoid aspiration

Tx/Mgmt:
1. Antibiotics: vancomycin plus third-generation cephalosporin (ceftazidime), a quinolone, or an aminoglycoside
2. surgical debridement
3. vacuum-assisted closure before delayed closure

Pleural Effusion

Buzz Words: Orthopnea, PND, blunted costophrenic angles (Fig. 7.8)

Clinical Presentation: Most cases of pleural effusions are indolent and therefore the patient is asymptomatic. If symptomatic, signs and symptoms include dyspnea on exertion, peripheral edema, orthopnea, PND, dullness to percussion, decreased breath sounds, and decreased tactile fremitus.

MoD: Pleural effusions are caused by an increased drainage of fluid into the pleural space, increased fluid production in the pleural space, or decreased drainage from the pleural space. The causes of pleural effusions are broken down into two categories, transudative or exudative, based on Light's criteria (Box 7.3). Transudative effusions are caused by increased hydrostatic pressure or decreased plasma or intrapleural oncotic pressures. On the other hand, exudative effusions are due to increased capillary or pleural membrane permeability.

Dx:
1. Chest x-ray (lateral decubitis films more reliable for detecting small effusions)
2. Thoracentesis/analysis of pleural effusion (see Box 7.2, Table 7.2)

Tx/Mgmt: Therapeutic thoracentesis if symptomatic

QUICK TIPS

The most common causes of transudative pleural effusions include: CHF, constrictive pericarditis, cirrhosis, PE, nephrotic syndrome, hypoalbuminemia, and atelectasis.

QUICK TIPS

The most common causes of exudative pleural effusions include: bacteria pneumonia, tuberculosis, malignancy, PE, and collagen vascular disorder.

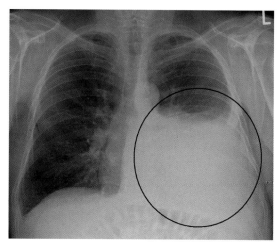

FIG. 7.8 X-ray of pleural effusion. (From Wikimedia Commons: https://commons.wikimedia.org/wiki/File:Effusionhalf.PNG. Created by James Heilman, MD. Used under Creative Commons Attribution-Share Alike 3.0 Unported license: https://creativecommons.org/licenses/by-sa/3.0/deed.en.)

BOX 7.3 Light's Criteria Rule for Exudative Fluid

Must meet at least one of the following:
Pleural fluid protein/serum protein ratio >0.5
Pleural fluid LDH/serum LDH ratio >0.6
Pleural fluid LDH greater than two-thirds the upper limits of the normal serum LDH

LDH, Lactic acid dehydrogenase.

TABLE 7.2 Pleural Effusion Clues

Description	Likely Diagnoses
Elevated pleural fluid amylase	Esophageal rupture, pancreatitis, or malignancy
Milky fluid	Chylothorax
Frank pus	Empyema
Bloody effusion	Malignancy
Exudative and primarily lymphocytic	TB
pH <7.2	Parapneumonic effusion or empyema
Glucose <60	Rheumatoid arthritis, TB, esophageal rupture, malignancy, or lupus

TB, Tuberculosis.

Pleuritis

Buzz Words: Sharp pain, worse with breathing

Clinical Presentation: Sharp, stabbing pain that worsens with deep breathing.

PPx: Early treatment of pneumonia

MoD: Inflammation of the lung pleura most often due to autoimmune diseases, complicated pneumonia, and drugs

Dx: Chest x-ray, ECG

Tx/Mgmt:

1. Pain management
2. Treat underlying cause
3. Screen for SLE: ANA, anti-ds DNA Ab, anti-Sm Ab, antihistone Ab
4. Screen for RA: RF, anticitrullinated peptide/protein Ab (ACPA)

QUICK TIPS
Autoimmune diseases that may causes pleuritis: systemic lupus erythematosus (SLE) or rheumatoid arthritis (RA).

QUICK TIPS
Drugs that may cause pleuritis: procainamide, hydralazine, and isoniazid.

Spontaneous Pneumothorax

Buzz Words: Tall, lean, young men, acute respiratory distress

Clinical Presentation: The patient presents with tachypnea, pleuritic chest pain, hypoxia, unilateral diminished or absent breath sounds, and unilateral hyperresonance to percussion. Primary spontaneous pneumothorax is more common in tall, lean, young men, and in smokers.

PPx: Smoking cessation

MoD: Pneumothorax is an abnormal collection of air in the pleural spaces that leads to an uncoupling of the lung from the chest wall. This leads to decreased lung volume and therefore hypoxia. Spontaneous pneumothorax may be classified as primary or secondary. Primary spontaneous pneumothorax occurs due to rupture of subpleural blebs without a precipitating event in a person who does not have lung disease. Secondary pneumothorax occurs in patients with underlying lung disease

Dx: Chest x-ray, chest CT scan

Tx/Mgmt:

1. Supplemental oxygen if patient stable and small pneumothorax
2. Chest tube if clinical unstable pneumothorax
3. Pleurodesis via VATS for recurrent cases

QUICK TIPS
Causes of secondary spontaneous pneumothorax: COPD, asthma, interstitial lung disease, neoplasm, cystic fibrosis, and tuberculosis.

Traumatic and Mechanical Disorders

Upper Airways

Epistaxis

Buzz Words: Nosebleed, fall/winter season

Clinical Presentation: Patient presents with a nosebleed, a common occurrence that most patients do not seek care for.

MoD: Epistaxis can be broken down into two categories: anterior bleeds and posterior bleeds.

Anterior nosebleeds are often a result of mucosal trauma, such as nose picking, but can also be due to low

QUICK TIPS
Anterior bleeds are by far the most common with 90% occurring within the vascular watershed area of the nasal septum known as Kiesselbach's plexus.

moisture. Posterior nosebleeds arise from the posterolateral branches of the sphenopalatine artery. Anterior and posterior nosebleeds may be associated with the following conditions: anticoagulation, hereditary hemorrhagic telangiectasia, platelet disorders, and aneurysm of the carotid artery.

Dx: Clinical diagnosis, coagulation studies if suspiciously recurrent

Tx/Mgmt:
1. Nasal packing
2. Balloon catheter for continuous posterior bleeding

Barotrauma

Buzz Words: Respiratory distress, mechanical ventilation

Clinical Presentation: May range from asymptomatic to tachypnea, tachycardia, acute respiratory distress, hypoxemia, and hemodynamic collapse.

PPx: Protective ventilator practices, such as limiting plateau pressure, using low tidal volume, and cautious use of PEEP.

MoD: Most often it is due to alveolar rupture from mechanical ventilation, leading to release of air into extra-alveolar areas.

Dx:
- Chest x-ray
- Chest CT scan
- Chest ultrasound

Tx/Mgmt:
- Manage ventilatory settings: lower tidal volume and/or PEEP
- Tube thoracostomy for pneumothorax
- Supportive measures for pneumoperitoneum, pneumomediastinum, and subcutaneous emphysema as they tend to be self-limiting in such cases.

Laryngeal/Pharyngeal Obstruction

Buzz Words: Acute respiratory distress

Clinical Presentation: Respiratory distress occurs with dyspnea, tachypnea, wheezing, tachycardia, and hypoxemia; decreased breath sounds.

MoD: Narrowing or blocking of upper airways is due to many causes including: allergic reactions, foreign bodies, chemical burns, epiglottitis, peritonsillar abscess, retropharyngeal abscess, and neoplasm.

Dx:
- Chest/neck x-ray
- Laryngoscopy/pharyngoscopy

QUICK TIPS

Barotrauma may lead to pneumothorax, pneumomediastinum, pneumoperitoneum, and subcutaneous emphysema.

Tx/Mgmt:
- Manage airway
- Removal of foreign body via laryngoscopy/pharyngoscopy
- Treat underlying condition

Tracheal Stenosis
Buzz Words: Dyspnea, multiple intubations, congenital

Clinical Presentation: Gradual onset of symptoms, which can usually be mistaken for other disorders, such as difficult to treat adult asthma. Patient presents with cough, dyspnea, hypoxia, wheezing, stridor, and fatigue.

MoD: Narrowing or constriction of trachea: Most cases develop as a result of tracheal injury after prolonged intubation or from a tracheostomy. Rarely, it may be congenital.

Dx:
1. Chest x-ray
2. Chest CT scan
3. Fluoroscopy
4. Bronchoscopy

Tx/Mgmt:
1. Surgical correction: tracheal resection and reconstruction, tracheal laser surgery (breaks up scar tissue)
2. Tracheal dilation with either balloon or tracheal dilators
3. Tracheobronchial airway stent

Tracheomalacia
Buzz Words: Dyspnea, positional wheezing

Clinical Presentation: It may be asymptomatic. However, as the severity of airway narrowing due to tracheomalacia increases, patients may present with dyspnea, cough, and sputum retention. Wheezing and stridor may also be recurring events in such patients. Certain maneuvers can elicit signs of tracheomalacia, including forced expiration, cough, Valsalva maneuver, and laying down.

MoD: It is caused by diffuse of segmental tracheal weakness. The acquired causes of tracheomalacia includes: damage via tracheostomy or endotracheal intubation, external chest trauma, thoracic surgery, chronic compression of trachea (commonly due to a benign goiter), chronic inflammation from smoking and severe emphysema, and recurrent infections, such as those seen in chronic bronchitis and cystic fibrosis patients. It may also be congenital.

Dx:
- Bronchoscopy
- Chest CT scan
- Pulmonary functional tests

QUICK TIPS

Other less common causes of tracheal stenosis include trauma, radiotherapy, neoplasm, and autoimmune conditions, such as sarcoidosis or Wegener's granulomatosis.

Tx/Mgmt:
1. No treatment for asymptomatic patients
2. Continuous positive airway pressure (CPAP) if in respiratory distress
3. Surgery—tracheobronchoplasty with polypropylene mesh for patients who improve with stenting and are surgical candidates
4. Long-term stenting for nonsurgical candidates

Blunt Tracheal Injury

Buzz Words: Motor vehicle collision (MVC), respiratory distress, subcutaneous emphysema

Clinical Presentation: Blunt trauma more commonly affects the intrathoracic trachea. Diagnosis is often delayed, as intrathoracic injury may be subtle and indolent, presenting with retained secretions, recurrent pneumothoraces, and obstruction. The telltale sign of blunt tracheal injury is a pneumothorax or pneumomediastinum that reoccurs despite tube thoracostomy. Radiographic signs include subcutaneous emphysema, rising of the larynx above the third cervical vertebra, and abnormal location of endotracheal tube.

MoD: Blunt tracheal injury post MVC is a rare occurrence, occurring in less than 1% of patients with blunt thoracic trauma. This is the case because the trachea is protected from injury by its position relative to the mandible, sternum, and its relative elasticity. Most of the patients who do have blunt trauma to the trachea die at the scene.

Dx:
1. Chest x-ray
2. Chest CT scan
3. Bronchoscopy
4. Visualization during surgery

Tx/Mgmt:
1. Manage airway
2. Primary surgical repair with possible lung resection

Penetrating Neck/Tracheal Injury

Buzz Words: Gunshot or stab wound in the neck, respiratory distress

Clinical Presentation: Tracheal injuries due to penetrating wounds are predominantly confined to the cervical trachea. Patients present with respiratory distress, stridor, subcutaneous air, hemoptysis, odynophagia, dysphonia, or anterior neck tenderness. Patients may appear stable initially, but may quickly decompensate.

Anatomical zones of the neck

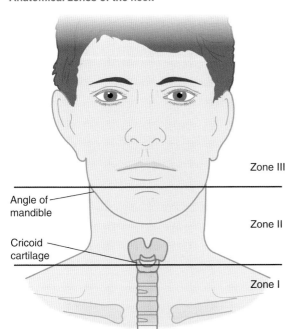

FIG. 7.9 Neck zones. (From Martin T. "Neck Trauma Management". Surgery (Oxford)<http://www.sciencedirect.com/science/journal/02639319> Volume 33, Issue 9<http://www.sciencedirect.com/science/journal/02639319/33/9>, September 2015, Pages 449-454, Figure 1, Elsevier https://doi.org/10.1016/j.mpsur.2015.07.002.)

MoD: Gunshot wounds, stab wounds, or penetrating debris such as glass or shrapnel: Penetrating neck injuries are defined as any injury that penetrates the platysma.

Dx:

1. Primary assessment with a focus on airway, breathing, and circulation (ABCs)
2. Secondary evaluation via a head-to-toe exam with a focus on determining if the platysma has been penetrated, what zones of the neck are involved (Fig. 7.9, Box 7.4), and hard versus soft signs of penetrating neck injury (Box 7.5)
3. Head/neck x-ray
4. CT with angiography (multidetector computed tomography [MDCT]-A)
5. Nasopharyngoscopy/laryngoscopy/bronchoscopy

Tx/Mgmt:

1. Manage ABCs: Secure airway, ensure adequate ventilation, control bleeding, two large-bore intravenous (IV) catheters.

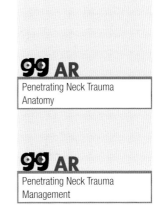

gg AR

Penetrating Neck Trauma Anatomy

gg AR

Penetrating Neck Trauma Management

BOX 7.4 Neck Anatomy: Structures Within Each Zone

Zone I: From Sternal Notch to Cricoid Cartilage	Zone II: From Cricoid Cartilage to Angle of the Mandible	Zone III: From Angle of the Mandible to the Base of the Skull
Subclavian arteries and veins Internal jugular veins Proximal carotid arteries Vertebral artery Apices of the lungs Trachea Esophagus Spinal cord Thoracic duct Thyroid gland	Common carotid arteries Internal and external branches of carotid arteries Vertebral arteries Jugular veins Trachea Esophagus Larynx Pharynx Spinal cord Vagus and recurrent laryngeal nerves	Distal portion of the internal carotid arteries Vertebral arteries Jugular veins Pharynx Spinal cord Cranial nerves IX, X, XI, XII Sympathetic chain

BOX 7.5 Hard and Soft Signs of Penetrating Neck Injury

Hard Signs	Soft Signs
Severe hemorrhage Large, expanding, or pulsatile hematoma Thrills or bruits Shock unresponsive to fluids Absent or diminished radial pulse Neurologic deficit Air bubbles from a wound Massive hemoptysis or hematemesis Respiratory distress	Proximity wounds Minor hemorrhage Mild hypotension responsive to fluids Minor hemoptysis or hematemesis Subcutaneous or mediastinal air Non-pulsatile, non-expanding hematoma Dysphonia Dysphagia

2. No-zone approach: Surgical exploration/intervention for unstable patients regardless of which zone was injured (patients with hard signs). MDCT-A for stable patients (patients with soft signs), treat underlying injuries accordingly.
3. Zone approach: Surgical exploration/intervention for injuries located in zone II, MDCT-A for patients with injuries located in zone I or III.

Foreign Body Aspiration (Pharynx, Larynx, and Trachea)
Buzz Words: Acute asphyxiation, cyanosis

Clinical Presentation: Unlike foreign bodies in the lower airways, obstruction of the upper airway is more likely to present as choking with acute asphyxiation leading to respiratory distress. Monophasic wheeze and/or stridor may be present due to tracheal foreign body aspiration. It is more common in children, psychiatric patients, and the elderly.

PPx: Chewing food thoroughly, not leaving small children unattended

MoD: Aspiration of foreign body: In adults, commonly inhaled objects include incompletely chewed foods, nails, pins, and dental debris/prostheses. In children, nuts, seeds, and other foods account for the majority of cases of foreign body aspiration. Majority of foreign bodies are radiolucent. One-third of aspiration presenting with acute asphyxiation is located in the supraglottic position.

Dx:
1. Assess ABCs
2. Neck x-ray
3. Chest CT scan
4. Laryngoscopy or bronchoscopy

Tx/Mgmt:
1. Secure airway in acute asphyxiation: Heimlich maneuver, proper oxygenation, cricothyrotomy, or tracheotomy
2. Retrieve foreign body via laryngoscopy or bronchoscopy

Nasal Cavity/Sinuses

Septal Perforation

Buzz Words: Young adult, nasal erythema and discharge

Clinical Presentation: It may be asymptomatic with only minor erythema. Small perforations may present with whistling noise. Larger perforations may lead to more severe symptoms, such as crusting, bloody discharge, pressure, and nasal discomfort

PPx: Cessation of nasal cocaine

MoD: Septal perforation is a condition often seen with intranasal cocaine use. Other causes include: septal surgery, atrophic rhinitis, rheumatologic disorders, and granulomatosis with polyangiitis

Dx: Clinical diagnosis

Tx/Mgmt:
1. Humidification
2. Observation for asymptomatic patients
3. Surgical closure for symptomatic patients
4. Tox screen

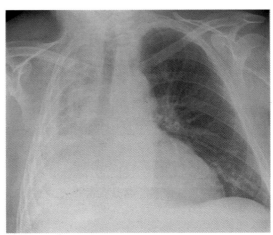

FIG. 7.10 Atelectasis. (From Wikimedia Commons: https://commons.wikimedia.org/wiki/File:Atelectasia1.jpg. Used under Creative Commons Attribution-Share Alike 3.0 Unported license: https://creativecommons.org/licenses/by-sa/3.0/deed.en.)

99 AR

| Review of postop fever |

Lower Airways and Pleura

Atelectasis

Buzz Words: Fever, hypoxemia, postoperative day 2 (Fig. 7.10)

Clinical Presentation: Increased work of breathing, hypoxemia, and fever usually occurring on postoperative day 2. Atelectasis is one of the most common postoperative pulmonary complications, especially following abdominal and thoracoabdominal procedures.

PPx: Smoking cessation at least 8 weeks before surgery, deep breathing, incentive spirometry, early mobilization, adequate pain control (epidural analgesia or intercostal nerve blocks), CPAP.

MoD: Collapse of lung tissue leads to loss of lung volume. Caused by decreased compliance of lung tissue, impaired regional ventilation, retained secretions, and pain interfering with deep breathing and coughing.

Dx: Chest x-ray

Tx/Mgmt: Chest physiotherapy and suctioning

Blunt Chest Wall and Diaphragm Injury

Buzz Words: MVCs, respiratory distress, seatbelt sign

Clinical Presentation: The common presentation of blunt chest wall and diaphragm injury consists of respiratory distress, signs of shock, and possibly hypoxia. The remainder of the Clinical Presentation: depends on the specific injury sustained. Patients with clavicular fracture will often present with a complaint of pain exacerbated by shoulder movement, and will have a palpable deformity of the clavicle. Patients with sternal fracture will often present with severe pain localized to the sternum (may have pleuritic component) and have a palpable deformity of the sternum. Patients with rib fractures will have focal tenderness and palpable deformities. On the other hand, patients with flail chest will depict a paradoxical motion with breathing (opposite motion of the uninjured chest wall). Lastly, patients with diaphragmatic rupture will often present with abdominal pain along with referred shoulder pain.

MoD: The most common mechanism of injury leading to blunt chest wall and diaphragm injury is MVCs. Blunt trauma to the thoracic region has the potential to cause various injuries to the chest wall and diaphragm including: clavicle fracture, sternum fracture, rib fracture, flail chest, diaphragmatic rupture, pneumothorax, and pulmonary contusion. Of note, flail chest occurs due to three or more adjacent ribs being fractured in two different locations, creating a "floating" segment of ribs.

Dx:
1. Primary assessment with a focus on ABCs
2. Secondary evaluation via a head-to-toe exam
3. Extended focused assessment with sonography (E-FAST)
4. Chest and abdominal x-ray
5. Chest and abdominal CT scan

Tx/Mgmt:
1. Manage ABCs: Secure airway, ensure adequate ventilation, control bleeding, two large-bore IV catheters:
   - Clavicular fracture: Surgical open reduction and internal fixation if displaced, otherwise immobilization via sling
   - Sternal and rib: Adequate pain control and follow-up as the majority are non-displaced and heal on their own
   - Flail chest: Conservative management via ventilatory support or surgical open reduction and internal fixation
   - Diaphragmatic rupture: Surgical repair usually done via trauma laparotomy

Penetrating Chest Wound

Buzz Words: Respiratory distress, knife wound, gunshot wound

Clinical Presentation: We will focus on the general presentation and approach to penetrating chest wound, as individual injury to the respiratory system will be discussed separately. Presentation is variable from stable patients with few complaints to hemodynamically unstable patients.

The clinical picture depends on what structures were injured and its resulting pathophysiology. Serious injury to respiratory system will all present with respiratory distress, decreased breath sounds, and/or hemodynamically instability. Although less common than blunt trauma, penetrating chest trauma tends to be more deadly.

MoD: Penetrating trauma to thorax: Possible injuries include: pneumothorax, pulmonary contusion, hemothorax, tracheobronchial injury, pericardial tamponade, diaphragmatic rupture, and esophageal injury.

Dx:
1. Primary assessment with a focus on ABCs
2. Secondary evaluation via a head-to-toe exam
3. E-FAST
4. Chest and abdominal x-ray
5. Chest and abdominal CT scan
6. Esophagoscopy/bronchoscopy

Tx/Mgmt:
1. Manage ABCs: Secure airway, ensure adequate ventilation, control bleeding, two large-bore IV catheters
2. Urgent thoracotomy for cardiac tamponade, and significant hemorrhage, or a persistent air leak from a chest tube

Management of pneumothorax, pulmonary contusion, and hemothorax will be discussed separately.

Traumatic Pneumothorax/Tension Pneumothorax

Buzz Words: Respiratory distress, trauma, tracheal deviation (Fig. 7.11)

Clinical Presentation: Patient presents with tachypnea, chest pain, hypoxia, unilateral diminished or absent breath sounds, and unilateral hyperresonance to percussion. Tension pneumothorax leads to a more serious presentation consisting of severe respiratory distress, hypotension, distended neck veins, and tracheal deviation away from pneumothorax. This is an emergent condition.

PPx: Chest x-ray after procedures with potential to disrupt pleura

MoD: Pneumothorax is an abnormal collection of air in the pleural spaces the leads to an uncoupling of the lung from the chest wall. This leads to decreased lung volume and therefore hypoxia. Pneumothorax is a common serious injury associated with penetrating or blunt chest trauma. A tension pneumothorax occurs when tissues surround the opening into the pleural cavity act as a one-way valve allowing air to enter, but not to leave.

Dx: Clinical diagnosis, chest x-ray

QUICK TIPS

Pneumothorax can also be iatrogenic due to chest tube placement, thoracentesis, transthoracic needle aspiration, and central line placement.

Great review and images of tension pneumothorax

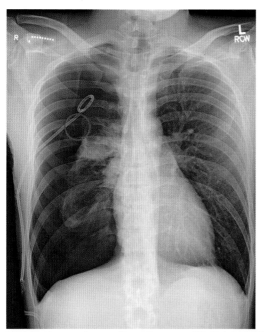

FIG. 7.11 Pneumothorax. (From Segraves JM, Dulohery MM: Primary spontaneous pneumothorax due to high bleb burden. *Respir Med Case Rep* 19:109–111, 2016.)

Tx/Mgmt:
1. Needle decompression in second intercostal space, midclavicular line for tension pneumothorax
2. Sterile occlusive dressing taped on three sides for open pneumothorax
3. Chest tube
4. Serial chest x-ray for small/asymptomatic pneumothorax

Hemothorax

Buzz Words: Respiratory distress, trauma, pleural effusion

Clinical Presentation: Patient presents with tachypnea, chest pain, hypoxia, unilateral diminished or absent breath sounds, and unilateral dullness to percussion.

MoD: Blood in the pleural space is most commonly a result of blunt chest trauma. Injuries leading to hemothorax include aortic rupture, myocardial rupture, injuries to hilar structures, injuries to lung parenchyma, and injuries to intercostal or mammary blood vessels.

Dx: Ultrasound, chest x-ray, chest CT scan

Tx/Mgmt:
1. Manage ABCs
2. Chest tube
3. Surgical thoracotomy for immediate bloody drainage of 1500 mL or shock with persistent, substantial bleeding (>3 mL/kg per hour)

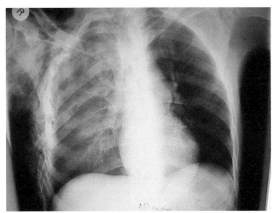

FIG. 7.12 Pulmonary contusion. (From Wikimedia Commons: https://commons.wikimedia.org/wiki/File:Pulmonary_contusion.jpg. Used under Creative Commons Attribution-Share Alike 3.0 Unported license: https://creativecommons.org/licenses/by-sa/3.0/deed.en.)

Pulmonary Contusion

Buzz Words: Respiratory distress, bilateral patchy, alveolar infiltrates, blunt trauma

Clinical Presentation: Tachypnea, chest pain, hypoxia usually occurs within 24 hours of trauma. Initial chest x-ray may not depict contusion. Symptoms worsen with fluids.

MoD: Bruising after lung trauma (blunt or penetrating) resulting in hemorrhage/edema within the lung parenchyma.

Dx: Chest x-ray, chest CT scan (Fig. 7.12)

Tx/Mgmt:
1. Manage ABCs
2. Pain control
3. Pulmonary toilet
4. Restrict fluids to euvolemia
5. Self-resolves within 7 days

Pneumomediastinum

Buzz Words: Chest crepitance, trauma

Clinical Presentation: Patient presents with dyspnea, chest pain, neck pain, tachycardia, tachypnea, or hypertension. Crepitus may be heard during physical exam.

MoD: Air occurs in the mediastinum. May be due to blunt/penetrating trauma, esophageal rupture, alveolar rupture, bowel rupture, or iatrogenic (esophagoscopy, barotrauma).

Dx: Chest x-ray. Chest CT scan.

Tx/Mgmt:
1. Manage ABCs
2. Treat underlying cause, air usually resorbs

BOX 7.6 Methods of Rewarming Hypothermic Patients		
Passive External Rewarming	**Active External Rewarming**	**Active Internal Core Rewarming**
Blankets	Warm blankets Radiant heat Forced warm air applied to skin	Warmed humidified oxygen via tracheal tube Intravenous of warmed crystalloid Irrigation of the peritoneum or thorax with warmed isotonic crystalloid Extracorporeal blood rewarming

Drowning/Near Drowning

Buzz Words: Unconscious, near body of water, alcohol use

Clinical Presentation: Patient is unconscious and hypothermic. Difficult to assess pulse due to hypothermia. Drowning is a common cause of accidental death. Risk factors include risk-taking behavior, use of alcohol and illicit drugs, and inadequate adult supervision.

PPx: Secure fencing and gating around swimming pools, adult supervision, swimming with partner, avoiding alcohol, and illicit drugs while swimming

MoD: Prolonged submersion causing hypoxemia ultimately producing widespread tissue hypoxia

Dx: Clinical diagnosis

Tx/Mgmt:
1. ACLS protocol with a focus on ventilation
2. Remove wet clothing and rewarm with passive and active external rewarming and possibly active internal core rewarming (Box 7.6)

Foreign Body Aspiration (Bronchi and Lungs)

Buzz Words: Recurrent pneumonia, unilateral wheeze

Clinical Presentation: Depends on the degree of obstruction as well as the location and length of time the foreign body has been in the airway. In adults, the clinical presentation is often subtle. Therefore, a chronic cough due to distal obstruction is the most common symptom followed by symptoms that may mimic pneumonia, such as fever, chest pain, and hemoptysis. Patient may not remember inhalation of foreign body. Dyspnea is an uncommon presentation for adults. Patient may have a unilateral wheeze from main stem or lobar obstruction. The most common site of aspiration is the right bronchus.

MoD: Aspiration of foreign body: In adults, commonly inhaled objects include incompletely chewed foods, nails, pins, and dental debris/prostheses. In children nuts, seeds, and other foods account for most cases of foreign body aspiration.

Dx:

1. Assess ABCs
2. Chest x-ray
3. Chest CT scan
4. Laryngoscopy or bronchoscopy

Tx/Mgmt:

1. Manage ABCs
2. Retrieve foreign body via bronchoscopy
3. Treat pneumonia if present

Upper and Lower Respiratory Tract

Obstructive Sleep Apnea

Buzz Words: Snoring, daytime somnolence, overweight

Clinical Presentation: Obstructive apneas, hypopneas, snoring, and resuscitative snorts occur. Daytime symptoms may include sleepiness, fatigue, or poor concentration. Risk factors include advanced age, male gender, obesity, and craniofacial or upper airway soft tissue abnormalities.

PPx: Weight loss

MoD: Recurrent, functional collapse during sleep of the velopharyngeal and/or oropharyngeal airway leading to reduced or complete cessation of airflow despite breathing efforts. Ultimately leads to hypercapnia and hypoxemia and fragmented sleep.

Dx:

1. In-laboratory polysomnography
2. Home sleep apnea testing

Tx/Mgmt:

1. Weight loss
2. CPAP
3. Oral appliances
4. Upper airway surgery to remove floppy tissue
5. Hypoglossal nerve stimulation

Central Sleep Apnea

Buzz Words: Cheyne-Stokes breathing, daytime somnolence, heart failure, stroke

Clinical Presentation: Symptoms of disrupted sleep, such as excessive daytime sleepiness, poor sleep quality, and poor concentration. Patient may also present with PND, morning headaches, and nocturnal angina. Patients with heart failure or previous stroke are more likely to exhibit central sleep apnea with Cheyne-Stokes breathing. Risk factors include advanced age, male sex, heart failure, stroke, and chronic opioid use.

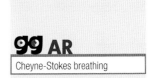
Cheyne-Stokes breathing

MoD: Central nerves system fails to transmit proper signals to respiratory muscles. The most common type of central sleep apnea is due to hyperventilation: Hypoxia (possibly due to secretions) triggers hyperpnea during sleep. This causes a ventilator overshoot leading to hypocapnia, which induces central apnea.

Dx: In-laboratory polysomnography

Tx/Mgmt:
1. CPAP
2. Adaptive servo-ventilation (ASV) for patients without heart failure
3. Nocturnal oxygen
4. Medical management of heart failure

ASV

Obesity-Hypoventilation Syndrome

Buzz Words: Symptoms of OSA, signs of right-sided heart failure

Clinical Presentation: The majority of patients will have coexisting OSA and therefore the presentation is almost identical: obstructive apneas, hypopneas, snoring, and resuscitative snorts. Daytime symptoms may include sleepiness, fatigue, or poor concentration. Patients will often have severe obesity (BMI >50 kg/m^2) and may have signs of right-sided heart failure. Untreated it can progress to acute, life-threatening cardiopulmonary compromise, and is associated with high mortality syndrome (Box 7.7)

QUICK TIPS

Signs of right-sided heart failure of elevated JVD, hepatomegaly, and peripheral edema

MoD: The result of the complex interaction of several physiologic abnormalities such as sleep-disordered breathing (OSA), altered pulmonary function, and altered ventilatory control.

Dx:
1. ABG
2. Pulmonary function tests
3. Serum bicarbonate in-laboratory polysomnography
4. Chest x-ray

BOX 7.7 Diagnosis Criteria of Obesity-Hypoventilation Syndrome

Obesity (body mass index >30 kg/m^2)
Awake alveolar hypoventilation (PaCO$_2$ >45 mm Hg)
An alternative cause cannot be identified

Tx/Mgmt:
1. Weight loss
2. CPAP
3. Abstain from alcohol and drugs that diminish respiratory drive, such as benzodiazepines, opioids, and barbiturates

Congenital Disorders

Bronchogenic Cysts

Buzz Words: Recurrent cough, pneumonia, second decade of life

Clinical Presentation: Recurrent cough, wheezing, and pneumonia occurs usually during the second decade of life. May also be detected as neck masses or incidental findings on imaging.

MoD: Arise from anomalous budding of the foregut during development and can occur at any point throughout the tracheobronchial tree.

Dx: Chest x-ray, chest CT scan

Tx/Mgmt: Surgical excision via partial or total lobectomy

Congenital Diaphragmatic Hernia

Buzz Words: Acute respiratory distress in neonates, PH (Fig. 7.13)

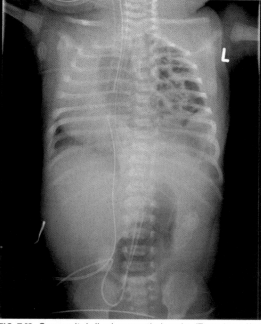

FIG. 7.13 Congenital diaphragmatic hernia. (From http://pediatrici-maging.wikispaces.com/White+-+001.)

Clinical Presentation: It is usually diagnosed prenatally. Neonates present in the first few hours of life with acute respiratory distress that may be mild or severe to the point of incompatibility with life. May also present with persistent PH of the newborn (PPHN) and adrenal insufficiency. May be isolated or associated with additional abnormalities including trisomy 18, 13, and 21.

MoD: Congenital defect of the diaphragm that allows the abdominal viscera to herniate into the chest. In most cases, the herniation occurs on the left. The herniation compresses the lungs during its development. This compression decreases bronchial and pulmonary artery branching, leading to increasing degrees of pulmonary hypoplasia. This hypoplasia is most severe on the ipsilateral side, but may also occur on the contralateral side due to a shift of the mediastinum. Hypoplasia may also lead to PPHN.

Dx:
1. Prenatal ultrasound
2. Ultrafast fetal MRI
3. Fetal echocardiography
4. Fetal genetic studies
5. Umbilical artery line for monitoring of blood gas and blood pressure

Tx/Mgmt:
1. Fetal monitoring via nonstress testing or biophysical profile testing at 33–34 weeks
2. Antenatal glucocorticoids
3. Intubation and ventilation
4. Nasogastric tube
5. Isotonic fluids, dopamine and/or dobutamine, and hydrocortisone for BP support
6. Surfactant
7. Inhaled nitric oxide

QUICK TIPS

NO decrease in pulmonary hypertension, viii. Extracorporeal membrane oxygenation (ECMO), ix. Surgical correction consisting of reduction of the abdominal viscera and primary closure of the defect.

Pulmonary Sequestration

Buzz Words: Respiratory distress, non-functioning lung mass

Clinical Presentation: It is usually diagnosed prenatally. Most affected neonates are asymptomatic; however, the minority that are symptomatic at birth present with respiratory distress. The patients that have intralobar sequestration tend to present later in life with symptoms of recurrent infections, such as fever, cough, hemoptysis, and chest pain. May be found as an accidental finding on imaging. Cases can be isolated or associated with congenital diaphragmatic hernia, vertebral anomalies, congenital heart disease, and colonic duplication.

QUICK TIPS
Pulmonary sequestration is characterized by its location, either intralobar (most common) or extralobar.

MoD: A rare abnormality of the lower airways consisting of a non-functioning mass of lung tissue. This abnormal lung receives its arterial blood supply from the systemic circulation tissue as it lacks normal communication with the tracheobronchial tree.

Dx:
1. Prenatal ultrasound
2. Chest x-ray
3. Chest CT scan

Tx/Mgmt:
1. Manage airway and ventilation
2. Surgical resection for symptomatic patients and asymptomatic patients with large lesions (occupies ≥20% of the lobe)
3. Observation for asymptomatic patients with small lesions

Immotile Cilia Syndrome/Primary Ciliary Dyskinesia

Buzz Words: Chronic rhinitis since childhood, infertility, bronchiectasis

Clinical Presentation: It is variable depending on the extent of ciliary defect. The most common presenting features are recurrent infections of the upper and lower respiratory tract with most patients presenting in childhood. Patients may also present with bronchiectasis manifesting as auscultatory crackles. Of note, men with this condition are infertile and women have decreased fertility and increased risk of ectopic pregnancy.

It is associated with cardiac abnormalities, pyloric stenosis, and epispadias.

QUICK TIPS
If a patient presents with situs inversus, chronic sinusitis, and bronchiectasis, he or she has Kartagener's syndrome (a subset of immotile cilia syndrome [ICS]).

MoD: Inherited autosomal recessive disease that leads to a congenital impairment of mucociliary clearance. A highly heterogeneous disease that can be caused by a defect in any of the many polypeptide species within the axoneme of cilia or of sperm flagella. The cilia may be unable to beat, unable to beat normally, or be absent altogether.

Dx:
1. Chest x-ray
2. Measuring nasal nitric oxide (low or absent in ICS)
3. Inhalation of tagged colloid albumin to measure mucocilliary transport
4. Biopsy with electron microscopy to assess ciliary motion and structure
5. Genetic testing

Tx/Mgmt:
1. Daily chest physiotherapy
2. Humidified air
3. Smoking cessation

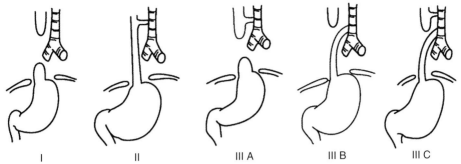

| I | II | III A | III B | III C |

FIG. 7.14 Types of TE fistula. (From Rasch DK, Ramamurthy, RS. "Tracheoesophageal Fistula (TEF)", Decision Making in Anesthesiology (Fourth Edition)<http://www.sciencedirect.com/science/book/9780323039383> An Algorithmic Approach, 2007, Pages 368–369, Figure 1, Mosby (https://doi.org/10.1016/B978-0-323-03938-3.50134-2.)

4. Amoxicillin-clavulanate for infections
5. Intranasal glucocorticoids
6. Surgery for debulking nasal polyposis
7. Vaccination against influenza and pneumococcus

Tracheoesophageal Fistula

Buzz Words: Excessive drooling in newborn, polyhydramnios, inability to feed

PPx: N/A

Clinical Presentation: Depends on the presence or absence of esophageal atresia (EA): In patients with EA (95%), polyhydramnios occurs in the gestational period. Infants with EA are symptomatic with excessive secretions causing drooling, choking, respiratory distress, and inability to feed. If a fistula between the trachea and distal esophagus is present, the infant can present with gastric distension and aspiration pneumonia.

MoD: A common congenital anomaly of the respiratory tract and typically occurs with EA. This malformation is characterized according to their anatomic configuration (Fig. 7.14).

Dx:
1. Attempt to pass a catheter into the stomach
2. Chest x-ray
3. Upper GI series with water-soluble contrast

Tx/Mgmt:
1. Manage airway
2. Surgical ligation of fistula with primary anastomosis of the esophageal segment if necessary
3. Staged procedures for long distance between esophagus and stomach, which includes elongation of the esophagus, interposition of the jejunum or colon, and gastric transposition

GUNNER PRACTICE

1. A 40-year-old male with a history of asthma, angina, and bipolar disorder presents to the clinic with a mild cough accompanied by shortness of breath and fever. His wife states he has had these symptoms for the past 3 weeks with no improvement. He is currently taking albuterol, nitro, and lithium. Of note, the patient quit smoking 20 years ago. His chest x-ray not only depicts a left lobar consolidation, but also a 4-cm nodule is visible on the peripheral right lower lobe. What is the best next step in management besides antibiotics for his pneumonia?
   A. Transthoracic biopsy
   B. Compare with older imaging
   C. Chest CT scan
   D. Surgical excision
   E. Follow-up in 2 months

2. A 25-year-old female presents to the emergency department after being involved in a motor vehicle crash. She has past medical history of anorexia, insulin-dependent diabetes, and a previous ACL tear. Examination depicts a dislocated shoulder, seat-belt sign, and crepitus over the sternum. Three hours after admission, she appears to be in respiratory distress with dyspnea and tachycardia. The patient has a temperature of 39°C, HR 100, BP 130/90, RR 24, pulse ox 85% on 2L via nasal cannula. What is a chest x-ray most likely to depict?
   A. Patchy, alveolar infiltrates
   B. Blunted costophrenic angle
   C. Air in the mediastinum
   D. Pulmonary nodule
   E. Lobar consolidation

3. A 45-year-old male, who is postoperative day 2 from an open reduction and internal fixation of his right femur following a traumatic fracture from a motorcycle accident, presents with confusion, acute dyspnea, tachycardia, elevated temperature, and hypoxemia. He also has a diffuse petechial rash over his mid-torso. What is the most likely cause of his symptoms?
   A. Pulmonary embolism
   B. ARDS
   C. Fat embolism
   D. Myocardial infarction
   E. Atelectasis

Notes

ANSWERS: What Would Gunner Jess/Jim Do?

1. WWGJD? A 40-year-old male with a history of asthma, angina, and bipolar disorder presents to clinic with a mild cough accompanied by shortness of breath and fever. His wife states he has had these symptoms for the past 3 weeks with no improvement. He is currently taking albuterol, nitro, and lithium. Of note, patient quit smoking 20 years ago. His chest x-ray not only depicts a left lobar consolidation, but also a 4 cm nodule is visible on the peripheral right lower lobe. What is the best next step in management besides antibiotics for his pneumonia?

Answer: B, Compare with older imaging.

   Explanation: This is a classic example of the presentation of an SPN. The patient often presents for a complaint that requires a chest x-ray; in this case a typical presentation of pneumonia. In such cases, you always want to compare the current imaging with a previous radiographical image.

   A. Transthoracic biopsy → Incorrect. Getting a biopsy is too aggressive for this point in time.

   C. Chest CT scan → Incorrect. A chest CT scan might be appropriate if, after looking at previous imaging, the nodule is not stable.

   D. Surgical excision → Incorrect. Too aggressive for this point in time.

   E. Follow-up in 2 months → Incorrect. Despite the low risk of malignancy in this patient (age <45, quit smoking ≥7 years prior, small nodule <0.5 cm) following up in 2 months would be inappropriate without looking at an old x-ray/CT scan.

2. WWGJD? A 25-year-old female presents to the emergency department after being involved in a motor vehicle crash. She has past medical history of anorexia, insulin-dependent diabetes, and a previous ACL tear. Examination depicts a dislocated shoulder, seat-belt sign, and crepitus over the sternum. Three hours after admission, she appears to be in respiratory distress with dyspnea and tachycardia. The patient has a temperature of 39°C, HR 100, BP 130/90, RR 24, pulse ox 85% on 2L via nasal cannula. What is a chest x-ray most likely to depict?

Answer: A, Patchy, alveolar infiltrates.

   Explanation: This patient is presenting with pulmonary contusion, which can have a delayed presentation after a motor vehicle crash. Her physical exam depicts a strong force to her chest wall (dislocated

shoulder, seat-belt sign) and a possible sternal fracture. All of which are associated with pulmonary contusion. It is possible that the x-ray was normal when she first arrived to the emergency department as the signs, symptoms, and radiographical depiction of pulmonary contusion may present hours after admission.
- B. Blunted costophrenic angle → Incorrect. A blunted costophrenic angle would be a sign of pleural effusion, which is less likely to present acutely 3 hours after the injury.
- C. Air in the mediastinum → Incorrect. Air in the mediastinum may be due to a rupture of the bronchus or trachea, a very rare injury.
- D. Pulmonary nodule → Incorrect. A pulmonary nodule is clearly not applicable to this case.
- E. Lobar consolidation → Incorrect. Lobar consolidation is clearly not applicable to this case.

3. WWGJD? A 45-year-old male, who is postoperative day 2 from an open reduction and internal fixation of his right femur following a traumatic fracture from a motorcycle accident, presents with confusion, acute dyspnea, tachycardia, elevated temperature, and hypoxemia. He also has a diffuse petechial rash over his mid-torso. What is the most likely cause of his symptoms?

Answer: C, Fat embolism.

Explanation: It is a classic presentation of fat embolism in a patient that underwent an orthopedic procedure. What truly makes this diagnosis likely is the petechial rash, which is not found with other common causes of respiratory distress in a postoperative patient, such as pulmonary embolism, ARDS, or atelectasis.
- A. Pulmonary embolism → Incorrect. Petechial rash is not found with pulmonary embolism.
- B. ARDS → Incorrect. Petechial rash is not found with ARDS.
- D. Myocardial infarction → Incorrect. Myocardial infarction (MI) is a very unlikely for this patient's presentation as he has no risk factors for MI.
- E. Atelectasis → Incorrect. Petechial rash is not found with atelectasis.

Notes

Nutritional and Digestive Disorders

Alejandro Suarez-Pierre, William Plum, Hao-Hua Wu,
Leo Wang, Drake LeBrun, Rebecca Gao, and Sean Harbison

CHAPTER

8

Introduction

The National Board of Medical Examiners (NBME) Surgery Shelf exam devotes 20%–25% of its questions to nutritional and digestive disorders, which makes it the most frequently tested subject.

This chapter gives structure to the myriad topics considered pertinent to your shelf exam and attempts to narrow down on frequently tested subjects. It is organized into (1) Infectious Disorders (bacterial, viral, fungal, parasitic); (2) Immunologic and Inflammatory Disorders; (3) Neoplasms; (4) Signs, Symptoms, and Ill-Defined Disorders; (5) Disorders of the Salivary Glands and Esophagus; (6) Disorders of the Stomach, Small Intestine, Colon, Rectum, and Anus; (7) Disorders of the Liver and Biliary System, Noninfectious; (8) Disorders of the Pancreas; (9) Traumatic and Mechanical Disorders; (10) Congenital Disorders; (11) Adverse Drug Effects, and (12) Gunner Practice.

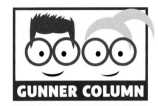

GUNNER COLUMN

Infectious Disorders

Bacterial

Pseudomembranous Colitis (Clostridium difficile)

Buzz Words: ICU patient who develops watery diarrhea while receiving broad-spectrum antibiotics, with obligate anaerobe gram-positive rods in stool.

Clinical Presentation: Classic presentation is secretory diarrhea. *C. difficile* is part of the normal gut flora. Patients who are exposed to antibiotics (most commonly clindamycin, quinolones, ampicillin) lose a significant portion of their flora, leading to colonization. Most common cause of nosocomial and health care–associated diarrhea.

Prophylaxis (PPx): Avoid abuse of broad-spectrum antibiotics

Mechanism of Disease (MoD): Exotoxins A and B alter the structural integrity of actin filaments, leading to increased permeability of tight junctions and promoting watery diarrhea; these cells end up undergoing apoptosis due to caspase activation and Rho protein inactivation. Exotoxin damage leads to the formation of a shaggy layer of fibrin and dead epithelial cells (pseudomembrane), which cover the mucosal lining.

Diagnostic Steps (Dx):
1. Cytotoxins can be detected in diarrhea
2. Glutamate dehydrogenase antigen test is also used and has excellent sensitivity and specificity

Treatment and Management Steps (Tx/Mgmt):
1. IV metronidazole first-line
2. Oral vancomycin if it fails (produces resistant strains)

Enteric Infections

Staphylococcus aureus

Buzz Words: Nausea and vomiting + abdominal pain + recent ingestion of dairy product (e.g., old mayonnaise)

Clinical Presentation: Fast onset (1–6 hours) of food poisoning occurs; nausea, vomiting, abdominal cramps.

PPx: Adequate refrigeration of food products, hand hygiene

MoD: Heat-stable enterotoxin B acts as a superantigen by forming a bridge between MHC-II on antigen-presenting cells and T-cell receptors on T cells. Growth occurs in dairy products, meats, and salads kept at room temperature. Beta-hemolytic, catalase-positive, coagulase-positive, gram-positive coccus.

Dx: Clinical diagnosis

Tx/Mgmt: Self-limited, offer supportive therapy

Escherichia coli

Buzz Words: Hemolytic uremic syndrome (HUS) + schistocytes + hemorrhagic diarrhea + recently ate undercooked meat (e.g., hamburgers) → EHEC

Clinical Presentation: There are four types of *E. coli* that can be tested by the National Board of Medical Education (NBME) (Table 8.1). Of the four, EHEC is the most high-yield. If pressed for time, skip EPEC, ETEC, and EIEC:
1. Enterohemorrhagic *E. coli* (EHEC)—shiga-like toxin from undercooked meat leading to HUS, most commonly tested
2. Enteropathogenic *E. coli* (EPEC)—Predominates in children (Peds), nonbloody diarrhea
3. Enterotoxifenic *E. coli* (ETEC)—Travelers' diarrhea, nonbloody diarrhea, second most commonly tested
4. Enteroinvasive *E. coli* (EIEC)—Inflammatory bowel, blood diarrhea

TABLE 8.1 Most Common Diarrheal Illnesses Caused by *Escherichia coli*

	ETEC (i.e., Traveler's Diarrhea)	EHEC *(O157:H7 Serotype)*	EIEC
Presentation	Watery diarrhea	Hemorrhagic colitis and HUS in 8% of cases	Dysentery 12–72 h after ingestion
MoD	Heat-labile (LT) and heat-stable (ST) toxins activate adenylate and guanylate cyclase respectively → secretory diarrhea	Shiga toxin (verotoxin) → inactivates ribosomal 60S component → endothelial damage (gut, kidney, lung) → hemorrhage	Mucosal cell invasion causing membrane disruption
Clinical cues	Travelers and children age <5	Children and elderly; transmitted through undercooked ground beef	Developing countries; invasion rarely goes beyond submucosa
Management	Fluid replacement Ciprofloxacin	Fluid replacement *Avoid antibiotics!* These may precipitate HUS	Fluid replacement

EHEC, Enterohemorrhagic *E. coli*; *EIEC*, enteroinvasive *E. coli*; *ETEC*, enterotoxifenic *E. coli*; *HUS*, hemolytic uremic syndrome; *MoD*, mechanism of disease.

PPx: Handwashing, adequate sanitization of water, and avoiding food contamination

ETEC causes secretory diarrhea. Patients traveling to endemic areas can take antibiotics (fluoroquinolones first-line, azithromycin if going to Asia) and use them in case of developing diarrhea during their trip; these decrease duration of symptoms.

MoD:
- *For EHEC:* Shiga toxin (verotoxin) → inactivates ribosomal 60S component → endothelial damage (gut, kidney, lung) → hemorrhage
- EHEC and EIEC → bloody diarrhea = bacteria invade mucosa
- ETEC and EPEC do not invade and inflame gut mucosa

Dx:
1. Blood culture and Gram stain (motile, encapsulated gram-negative rod, catalase-positive, and oxidase-negative)
2. MacConkey agar (pink; lactose fermenter)
3. DNA assays, enzyme immunoassays for toxin

Tx/Mgmt:
1. Supportive therapy (i.e., fluids)
2. Avoid antiperistaltic agents (loperamide), as these might prolong duration of infection
3. For EHEC: fluid replacement and avoid antibiotics, which may precipitate HUS

Listeria monocytogenes

Buzz Words: Pasteurized milk + dark/cloudy amniotic fluid + newborn meningitis

Clinical Presentation: Febrile gastroenteritis is present, which might progress to systemic disease in pregnant patients, during steroid therapy, or in the immunosuppressed. *Listeria* is also the third most common cause of meningitis in newborns and is the reason why **ampicillin** is added to the treatment regimen at times in ≤6-month olds with sepsis.

MoD: It is motile by actin filament polymerization and transmitted through contaminated dairy products and deli meat. The organism can survive refrigerator temperatures and a wide range of pH.

Dx: Stool culture and Gram stain—shows tumbling motility; catalase-positive, gram-positive; facultative anaerobe

Tx/Mgmt: Ampicillin, trimethoprim-sulfamethoxazole (TMP-SMX) (antibiotic resistance is rare)

Yersinia enterocolitica

Buzz Words: Gram-negative coccobacillus with bipolar staining ("safety-pin" appearance), resistant to cold temperatures

Clinical Presentation: Enterocolitis in children may be accompanied by pharyngitis (no other cause of bacterial diarrhea). Mesenteric lymphadenitis that simulates acute appendicitis. Associated with HLA-B27 tissue type (seronegative spondyloarthropathies), may have erythema nodosum and reactive arthritis as sequelae.

PPx: Avoid contact with canine feces and ensure handwashing after exposure to swine products. Administer killer vaccine.

MoD: Organism courses through the stomach, attaches and invades the gut wall, ends up localizing in regional lymphoid tissue.

Dx: Culture isolation from stool, pharynx, or mesenteric nodes

Tx/Mgmt: Ciprofloxacin (adults) or TMP-SMX (children) in patients with severe disease only

MNEMONIC

Diseases associated with HLA-B27 subtype (**PAIR**): **P**soriasis, **A**nkylosing spondylitis, **I**nflammatory bowel disease, and **R**eactive arthritis

Campylobacter spp

Buzz Words: Bloody diarrhea, fever, and cramping periumbilical abdominal pain

Clinical Presentation: Bloody diarrhea, fever, and cramping periumbilical abdominal pain occurs. Children may manifest abdominal pain that mimics appendicitis or colitis. Guillain-Barré syndrome (ascending paralysis), HUS, and reactive arthritis are late complications.

PPx: Avoid eating raw/undercooked meat

MoD: It is invasive with a low infective dose (~500 bacteria). Poultry is a reservoir. Puppies are the most common source of infection for children. Produces crypt abscesses resembling ulcerative colitis. Disease is self-limited with a mean duration of 7 days.

Dx: Stool culture: Serologic test may be used to detect recent infection once the organism is no longer in the stool.

Tx/Mgmt:
1. Supportive therapy
2. Fluoroquinolones, azithromycin, or erythromycin in setting of severe diarrhea

Vibrio cholerae

Buzz Words: Rice-water stools, comma-shaped gram-negative rod, acid-labile, oxidase-positive

Clinical Presentation: High-volume secretory diarrhea (up to 10 L/day) ± vomiting, significant hypovolemia, electrolyte abnormalities, which may occur hours after onset of disease.

PPx: Adequate hygiene and keeping a clean water supply

MoD: Fimbriae allow attachment to gut wall. Toxin attaches to GM1 ganglioside → activates G_s pathway → increases cAMP → opens CFTR Cl^- channels → secretory diarrhea.

Dx: Clinical diagnosis

Tx/Mgmt:
1. Aggressive oral rehydration therapy
2. IV fluids for patients in hypovolemic shock
3. Supplement zinc and vitamin A in children

Salmonella spp

Buzz Words:
- Fever + abdominal cramps + diarrhea + chicken + fever + 60% lymphs
- Sickle cell patient + osteomyelitis

Clinical Presentation: Inflammatory diarrhea, nausea, vomiting, fever, and abdominal cramps occur. It is an important cause of osteomyelitis in patients with sickle cell disease.

PPx: Adequeate hygiene, live-attenuated (Ty21a) or Vi capsular vaccines exist

MoD: It is transmitted through ingestion of poultry, eggs, and milk products. The organism invades the intestinal wall and submucosal lymphoid system, reaches the circulation, and finally finds shelter within macrophages of the reticuloendothelial system. Type III secretion system and lipid A are the two main virulence factors. Chronic carriage state (>1 year) most usually occurs in elderly patients with biliary tract abnormalities (gallstones most commonly).

Dx: Stool culture (H2S+, motile, acid-labile, capsulated, gram-negative bacilli, black colonies on Hektoen agar, pea-soup diarrhea)

Tx/Mgmt:
1. Supportive therapy
2. Antibiotic therapy (fluoroquinolones) is warranted only for severe infection or patients with risk factors.

Shigella spp

Buzz Words: Bloody diarrhea + day-care center, mental institution + beef ingestion

Clinical Presentation: Patient has frequent small-volume, bloody stools with fever, abdominal cramps, and tenesmus. Intestinal complications involve toxic megacolon, colonic perforation, intestinal obstruction, proctitis, and rectal prolapse. Thrombocytopenia and HUS are common in young children (similar to EHEC); other systemic complications include protein-loss enteropathy, leukemoid reaction, neurologic manifestation, and reactive arthritis.

PPx: Adequate hygiene

MoD: Invasion of M cells occurs. Toxin inactivates ribosomal 60S subunit (similar to verotoxin in EHEC). Glomerular damage; spread is via fecal-oral, hand-hand.

Dx: Stool culture to isolate bacteria (acid-stable, immotile, gram-negative bacilli; green colonies on Hektoen agar)

Tx/Mgmt:
1. Supportive therapy; self-limited infection
2. Antibiotics (ceftriaxone or azithromycin) are appropriate for children and immunosuppressed patients.

Hepatic Abscess

Pyogenic

Buzz Words: History of appendicitis or diverticulitis

Clinical Presentation: A patient who had peritonitis and developed leakage of bowel contents and develops right upper quadrant (RUQ) pain, fever, leukocytosis and elevated alkaline phosphatase.

PPx: Adequate antibiotic therapy in gastrointestinal (GI)/biliary tract infections

MoD: Bacteria usually find their way to the liver from a GI or biliary tract source of infection. Nonetheless, hematogenous seeding may also be etiology in the setting of bacteremia.

Dx:

1. Ultrasound shows hypoechoic mass with a hyperechoic wall.
2. Computed tomography shows a well-demarcated, encapsulated fluid lesion.

Tx/Mgmt:

1. Percutaneous catheter drainage (when >5 cm), the catheter should remain in place until drainage ceases (~7 days).
2. Bacterial cultures on collected fluid are done to narrow down on antimicrobial therapy.
3. Surgical drainage should be considered in the setting of multiple abscesses, loculated abscesses, viscous contents, and inadequate clearing with drainage.

Amebic Abscess

Buzz Words: Immigrant/recent travel to Central or South America, abscess containing "anchovy paste"–appearing fluid

Clinical Presentation: Adult male presents with 1–2 weeks of RUQ and fever ± diarrhea. Hepatosplenomegaly and point tenderness occurs over the liver on abdominal exam.

MoD: *Entamoeba histolytica* trophozoites invade the colon wall and migrate to the liver through the portal circulation. Liver abscesses occur in 10% of patients with amebiasis. Although most occur in the right lobe, lesions in the left hepatic lobe are at higher risk of spontaneous rupture.

Dx:

1. Ultrasound-guided percutaneous aspiration, sterile fluid with anchovy-paste appearance
2. Antiamebic antibodies useful in patients who are not from endemic areas (individuals from endemic areas will test positive even in absence of infection)

Tx/Mgmt:

1. Metronidazole or tinidazol
2. Subsequent treatment with paromomycin to eliminate intraluminal cysts
3. Surgical drainage is required in the setting of rupture of secondary bacterial infection.

Echinococcus

Buzz Words: Sheep + dogs + cystic mass in liver + abdominal pain + fever + eosinophilia

Clinical Presentation: *Echinococcus* causes a parasitic infection that forms hydatid cysts in the liver and can lead to anaphylaxis if cystic contents leak out through biopsy. Thus biopsy or rupture of cysts is avoided. It is associated with sheep and dogs.

PPx:
1. Avoid sheep/dogs
2. Avoid biopsy (leakage of fluid in cysts →
   anaphylaxis)

MoD: *Echinococcus granulosus* infection, carried by sheep and dog feces

Dx:
1. CBC (eosinophilia)
2. Casoni skin test positive

Tx/Mgmt:
1. Albendazol
2. Surgical removal of entire cysts (don't rupture them)

Peritonitis

Definition: Peritonitis is defined as an acute inflammatory process involving the peritoneum, most commonly (but not exclusively) due to infection. Inflammation causes increased regional blood flow, permeability, and the formation of fibrinous exudates, making the surrounding loops of bowel slow down, causing ileus and allowing the omentum to adhere. Intra-abdominal infections represent a major cause of morbidity and mortality. In general, peritonitis has the following Buzz Words and Clinical Presentation:

Buzz Words: "Washboard" abdomen + Blumberg sign (rebound tenderness) + involuntary guarding + tenderness to percussion

Clinical Presentation: Diffuse, poorly defined pain should make you think of inflammation of the visceral peritoneal layer. Divided by embryological derivatives, it is epigastrium—foregut, periumbilical—midgut, hypogastrium—hindgut. Pinpoint and well-localized pain should make you think of inflammation of the parietal peritoneal layer. Progression from the first to the second is a valuable clue to identifying progression of peritonitis (e.g., appendicitis). More specific types of peritonitis are mentioned below.

Primary Peritonitis

Buzz Words: Spontaneous bacterial peritonitis (SBP)

Clinical Presentation: Most commonly occurs in the setting of chronic liver disease and ascites (10% of patients with ascites); nonetheless it may also occur in nephrotic syndrome, acute viral hepatitis, malignancy, and systemic lupus erythematosus (SLE). Clinical cues are fever, altered mental status, and diffuse abdominal pain.

PPx: Antibiotics (i.e., TMP-SMX, ciprofloxacin, or norfloxacin) in patients at high risk for developing SBP (grade 1A evidence supports this). High-risk patients:
- Patients who had SBP (recurrence rate is 70% at 1 year)
- Cirrhosis + GI bleed
- Ascitic fluid protein less than 1.5 g/dL + impaired renal function OR liver failure

MoD: Occurs in the absence of an evident intraabdominal source of infection. Route of infection is usually hematogenous. Most common contaminating pathogens: *E. coli*, *Klebsiella*, and *Steptococcus* spp.

Dx: Paracentesis prior to initiating antibiotics (ascitic fluid absolute polymorphonuclear neutrophil [PMN] count ≥250/mm^3 and positive fluid culture). The fluid separates the visceral and parietal surfaces, preventing the development of a rigid abdomen; therefore some patients are asymptomatic at time of diagnosis.

Tx/Mgmt:
1. Cefotaxime as empiric therapy, narrow spectrum once culture and sensitivities come back
2. Start albumin infusion on patients with borderline renal function (decreased risk of developing renal failure)
3. Discontinue nonselective beta blockers (associated with worst transplant-free survival, greater incidence of hepatorenal syndrome, and prolonged hospitalization)

Secondary Peritonitis

Buzz Words: Free air in the belly, anastomotic dehiscence

Clinical Presentation: Very rare when compared with SBP. Manifestations may also be subtle and identification of symptoms requires high clinical suspicion.

MoD: Ascitic fluid infection occurs in the setting of a surgically treatable source of infection. Secondary bacterial peritonitis is lethal when treatment consists only of antibiotics and no surgery. The mortality for an unnecessary laparotomy in the setting of SBP is ~80%.

QUICK TIPS

Secondary bacterial peritonitis w/o surgical treatment is lethal!

Dx: Paracentesis: Infection is usually polymicrobial. On analysis of ascitic fluid, Ruyon criteria (2 of 3 findings) are indicative of secondary bacterial peritonitis:
- Total protein >1 g/dL
- Glucose <50 mg/dL
- Lactate dehydrogenase (LDH) greater than upper limit of normal for serum

Tx/Mgmt:
1. Empiric antibiotics
2. Exploratory laparotomy should be done emergently in the setting of "free air" or if a surgically treatable source of infection is found
3. Repeat paracentesis at 48 hours to assess response to treatment

Whipple Disease

Clinical Presentation: Middle-aged patient (male > female) who has intermittent steatorrhea, colicky abdominal pain, fever, recurrent polyarthritis, generalized lymphadenopathy, and increased skin pigmentation. Central nervous system (CNS) involvement may present as cognitive dysfunction and confusion. Can ultimately lead to severe wasting syndrome.

MoD: *Trypheryma whippelii* enters macrophage → macrophage unable to digest *T. whippelii* → decreased lymphatic drainage and chylomicron transportation into the blood (similar MoD to apoB48 deficiency).

Dx:
1. Polymerase chain reaction (PCR) or stool test for *T. whippelii* (shows positive periodic acid–Schiff [PAS-positive], non–acid-fast, Gram-positive rod)
2. Esophagogastroduodenoscopy (EGD) with small intestine biopsy (PAS-positive foamy macrophages)

Tx/Mgmt: Long-term antibiotics (6–12 months); ceftriaxone and maintenance with TMP-SMX or doxycycline plus hydroxychloroquine

Viral Infections of the Gastrointestinal Tract

Infectious Esophagitis

Buzz Words: Esophageal erosions on EGD

Clinical Presentation: Immunosuppressed patient presents with odynophagia and dysphagia.

PPx: Maintain high clinical suspicion for immunosuppressed patients.

MoD: Most common viral agents are herpes simplex virus (HSV) and cytomegalovirus (CMV). CMV usually damages the colon as well.

Dx: EGD to take biopsies or brushing from the edge of the ulcer.

Tx/Mgmt:
- HSV-esophagitis: acyclovir PO during 1 week for immunocompetent and 2–3 weeks for immunosuppressed patients
- CMV-esophagitis: ganciclovir

Hepatitis A

Buzz Words: Travel to rural area or developing country + jaundice + elevated liver function tests (LFTs) + no history of hepatitis A virus (HAV) vaccine + ingestion of uncooked shellfish

Clinical Presentation: Patients who travel to endemic areas are at higher risk. It presents as jaundice in adults, anicteric hepatitis might present in children. One-month duration of symptoms. Infection develops aversion to smoking.

PPx:
1. Inactivated vaccine
2. Hygienic practices such as handwashing, heating food appropriately, and avoiding drinking tap water in areas of poor sanitation

MoD: Fecal-oral transmission: Uncooked shellfish is a common source of infection in developed countries.

Dx: Serum IgM anti-HAV antibodies: HAV RNA can be detected in stool prior to onset of symptoms.

Tx/Mgmt: Self-limiting infection, supportive therapy

Hepatitis B

Buzz Words: History of blood transfusion/IV drug use/ unprotected sex + painful hepatomegaly + polyarteritis nodosa/membranous glomerulonephritis (GN)/membranoproliferative GN + no history of vaccination.

Clinical Presentation: Variable fever, purpuric macules, painful hepatomegaly, profound malaise, and urticaria occur. Patient has polyarteritis nodosa and secondary kidney disease. It is associated with membranous and membranoproliferative GN. Second most common cause of fulminant hepatitis (7% of cases). Ten percent of adult infections progress to chronic infections and 90% of neonatal infections progress to chronic infections. It is associated with hepatocellular carcinoma (10%–15% of cases).

99 AR

Hep B serologies timeline

PPx: Immunization with recombinant vaccine

MoD: Uses a reverse transcriptase to infect hepatocytes. Spread is by maternal-fetal route, blood, or sexual activity.

Dx: Alanine aminotransferase (ALT) rises during adult symptomatic infection (ALT > aspartate aminotransferase [AST]) but does not vary significantly in children (Table 8.2).

Tx/Mgmt: Interferon-alpha, lamivudine, nucleoside reverse transcriptase inhibitors (NRTIs), and liver transplantation

Hepatitis C

Buzz Words:
- **Acute:** Elderly adult w blood transfusion OR young adult w/IV drug use + elevated LFTs
- **Chronic:** Elderly adult w/blood transfusion OR young adult w/IV drug use + cirrhosis/hepatocellular carcinoma (HCC) + decreased LFTs

Clinical Presentation: Some 60%–80% will progress to a chronic infection. May lead to cirrhosis and HCC. It is the most common cause of fulminant hepatitis, hepatitis in health care workers, and main indication for liver transplantation in the United States.

PPx: Virus is usually transmitted parenterally; avoid needle sharing. Once infected, avoid habits known to accelerate progression of liver disease such as alcohol, marijuana, and obesity. Those who develop cirrhosis require abdominal ultrasound every 2 years for early detection of HCC.

MoD: Lacks proofreading enzymes (3'-5' exonuclease), which allows for significant antigenic variability of envelope. The virus has six different genotypes, which modify preferred therapy.

TABLE 8.2 Hepatitis B Virus Serologic Studies

Interpretation	HBsAg	HBV DNA	Anti-HBc IgM	Anti-HBc IgG	Anti-HBs
Early infection	+	–	–	–	–
Acute infection	+	+	+	–	–
Window phase	–	–	+	–	–
Recovery	–	–	–	+	+
Immunized	–	–	–	–	+
Healthy carrier	+	–	–	+	–
Infective carrier	+	+	–	+	–

HBV, hepatitis B virus.

Dx:
1. Anti–hepatitis C virus (HCV) antibodies or HCV RNA in serum
2. Alaninine aminotransferase (ALT) rises during symptomatic infection (ALT > aspartate aminotransferase [AST])
3. Chronic HCV infection is characterized by detectable viral titers for greater than 6 months. LFTs usually downtrend from the decreasing number of viable hepatocytes.

Tx/Mgmt: Combination therapy with ribavirin and/or interferon alpha

Hepatitis D

Buzz Words: Concomitant hepatitis B virus (HBV) and hepatitis D virus (HDV) infection

Clinical Presentation: Coinfection = HBV + HDV at the same time (usually transient and self-limited). Superinfection = chronic HBsAg carrier + HDV infection. Severity of infection is dependent on viral genotype. Genotype 1, which is most common in the western world, has a fulminant course with rapid progression toward cirrhosis. Infection tends to occur in children and young adults. Endemic in the Mediterranean region.

PPx: Mode of transmission is unclear.

MoD: Although HDV can replicate autonomously, it requires HBsAg for virion assembly and secretion.

Dx: Serum HDAg, HDV RNA, or anti-HDV antibodies (both IgM and IgG)

Tx/Mgmt: Pegylated interferon alpha

Hepatitis E

Buzz Words: Elevated LFTs + self-limited + pregnancy/preexisting disease

Clinical Presentation: It is a self-limited acute viral hepatitis. Fulminant hepatitis may occur in pregnant patients or those with preexisting liver disease.

PPx: Handwashing and avoiding consumption of untreated water

MoD: Fecal–oral transmission; outbreaks are associated with contaminated water sources.

Dx: Detection of hepatitis E virus (HEV) in serum or stool by PCR, anti-HEV IgM antibodies in serum

Tx/Mgmt: Supportive therapy

Rotavirus Enteritis

Buzz Words: Double-stranded RNA virus, 11 RNA segments, telescoping of the bowel

Clinical Presentation: Secretory diarrhea, nausea, low-grade fever, and vomiting are seen in small children. Occurs most frequently in the winter months.

PPx: Oral live-attenuated vaccine exists; has been associated with intussusception.

MoD: Most common cause of severe diarrhea in children. NSP4 toxin causes chloride permeability through the intestinal cell membranes.

Dx: Rotazyme test on stool

Tx/Mgmt: Oral rehydration

Mumps

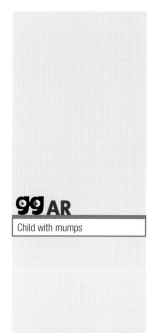

<99 AR

Child with mumps

MNEMONIC

Mumps gives you MOPs:
Meningitis, Orchitis, Parotitis

Buzz Words: Chipmunk facies (bilateral parotitis) + orchitis + fever/headache + no vaccination history

Clinical Presentation: It is a vague viral prodrome consisting of low-grade fever, malaise, headache, myalgias, and anorexia. Bilateral parotitis occurs in 70% of cases. Unilateral orchitis occurs most commonly in an older child or adult.

PPx: MMR vaccine and isolation of any infected individual

MoD: Neuraminidase and hemagglutinin are the main virulence factors. It is caused by RNA paramyxovirus.

Dx:
1. CBC (leukopenia with a relative lymphocytosis)
2. Increased serum amylase (released from salivary glands)

Tx/Mgmt: Supportive therapy with analgesics and antipyretics

Gingivostomatitis, Herpetic

Buzz Words: Cowdry bodies, appearance of dewdrops on a rose petal, multinucleated giant cells in Tzanck smear/prep, dsDNA virus

Clinical Presentation: Viral prodrome (fever + constitutional symptoms) that is followed by oral lesions (initially vesicles on erythematous base → painful ulcers cover by grayish membrane), halitosis, refusal to drink, anorexia, and regional lymphadenitis. Affected age group 6 months–5 years.

PPx: Contact precautions with affected children

MoD: Herpes simplex virus type 1 (HSV-1): After resolution of symptoms the virus migrates to the trigeminal ganglion to establish latent infection. Reactivation can be induced by exposure to sunlight, trauma, cold, stress, or immunosuppression.

Dx: Clinical diagnosis

Tx/Mgmt: Supportive therapy, acyclovir if disease is prolonged (>72 hours).

Fungal

Thrush

Buzz Words: White plaques that are easy to scrape from oral mucosa

Clinical Presentation: Fuzzy white plaques on oral mucous membranes that come off by scraping with a tongue depressor, revealing inflamed and friable mucosa. Differentiate from hairy leukoplakia (Epstein-Barr virus [EBV]), which does not come off by scraping and is usually associated with human immunodeficiency virus (HIV).

MoD: Oropharyngeal colonization of *Candida albicans*: May happen in the immunocompetent neonate or immunocompromised adult. Infection can be transmitted by passage through the birth canal, from the mother's nipple, or from the environment.

Dx: Physical examination is adequate. May also confirm by KOH smear or fungal culture.

Tx/Mgmt:
   1. Topical nystatin or fluconazole
   2. If the mother's breasts are also infected, treat at the same time

Parasitic

Most of the parasitic organisms that produce enterocolitis are opportunistic (acquired immunodeficiency syndrome [AIDS] <50/mm^3). Tend to present as patients who have traveled or migrated from endemic regions and have had diarrhea >7 days.

Cryptosporidium

Buzz Words: AIDS patient with <100/mm^3 CD$_4$ cells + intracellular protozoan + banana-shaped motile sporozoites

Clinical Presentation: Most common cause of diarrhea in AIDS and diarrhea from swimming in municipal pools. Also associated with children who attend day care.

PPx: Strict handwashing and avoiding consumption of untreated water and undercooked food when traveling to endemic regions.

MoD: Organisms can be present in stool, duodenal aspirates, and bile or respiratory secretions.

Dx:
   1. Stool antigen test (high sensitivity and specificity)
   2. Modified acid-fast stain
   3. Alkaline phosphatase (ALP) may be elevated in patients with biliary tract involvement

Tx/Mgmt:

- Nitazoxanide in immunocompetent patients (less effective in immunodeficient) who have had symptoms more than 2 weeks.
- For AIDS patients, antiretroviral therapy should be initiated in association with supportive therapy.

Cyclospora

Buzz Words: AIDS patient or international traveler to endemic area + pink acid-fast oocysts

Clinical Presentation: Patient presents with low-grade fever, diarrhea, abdominal cramping, flatulence, anorexia, and nausea.

PPx: Strict handwashing and avoiding consumption of untreated water and undercooked food when traveling to endemic regions.

MoD: Oocysts passed in the stool are shed in a noninfective form and require several days before they become infectious. Low infectious doses (10–100 organisms). Causes food- and water-borne infection.

Dx: Stool microscopy with acid-fast staining (oocysts are larger than cryptosporidium oocysts, which are also acid-fast).

Tx/Mgmt: TMP-SMX

Entamoeba histolytica

Buzz Words: Flask-shaped ulcers in the patient who recently visited or migrated from a developing country + bloody diarrhea + spherical cysts

Clinical Presentation: Symptoms range from mild diarrhea to dysentery with severe abdominal pain and bloody stools. Fulminant colitis or toxic megacolon with bowel perforation can also occur.

PPx: Strict handwashing and avoiding consumption of untreated water and undercooked food when traveling to endemic regions.

MoD: Transmission by ingestion of cysts in contaminated food/water; cysts become trophozoites in the cecum and secrete histolytic agents, which produce flask-shaped ulcers. Trophozoites can invade hepatic veins and produce a liver abscess (discussed earlier) or systemic disease.

Dx: Stool antigen test

Tx/Mgmt:

1. Metronidazole for symptomatic patients
2. Paromomycin (eliminated intraluminal cysts) for asymptomatic carriers

QUICK TIPS

Be able to differentiate *Giardia lamblia* cysts, which are oval-shaped and cause **nonbloody** diarrhea.

QUICK TIPS

Be able to differentiate *Echinococcus* vs. *Entamoeba*; former presents 3 mo postinfection; latter presents 1–2 weeks postinfection w/abdominal pain.

Giardia

Buzz Words: Camper or hiker with **nonbloody** diarrhea + oval cysts in liver

Clinical Presentation: Steatorrhea with frequent burping, bloating, distention, and flatus (i.e., malabsorption) occur. Malaise and weight loss can occur when with chronic infection.

PPx: Strict handwashing and avoiding consumption of untreated water and undercooked food when traveling to endemic regions.

MoD: *Giardia lamblia* is a flagellated protozoan that produces a water-borne infection. Conditions with absent immunoglobulin (Ig)A production (IgA deficiency, Bruton agammaglobulinemia) make the perfect setting for giardiasis in a test question.

Dx: O&P, enzyme-linked immunosorbent assay (ELISA) stool antigen test, and nucleic acid detection assays

Tx/Mgmt: Metronidazole, tinidazole, or nitazoxanide for symptomatic patients. Treatment is warranted for asymptomatic patients who are food handlers, in contact with pregnant women, immunocompromised patients, or children in day care.

Cystoisospora (isospora) belli

Buzz Words: Partially acid-fast, opportunistic protozoan + watery diarrhea

Clinical Presentation: In the immunocompetent, it presents with self-limited, watery diarrhea. In AIDS patients (CD4 cells <50/mm^3), severe debilitating chronic diarrhea and wasting occur. Severe diarrhea may progress to hypokalemia, hypomagnesemia, and bicarbonate wasting.

PPx: Adequately sanitizing food and water sources, prophylactic antibiotics (TMPX-SMX) in AIDS patients with CD4 cells less than 200/mm^3

MoD: Acquired by ingestion of sporulated oocysts (fecal-oral). It is a common pathogen in AIDS diarrhea along with *Cyclospora* and microsporidia.

Dx: Detection of oocysts in feces through acid-fast staining

Tx/Mgmt:
1. Aggressive fluid and electrolyte replacement
2. For the immunosuppressed, TMP-SMX is the preferred treatment and prophylactic

Strongyloides stercoralis

Buzz Words: Abdominal pain + worm infection after walking barefoot ± AIDS patient

Clinical Presentation: Immunosuppressed patient has waxing and waning GI (abdominal pain and diarrhea), cutaneous, and respiratory symptoms (cough and wheezing) that persist for years.

PPx: Strict handwashing and avoiding consumption of untreated water and undercooked food when traveling to endemic regions.

MoD: Intestinal nematode that has a peculiar mode of transmission: larvae penetrate feet → larvae migrate to the lungs and ascend the airway to be swallowed → molt into adult form, which penetrate intestinal mucosa and lay eggs → eggs hatch and rhabditiform larvae go back into the stool → develop into filarial form, which is infective. Autoinfection may occur, which significantly increases the burden of adult worms.

Dx: Eosinophilia, stool sampling for rhabditiform larvae, or serologic testing

Tx/Mgmt: Ivermectin

Immunologic and Inflammatory Disorders

Autoimmune Hepatitis

Buzz Words: Abnormal LFTs + antinuclear antibodies + anti–smooth muscle antibodies

Clinical Presentation: It has a broad range of presentations from abnormal LFTs to fulminant hepatitis and cirrhosis. Most commonly occurs in young women. May be associated with other autoimmune disorders such as Graves disease or Hashimoto thyroiditis.

MoD: Two types exist: type 1 is the most common in the United States. It is associated with HLA DR3 and DR4.

Dx:
1. Anti–smooth muscle antibodies in serum (>85% of cases) and antinuclear antibodies (>60% of cases)
2. Liver biopsy is the most accurate test
3. Decreased serum albumin and prolonged prothrombin time (PT) in severe disease

Tx/Mgmt:
1. Steroids and azathioprine
2. Liver transplantation if disease progresses to fulminant hepatitis

99 AR

Autoimmune hepatitis—definition and pathology

Celiac Disease

Buzz Words: Malabsorption in diabetic patient with skin lesions + flattened/atrophic intestinal villi

Clinical Presentation: Steatorrhea, weight loss, failure to thrive, microcytic (Fe^{2+} deficiency) anemia occur. Prevalence is 1% in the United States.

PPx: Gluten-free diet (avoid wheat, barley, and rye products)

MoD: Inappropriate T-cell and IgA-mediated response against gluten, more specifically gliadin, a breakdown product of gluten. Duodenum is the most commonly injured site. Significant clinical associations are dermatitis herpetiformis, type 1 diabetes mellitus (T1DM), IgA deficiency, small bowel lymphoma, Turner syndrome, Down syndrome, and other autoimmune diseases (Hashimoto and primary biliary cirrhosis [PBC]). Associated with HLA DQ2 (95% of cases) and HLA DQ8 (5% of cases).

Dx:
1. Anti–tissue transglutaminase and anti–endomysial antibodies have specificities greater than 95%
2. Antigliadin antibodies are usually also elevated
3. Mucosal biopsy will show villous atrophy, crypt hyperplasia, and intraepithelial lymphocytic infiltration

Tx/Mgmt: Prevention is key! Gluten-free diet and steroids in refractory cases.

99 AR

Celiac disease—symptoms and pathophysiology

Eosinophilic Esophagitis

Buzz Words: History of food impaction, persistent dysphagia or gastroesophageal reflux disease (GERD) refractory to medical therapy; "feline" esophagus

Clinical Presentation: Young man with history of atopy who presents with vomiting, abdominal pain, dysphagia, and food impactation. Esophageal perforation after dilation of a stricture is also a presentation that should trigger the thought of this disease.

PPx: Some patients might find success in preventing the disease by pursuing elimination diets (testing-directed, empiric, or elemental).

MoD: Chronic immune-mediated disease characterized by esophageal dysfunction with an eosinophil-predominant inflammatory process. Genetic defects of calpain-14 may predispose to disease.

Dx: EGD with mucosal biopsies (>15 Eos/HPF) after 2 months of proton-pump inhibitor (PPI) therapy. Common visual findings in EGD are stacked circular rings ("feline" esophagus), strictures, linear furrowing, and white papules (eosinophilic microabscesses).

Tx/Mgmt:
1. Topical steroids (i.e., fluticasone or budesonide) and elimination diet
2. Refractory cases may benefit from oral prednisone or esophageal dilation

Inflammatory Bowel Disease

Definition: *Inflammatory bowel disease* (IBD) is the collective term for Crohn disease (CD) and ulcerative colitis (UC). The etiology of both is poorly understood but their management is similar. See Table 8.3 for differences between CD and UC. In general, CD and UC share elements of presentation and treatment.

Clinical Presentation: Abdominal pain, diarrhea, blood and mucus in stool. Other relevant findings are joint involvement, uveitis, erythema nodosum, and pyoderma gangrenosum. Erythema nodosum is a panniculitis

TABLE 8.3 Differences Between Crohn Disease and Ulcerative Colitis

	Crohn Disease	Ulcerative Colitis
Epidemiology	Children > adults, Jews > non-Jews, smoking is a risk factor	Smoking is protective, lower incidence if appendectomy <age 20
Location	May occur anywhere along the gastrointestinal tract, most commonly affects ileum	Rectum with continuous extension into lower colon
Depth	Transmural	Mucosa and submucosa
Macroscopic findings	Thick wall, narrow lumen, aphthous ulcers, skip lesions, strictures, fistulas, "cobble-stone" pattern	Pseudopolyps, ulceration, hemorrhage
Microscopic findings	Noncaseating granulomas and lymphoid aggregates	Ulcers and crypt abscesses; dysplasia/cancer may be present; mononuclear infiltration isolated to mucosa
Clinical cues	Right lower quadrant colicky pain, diarrhea, and weight loss; ulcers in oral mucosa; perianal fistulas	Left-sided cramping, diarrhea with blood and mucus, fever, and tenesmus; non-gastrointestinal: primary sclerosing cholangitis, HLA B27–positive arthritis; p-ANCA antibodies present (>45% of cases)
Complications	Anal fistulas, calcium oxalate renal stones (increased absorption of oxalate through inflamed mucosa), malabsorption, megaloblastic (B_{12}) anemia	Mortality rate 50% Toxic megacolon and adenocarcinoma
Treatment	Tumor necrosis factor inhibitors for fistulas and surgery for bowel obstruction	Total colectomy with ileostomy can be curative

characterized by tender, erythematous nodules symmetrically involving the lower extremities. Pyoderma gangrenosum begins as a pustule that evolves into an ulcer with rolled, undermined borders.

Tx/Mgmt:

- Steroids are used for acute episodes.
- Other immunosuppressants (azathioprine/6-MP, 6-mercaptopurine) are used to wean off steroids.
- Sulfasalazine and mesalamine are used for maintenance and long-term therapy.
- A colonoscopy is required after 10 years with IBD. Any form of IBD is associated with an increased risk of developing colon cancer.

Crohn Disease

Buzz Words: Skip lesions on colonoscopy, noncaseating granulomas, *string*-sign in terminal ileum from narrowing

Clinical Presentation: Patient presents with postprandial diarrhea, weight loss, low-grade fever, abdominal pain, and palpable abdominal masses. Viscus perforation, perianal fistula, fissures, and abscesses are characteristic (help differentiate from ulcerative colitis).

PPx: Avoid smoking

MoD: Segmental, transmural inflammation that can occur anywhere along the GI tract. The terminal ileum is the most commonly affected segment. Fistulas develop from transmural granulomas; these can form between intestines, into the bladder, or through the skin. Immune-mediated free radical damage to the cells of the GI tract. May be triggered by pathogens such as *Mycobacterium paratuberculosis*, *Pseudomonas*, and *Listeria*. A frameshift mutation of the *NOD2/CAR15* gene predisposes to CD.

Dx:

1. Fecal occult blood test (FOBT)
2. Colonocopy
3. Biopsy

Tx/Mgmt: Anti–tumor necrosis factor (TNF) alpha drugs (adalimumab, infliximab, etanercept) are used when fistulas occur. Antibiotics like ciprofloxacin or metronidazole are used for perianal disease; these are preferred owing to their additional anti-inflammatory effect.

Ulcerative Colitis

Buzz Words: IBD symptomatology with tenesmus and rectal urgency, *lead-pipe* radiographical appearance, **sclerosing cholangitis**

99 AR

Crohn disease—symptoms and pathophysiology

QUICK TIPS

If the patient has sclerosing cholangitis in the question stem, she/he also has UC.

Clinical Presentation: Young woman presents with diarrhea, bright red blood per rectum, vague abdominal cramping, and tenesmus.

MoD: Continuous and circumferential mucosal inflammation that begins in the rectum and ascends the GI tract; usually confined to the colon.

Dx:
1. FOBT
2. Colonocopy
3. Biopsy

Tx/Mgmt: Initial management of mild presentation is with 5-ASA enema, steroid (hydrocortisone) foams, or suppositories. Acetylsalicylic acid (ASA) enemas have been shown to decrease relapses. Colectomy and ileostomy can be curative. Resistant cases should be managed with systemic steroids (oral prednisone).

Ulcerative colitis—definition, symptoms, and causes

Microscopic Colitis

Buzz Words: Patient with chronic diarrhea, negative stool cultures, and normal-appearing colonic mucosa

Clinical Presentation: Inflammatory disease characterized by chronic watery diarrhea. Other symptoms are fecal urgency, fecal incontinence, and abdominal pain. It most commonly occurs in middle-aged women.

PPx: Discontinue medications associated with microscopic colitis (nonsteroidal anti-inflammatory drugs [NSAIDs], such as aspirin, PPIs, ranitidine, sertraline, and clozapine, to name a few).

MoD: Multifactorial disease with poorly understood pathogenesis

Dx:
1. Mucosa appears normal on colonoscopy
2. Biopsy for definitive diagnosis

Tx/Mgmt:
1. Budesonide ± cholestyramine (depending on initial response)
2. Anti-TNF agents may be used for patients with disease refractory to treatment.

Toxic Megacolon

Buzz Words: Toxic-appearing patient with altered sensorium and abdominal distention

Clinical Presentation: Severe bloody diarrhea, abdominal distention, tenderness, fever, tachycardia, and shock occur.

PPx: Earlier management of etiologic condition

MoD: May occur as a complication of IBD (UC > CD), ischemia, volvulus, diverticulitis, infectious colitis, or obstructive colon cancer.

Dx: Megacolon can be identified by abdominal film showing dilation of the R colon greater than 6 cm in diameter, loss of haustral markings, and mucosal ulcerations. Toxic megacolon = colonic dilation + systemic involvement.

Tx/Mgmt:

1. Fluid replacement, management of electrolytes abnormalities, initiation of broad-spectrum antibiotics (vancomycin if *C. difficile* is the culprit), IV steroids, bowel rest and decompression (nasogastric/orogastric [NG/OG] tube)
2. Failure of medical therapy requires a subtotal colectomy with end-ileostomy.

Neoplasms

Benign Neoplasms

Polyps

Gastric Polyps

Buzz Words: Mucosal outgrowth

Clinical Presentation: Asymptomatic presentation, found incidentally in the majority of cases. Important association with *H. pylori* chronic infection. Hyperplastic polyps are the most common, have a hamartomatous architecture, and have no malignant potential. Adenomatous polyps are neoplastic and have potential for malignant transformation.

MoD: Mucosal protuberance, complication of chronic gastritis and achlorhydria

Dx: EGD/biopsy

Tx/Mgmt:

1. All gastric polyps should be biopsied and complete resection should be attempted during endoscopy.
2. *H. pylori* eradication therapy should be commenced (e.g., triple therapy with PPI).

Polyps of the Small and Large Bowel

Buzz Words: Mucosal outgrowth

Clinical Presentation: Usually asymptomatic, but may twist around their own stalks and bleed, cause tenesmus if they are located in the rectum, or produce intestinal obstruction of they are large.

MoD: Mucosal protuberance occurs from the normally flat mucosa. Nonneoplastic polyps are usually classified as hyperplastic, mucosal, inflammatory, hamartomatous, or submucosal.

Dx: Colonoscopy with biopsy of all the accompanying lesions

Tx/Mgmt:
1. Endoscopic resection
2. Surveillance should be repeated every 5–10 years in patients with nonneoplastic poylps.

Oral Leukoplakia

Buzz Words: White plaques in oral cavity that do not scrape off with tongue depressor

Clinical Presentation: White lesions that arise in trauma-prone regions of the oral cavity. Risk of progression to squamous cell carcinoma is 20% within 10 years.

PPx: Avoid consumption of tobacco products

MoD: Precancerous lesion of the oral mucosa; strong association with human papillomavirus (HPV)

Dx: Clinical diagnosis: Lesions should be biopsied to document the degree of dysplasia.

Tx/Mgmt: Topical retinoid compounds might aid in regression of the lesion.

Oral Cancer

Squamous Cell Carcinoma

Buzz Words: Nonhealing ulcer or nodule in oral cavity

Clinical Presentation: Squamous cell carcinoma (SCC) manifests as papules, plaques, or nodules, which may be associated with hyperkeratosis, ulceration, or hyperpigmentation. Lesion sites in descending order of frequency are the lower lip, floor of the mouth, and lateral border of the tongue. Metastasizes to superjugular node.

PPx: Known risk factors are light-colored skin, HPV (most common, vaccination is protective), use of tobacco products, alcohol abuse (synergistic with tobacco), irritation from dentures, and lichen planus.

MoD: Erythroplakia and oral leukoplakia are precursor lesions. Usually develops in sites of chronic inflammation or scarring.

Dx: Biopsy

Tx/Mgmt:
- For early lesions: surgical resection ± radiation

- An ipsilateral neck dissection is recommended for lesions greater than 3 mm or advanced stage (III and IV).
- For advanced lesions: surgical resection + modified radical neck dissection + postoperative radiation ± chemotherapy.

Salivary Gland Neoplasm

Buzz Words: Mucoepidermoid carcinoma + Bell palsy
Clinical Presentation: Painless mass or swelling that arises from a salivary gland. May manifest signs of peripheral facial nerve involvement (Bell palsy). Tumors of the submandibular and sublingual are more likely than parotid to be malignant.
PPx: Avoid exposure to radiation
MoD: Mucoepidermoid carcinoma is the most common malignant tumor of the salivary glands. It is composed of mucinous and squamous cells. Usually arises from parotid and involves CN VII (facial nerve).
Dx:
1. Fine-needle aspiration (FNA) or ultrasound-guided core needle biopsy
2. As with any other tumor, imaging studies (i.e., CT, MRI, PET/CT) aid in staging and assessment of surgical candidacy
Tx/Mgmt:
1. Surgical resection for region-confined lesions
2. Patients with nodal metastases should undergo modified radical neck dissection followed by adjuvant radiation therapy (RT) in most cases
3. Patients who are not considered adequate surgical candidates should receive definitive RT

Barrett Esophagus

Buzz Words: Gland with different types of epithelium, goblet cells in esophageal epithelium

Barrett esophagus overview

Clinical Presentation: It is similar to GERD; no difference in symptoms. Found when performing EGD and mucosal biopsies. Complications include stricture formation and glandular dysplasia with increased risk for adenocarcinoma.
PPx: Adequate treatment GERD and dietary modifications (less coffee, wine, mints, etc.)
MoD: Premalignant lesion of the distal esophagus caused by long-standing GERD (years). Constant exposure to

gastric acid induces metaplasia. Nonkeratinized, stratified, squamous epithelium (normal) to columnar, secretory epithelium (intestinal).

Dx: EGD with mucosal biopsy in the setting of long-standing GERD

Tx/Mgmt: PPI and repeat scoping every 2–3 years for early detection of adenocarcinoma.

Esophageal Cancer

Squamous Cell Carcinoma

Buzz Words: Nodular mass with central area of ulceration

Clinical Presentation: Dysphagia to solids, weight loss, anemia, and nontender supraclavicular nodes occur. May also manifest hemoptysis (tracheal invasion), hoarseness (recurrent laryngeal nerve [RLN] compression), odynophagia, hypercalcemia (PTHrP secretion similar to small cell carcinoma in the lung). Lesions in the proximal two-thirds of esophagus (but may also occur in distal third).

PPx: Avoid known risk factors; smoking, alcohol, achalasia, caustic injuries, HPV infection, and nitrosamine exposure

MoD: Poor prognosis, overall 5-year survival rate is 13%

Dx:

1. EGD with biopsy
2. CT scan and endoscopic ultrasonography are useful for initial staging of tumor
3. Integrated PET/CT scans are warranted for patient with metastasis

Tx/Mgmt:

- Surgery alone is recommended for superficial esophageal adenocarcinoma or SCC. 5-year survival rate for stage I is only 50%–70%.
- Trimodality approach (chemoradiotherapy followed by surgery) has proven to be superior to surgery alone for patient with stage I tumors that invade the adventitia.

Adenocarcinoma

Buzz Words: Raised lesion at the junction of the distal esophagus and proximal stomach

Clinical Presentation: White middle-aged male presents with dysphagia, weight loss, and anemia. Lesions occur in the distal third of the esophagus.

PPx: Adequate management of GERD

MoD: Barrett esophagus is a significant risk factor; other risk factors are smoking and high body mass index

(BMI). Involvement of celiac and perihepatic nodes is more common than in SCC. *H. pylori* does not increase the risk of developing adenocarcinoma.

Dx: Tumors greater than 5 cm away from EGD are considered gastric adenocarcinoma.

Tx/Mgmt:

- Surgery alone is recommended for superficial esophageal adenocarcinoma or SCC. Five-year survival rate for stage I is only 50%–70%.
- Trimodality approach (chemoradiotherapy followed by surgery) has proven to be superior to surgery alone for patient with stage I tumors that invade the adventitia.

Gastrinoma and Zollinger–Ellison Syndrome

Buzz Words: Multiple peptic ulcers or ulcer in unusual locations + recurrent epigastric pain refractory to PPI

Clinical Presentation: Patient has recurrent epigastric pain and diarrhea refractory to treatment with PPI.

MoD: Tumor arises from enteroendocrine gastrin-producing cells in the pancreas and/or small intestine. Hypergastrinemia results in excessive amount of gastric acid production, which accounts for ulcers and diarrhea.

Dx:

1. Serum gastrin level after the patient has been off PPIs for at least a week
2. Secretin stimulation test to differentiate gastrinoma and other causes of hypergastrinemia
3. Somatostatin receptor scintigraphy localizes and helps stage the tumor
4. CT, MRI, or somatostatin receptor scintigraphy to locate tumor:
   - Most common endoscopic finding is a solitary ulcer in the first portion of the duodenum, although multiple ulcers in unusual locations (i.e., third or fourth portions of the duodenum) are also common.

Tx/Mgmt: PPIs, ocreotide, and surgical excision; screen for MEN1 syndrome

Carcinoid Tumors

Buzz Words: Flushing + diarrhea + wheezing + R-sided valvular disease → carcinoid tumor

Clinical Presentation: Carcinoid syndrome is the most common manifestation; described as flushing, cramps,

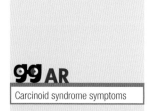

diarrhea (from hypermotility), intermittent wheezing, dyspnea, telangiectasia, and R-sided valvular disease (i.e., tricuspid regurgitation or pulmonary stenosis). Foregut and hindgut carcinoid tumors invade but rarely metastasize, while midgut carcinoid tumors invade and metastasize. The most common sites are the vermiform appendix (40% of cases) and terminal ileum.

MoD: Small bowel is the most common site of carcinoid tumors; however, these do not cause carcinoid syndrome because serotonin is metabolized by first-pass metabolism in the liver. Metastasis to the liver or lungs result in carcinoid syndrome.

Dx:

1. Urine levels of 5-hydroxyindoleacetic acid (5-HIAA)
2. Abdominal CT scan to find metastasis
3. Neurosecretory granules visible on electron microscopy
4. Bright yellow tumor intraoperatively

Tx/Mgmt:

1. Octreotide to manage diarrhea and flushing
2. Surgical resection of primary tumor ± chemotherapy for metastatic disease

Gastrointestinal Stromal Tumors

Buzz Words: Patient >40 y/o + skin hyperpigmentation + dysphagia

Clinical Presentation: Varies with site of lesion, depth of penetration, and stage of tumor progression. Most common age group is greater than 40 y/o and the most common site is the stomach. Some of these might involve dysphagia, skin hyperpigmentation, or be accompanied by paragangliomas.

MoD: Mutation of *c-kit* proto-oncogene, which activates KIT, a receptor tyrosine kinase. Gastrointestinal stromal tumors (GISTs) show a broad array of behaviors from benign to malignant, aggressive tumors. Mesenchymal spindle-cell neoplasms, CD117-positive.

Dx:

1. Contrast-enhanced CT for screening and staging
2. Biopsy (endoscopic US-guided FNA) is recommended only when metastatic disease is suspected or if preoperative imatinib is considered.
3. Fluorodeoxyglucose positron emission tomography (FDG-PET) is the best method to assess for metastatic disease.

Tx/Mgmt:
- Surgical resection of any tumor ≥2 cm in size through visceral resection; regional lymphadenectomy is not warranted.
- Imatinib (TK inhibitor) may be used as initial therapy for locally advanced or borderline resectable tumors.

Stomach

Adenocarcinoma

Buzz Words: *Signet ring* cells, Sister Mary Joseph nodule

Clinical Presentation: Epigastric pain, weight loss, vomit ± melena occur. Increased incidence is found in Japanese and blood group A individuals. Most commonly located in lesser curvature (~50% of tumors), followed by cardia, body, and fundus. Paraneoplastic skin findings: seborrheic keratosis (Leser-Trélat sign) and acanthosis nigricans.

PPx: Modifiable risk factors are dietary (high-sodium and low vegetable, smoked foods, nitrosamines) and substance abuse (i.e., alcohol and smoking). Adequate management of *H. pylori* infection is protective.

MoD: Gastric ulcer, adenomatous polyps, type A chronic atrophic gastritis, and intestinal metaplasia are associated with a higher risk of gastric cancer.

Dx: Endoscopic ultrasound-guided FNA to biopsy lesion, CT scan for staging. Serum tumor markers (i.e., CEA and CA-125) add little to the management. Most common sites of metastasis are liver, lung, and ovaries. Hematogenous spread of signet ring cells to ovaries produces Krukenberg tumors.

Tx/Mgmt: Surgery, radiation, and chemotherapy: Open total gastrectomy is preferred for tumors involving the proximal third of the stomach, while a distal gastrectomy can be performed for tumors in the distal two-thirds of the stomach.

Gastric Lymphoma

Buzz Words: Sheets of neoplastic small lymphoid cells in gastric wall, lymphoepithelial lesions

Clinical Presentation: Epigastric pain, anorexia, weight loss, nausea, vomiting, occult GI bleed, and early satiety occur. The majority are non-Hodgkin lymphomas with the stomach as the most common site (70% of cases), followed by small bowel, colon, rectum, and esophagus.

MoD: Gastric lymphomas are divided into extranodal marginal-zone B-cell lymphoma of mucosa-associated lymphoid tissue (i.e., MALToma) and diffuse large B-cell lymphoma (DLBL).

Dx: EGD findings are diverse and may range between mucosal erythema, ulceration, nodule, and a cerebroid mass. Characteristic translocation t(11;18) and fusion protein IAP2(API2)/MALT1. Neoplastic cells will be positive for B-cell markers (i.e., CD19, CD20, CD22).

Tx/Mgmt: For patients with *H. pylori*–positive MALToma, eradication therapy (Table 8.4) could induce regression in 50% of cases. *H. pylori*–negative MALToma requires local radiotherapy. DLBL requires chemotherapy + immunotherapy (i.e., rituximab) ± RT.

Colon, Rectum, Anus

See *Table 8.5*

Hereditary Colon Cancer Syndromes
Familial Adenomatous Polyposis

Buzz Words: Hundreds of colorectal polyps

TABLE 8.4 Simplified *Helicobacter pylori* Eradication Regimens

Consideration	Duration: 10–14 days
First-line	PPI + clarithromycin 500 mg bid + amoxicillin 1000 mg bid
Penicillin allergy	PPI + clarithromycin 500 mg bid + metronidazole 500 mg bid
Failed any of the regimens above	PPI + bismuth subsalicylate 525 mg qid + metronidazole 250 mg qid + tetracycline 500 mg qid

PPI, Proton-pump inhibitor.

TABLE 8.5 Colonoscopy Screening Recommendations

Group	Recommendation
No risk factors	Age >50 years — screen q10 years
First-degree relative w/ colon cancer	Age >40 years or 10 years earlier than family member — screen q10 years
Hereditary nonpolyposis colon cancer	Age >25 years — screen q1–2 years
Familial adenomatous polyposis	Age >10 years — screen every year

Clinical Presentation: Colorectal cancer from malignant transformation of polyps, usually develops by 45 years of age. Polyps begin to develop in second decade with malignant transformation in the fourth decade. Also incidence of duodenal adenomas, duodenal cancer, papillary thyroid cancer, medulloblastomas, desmoid tumors, and congenital hypertrophy of retinal pigment epithelium increases.

PPx: Preimplantation genetic diagnosis during preconception counseling for individuals with familial adenomatous polyposis (FAP)

MoD: Inactivation of the adenomatous polyposis coli (APC) tumor suppressor gene on chromosome 5q, autosomal dominant inheritance

Dx: Genetic testing and counseling for patient and family members

Tx/Mgmt: Aggressive screening for colon, duodenal, and other extraintestinal cancer is warranted. Eventually all patients will require a total colectomy; indications to perform the procedure include:
- Adenoma with high-grade dysplasia
- Concerning symptoms (i.e., GI bleed, weight loss, etc.)
- Marked increase in polyp number from one exam to the next

Hereditary Nonpolyposis Colon Cancer (Lynch Syndrome)

Buzz Words: Colorectal cancer and/or female reproductive tract cancer + family history + mutated mismatch repair genes

Clinical Presentation: Lynch syndrome is the most commonly inherited genetic syndrome that predisposes one to early colorectal cancer. It is a syndrome characterized by mutations to the mismatch repair family (e.g., *MLH1, MSH2, MSH6*, and *PMS2*) that is autosomal-dominant. There are two types to be aware of: Lynch syndrome I specific for only CRC and Lynch syndrome II, which has all features of Lynch syndrome I with increased occurrence of other cancers of female reproductive tract, GI tract, breast, brain, and skin.

PPx:
1. Aspirin has a protective effect against the incidence of cancer in these patients
2. Early screening for CRC

MoD: Germline mutation inactivates DNA mismatch repair genes *(MLH1, MSH2, MSH6, PMS2)*, which causes a microsatellite repeat replication error (i.e., microsatellite instability). This leads to frameshift mutations affecting tumor suppressor genes.

Dx: Loss of staining of mismatch repair proteins on immunohistochemistry

Tx/Mgmt:
1. Early screening for colorectal cancer
2. Surgery to remove precancerous lesions
3. After colorectal cancer dx: total colectomy with ileorectal anastomosis + yearly endoscopic surveillance

Peutz–Jeghers Syndrome

Peutz-Jeghers syndrome overview

Buzz Words: Perioral pigmentation + intestinal polyps

Clinical Presentation: Hamartomatous polyps predominate in the small intestine. Pigmentation macules occur on buccal mucosa and lips (95% of cases). Risk for colorectal, pancreas, breast, and gynecologic (ovarian sex cord tumors) cancer increases. Mean age at the time of cancer diagnosis is 42 years.

PPx: Preimplantation genetic diagnosis during preconception counseling for individuals with Peutz–Jeghers syndrome (PJS): See Tx/Mgmt for screening guidelines

MoD: Inactivation of the serine/threonine kinase 11 (STK11) tumor suppressor gene in chromosome 19p, autosomal dominant inheritance

Dx: Genetic testing for STK11 mutations

Tx/Mgmt:

Aggressive cancer screening:
- GI tract: EGD, video capsule endoscopy, and colonoscopy at 8 years of age; to repeat every 3 years if polyps are found.
- Gonads: Annual testicle exam (from birth for men) or pelvic exam + Pap smear (from 21 years of age for women).
- Breast: Monthly breast exams and annual mammograms starting at 18 and 25 years of age respectively.
- Pancreas: Endoscopic retrograde cholangiopancreatography (ERCP)/magnetic resonance cholangiopancreatography (MRCP) every 1–2 years starting at 30 years of age.

Gardner Syndrome

Buzz Words: Supernumerary teeth, bone osteomas, increased retinal pigmentation

Clinical Presentation: It has a constellation of colonic polyposis + extracolonic lesions. Benign osteomas, desmoid tumors, dental abnormalities, cutaneous lesions, adrenal adenomas, and nasal angiofibromas occur. Patients are at risk for neoplasms of pancreas, liver, thyroid, gallbladder, and biliary tract.

PPx: Preimplantation genetic diagnosis during preconception counseling for individuals with Gardner syndrome

MoD: Also associated with loss-of-function mutations to the APC gene, autosomal dominant inheritance

Dx: Genetic testing

Tx/Mgmt:
1. Aggressive cancer screening
2. Total colectomy upon any of the indications for FAP

Turcot Syndrome

Historic term used to describe association between inherited colonic polyposis and brain cancer.

MUTYH-Associated Polyposis

Buzz Words: 10–100 colonic polyps and ruled out APC mutation

Clinical Presentation: Colonic polyposis in individual with greater than 10 adenomatous polyps which might be accompanied by dental cysts, desmoids, osteomas, or sebaceous hyperplasia. Lifetime risk of colorectal carcinoma is 75%. Also increased risk for duodenal, ovarian, bladder, thyroid, and skin cancer.

MoD: The MUYTH gene codes for a glycosylase involved in DNA (base excision) repair. Autosomal recessive inheritance.

Dx: Genetic testing for biallelic germline mutations of MUTYH gene

Tx/Mgmt: Colonoscopy every 1–2 years starting at 25 years of age. Same indications for colectomy + ileorectal anastomosis as in FAP (see earlier).

Biliary Tract

Gallbladder Adenocarcinoma

Buzz Words: Porcelain gallbladder

Clinical Presentation: Patients are usually asymptomatic. Usually affects elderly Japanese women. Very uncommon but highly fatal malignancy.

MoD: Chronic cholecystitis, porcelain gallbladder, and development of gallstones at any point in life increases the risk significantly. Some hereditary neoplastic syndromes like Gardner and neurofibromatosis have also been associated.

Dx: CT, endoscopic ultrasound, and MRCP are the preferred imaging studies.

Tx/Mgmt: Cholecystectomy ± RT

Cholangiocarcinoma

Buzz Words: History of primary sclerosing cholangitis (PSC) + elevated CEA, AFP, or CA-19-9 + palpable gallbladder + elevated bili

Clinical Presentation: Extrahepatic cholestasis, Courvoisier sign (palpable gallbladder), and hepatomegaly occur. The tumor may be present anywhere along the extrahepatic biliary tract. Most common malignancy of the biliary tree.

MoD: PSC, *Clonorchis sinensis*, exposure to thorium dioxide, choledochal cysts, and Caroli disease are the most common causes of cholangiocarcinoma.

Dx:
1. Liver panel
2. MRI, MRCP, or multidetector-row CT
3. Tumor markers: CEA, AFP, or CA 19-9 may be elevated (Table 8.6).

Tx/Mgmt:
- Surgical resection should be attempted (only cure).
- Advanced disease, resections with positive margins, or positive regional lymph nodes should be treated with postoperative RT and chemotherapy.

Adenocarcinoma of the Ampulla of Vater

Buzz Words: FAP + acute pancreatitis + jaundice + palpable gallbladder

TABLE 8.6 Tumor Cancer Markers Versus Type of Cancer

Tumor Cancer Markers	Type of Cancer
CEA	Colon cancer
AFP	HCC
Ferritin	HCC
CA 19-9	Pancreatic cancer
CA-50	Pancreatic cancer
Beta-hCG	Testicular cancer + choriocarcinoma (fast-growing cancer of uterus)
CA-125	Ovarian cancer
Neuron-specific enolase	Small cell lung cancer
CA 15-3	Breast cancer

AFP, Alpha-fetoprotein; *CA,* cancer antigen; *CEA,* carcinoembryonic antigen; *HCC,* hepatocellular carcinoma; *hCG,* human chorionic gonadotropin.

Clinical Presentation: Presentation is similar to cholangio-carcinoma with obstruction of the biliary tree + possible complications from obstruction of the pancreatic ducts (i.e., acute pancreatitis). Males > females: Almost half of patients have developed lymph node metastasis at the time of diagnosis.

MoD: *K-ras* mutations may play a role in pathogenesis, associated with FAP.

Dx:

1. Liver panel
2. MRI, MRCP, or multidetector-row CT

Tx/Mgmt: Whipple procedure (pancreaticoduodenectomy)

Liver

Cavernous Hemangioma

Buzz Words: Contrast enhancement + mass in liver + asymptomatic → cavernous hemangioma

Clinical Presentation: Benign neoplasms of small blood vessel endothelial cells occur. It is the most common benign lesion of the liver. Focal, well-circumscribed, encapsulated, hypervascular lesion in liver parenchyma w/ spongy consistency. Can rarely rupture and produce intraperitoneal hemorrhage. It has no malignant potential.

PPx: **Avoid biopsy** to ppx against hemorrhage

MoD: Etiology incompletely understood, formed through ectasia of vasculature

Dx:

1. CT scan w/contrast
2. MRI or tagged RBC scan
3. Angiography

Tx/Mgmt: Observation: Surgical resection is done if painful or symptoms suggesting mass effect.

Focal Nodular Hyperplasia

Buzz Words: Central scar on CT + asymptomatic + discovered incidentally

Clinical Presentation: Focal nodular hyperplasia (FNH) is a common nonmalignant hyperplastic response to anomalous arteries. Females > males: Associated with hereditary hemorrhagic telangiectasia (Osler-Weber-Rendu disease). NOT associated with use of oral contraceptive pill (OCP). There is no malignant potential. It is the second most common benign liver tumor.

MoD: Nonmalignant localized aggregates of rapidly reproducing liver cells

Dx:
1. CT (central scar, hypervascular mass with arteriovenous [AV] connections)
2. Angiography
3. Biopsy shows Kupffer cells and sinuosoids (vs. hepatic adenoma, which shows glycogen and lipid)

Tx/Mgmt: Treatment is unnecessary unless the lesion is producing pain.

Hepatic Adenoma

Buzz Words: Young woman + OCP use + normal AFP + glycogen/lipids on biopsy

Clinical Presentation: Females > males: Most common cause is use of OCPs, followed by anabolic steroids and Von Gierke disease.

PPx: Avoid OCPs

MoD: Benign epithelial tumor, is frequently located in the R hepatic lobe. Highly vascular with a tendency to rupture during pregnancy (growth secondary to hyperestrogenemia), producing intraperitoneal hemorrhage.

Dx: CT

Tx/Mgmt:
- Emergent surgery if ruptured/bleeding
- Resection if >4 cm or patient desires pregnancy
- If <4 cm, d/c OCPs and monitor with serial CTs

Hepatocellular Carcinoma

Buzz Words: Cirrhosis + RUQ discomfort + weight loss + elevated AFP + HBV, HCV, afltoxin, CCl4 exposure

Clinical Presentation: Patient presents with previously compensated cirrhosis with decompensation (jaundice, encephalopathy, ascites). Might also manifest weight loss, early satiety, expending hepatomegaly, and abdominal pain. It is the most common primary liver cancer. Ectopic hormones such as erythropoietin (EPO), PTH-related protein, and insulin-like growth factor are produced. Lungs are the most common metastatic site. Males > females. Causes in order of frequency: HCV, alcoholic cirrhosis, HBV. Other minor causes of HCC: hemochromatosis, Wilson disease, aflatoxin-B1 (from *Aspergillus*), primary biliary cirrhosis, and alpha-1 antitrypsin deficiency. Second most common cause of death related to cancer worldwide (after lung).

PPx: US surveillance (every 6 months) in patients with high-risk profiles

99 AR
Benign liver tumors video—pathophysiology and symptoms

MoD: Associated with preexisting cirrhosis and states of constant damage–repair. Portal and hepatic vein invasion is common.

Dx:
1. Liver panel (elevated AFP, ALP and gamma-glutamyl transferase [GGT])
2. CT and ultrasound would show lesion with hypervascularity and venous invasion
3. CEA level to r/o mets from colon
4. Laparoscopic ultrasound is the gold standard.

Tx/Mgmt:
1. Single mass → resection
2. Multiple masses → radiation + cryoablation

Malignant liver tumors video—pathophysiology and symptoms

Peritoneal Cancer

Clinical Presentation: Abdominal pain, ascites, weight loss, and palpable abdominal mass or masses occur.

MoD: Malignant mesothelioma is the most common primary peritoneal cancer. Nonetheless, metastasis and seeding from other tumors (i.e., ovarian) are also common.

Dx: Peritoneal lavage through percutaneous technique or at time of surgical exploration. Ultrasound is the imaging study with the highest sensitivity due the peritoneum's close proximity to the abdominal wall.

Tx/Mgmt: Multimodal therapy, which consists of surgical resection to decrease the tumor load (± hysterectomy and b/l salpingo-oophorectomy), intraperitoneal administration of chemotherapy, and hyperthermia.

Pancreas

Neoplasms of the pancreas can be divided into two types. First, there are neoplasms of the exocrine pancreas, which do not produce hormones but lead to symptoms secondary to mass effect. Second, there are neoplasms of the endocrine pancreas (e.g., VIPoma, gastrinoma), which do lead to disorders of hormonal production. Buzz Words for the latter are high-yield for the shelf.

Exocrine Pancreas, Pancreatic Carcinoma (Table 8.7)

Buzz Words:
- Adenocarcinoma of the head of the pancreas: Obstructive jaundice + recently diagnosed diabetes + weight loss + abdominal pain + gastric outlet obstruction

TABLE 8.7 Endocrine Pancreatic Tumors

Tumor	Summary
Insulinoma (beta cells)	Most common islet cell tumor. Association with MEN I syndrome (80% of tumors). Fasting hypoglycemia. High levels of insulin and C-peptide. Treatment: surgical excision of mass. Streptozotocin may also be used (highly toxic to beta and delta cells).
Glucagonoma (alpha cells)	Hyperglycemia and rash (necrolytic migratory erythema) are the most common manifestations. Treatment: surgical excision. Ocreotide may also be used.
Somatostatinoma (delta cells)	Somatostatin inhibits the effects of gastrin, CCK, GIP, and secretin. Manifestation: achlorhydria, cholelithiasis, steatorrhea, and DM. Treatment: surgical excision of mass. Streptozotocin may also be used (highly toxic to beta and delta cells).
VIPoma	Excessive secretion of vasoactive intestinal peptide that produces secretory diarrhea (pancreatic cholera) and achlorhydria. Dx: metabolic acidosis due to loss of HCO_3 in stool and hypokalemia. Treatment: surgical excision. Ocreotide may also be used.
Zollinger-Ellison (gastrinoma)	Peptic ulcer refractory to PPI and triple therapy + high gastrin even after secretin administration and calcium infusion. Dx: (1) CT, (2) somatostatin radionuclide scan. Tx/Mgmt: (1) surgical removal, (2) omeprazole for mets.

CCK, cholecystokinin; *CT,* computed tomography; *DM,* diabetes mellitus; *GIP,* gastric inhibitory peptide; *PPI,* proton-pump inhibitor.

- **Malignant extrahepatic biliary obstruction:** Painless jaundice + palpable nontender gallbladder
- **Cystic adenocarcinoma (aka cystadenoma):** Mass in pancreas + subtle symptoms + elevated carcinoembryonic antigen (CEA) + no weight loss or diabetes:
  - Cystic cancer of the pancreas can be **resected,** leading to a much better survival rate!
  - Cystadenoma of the pancreas → distal pancreatectomy (or just resect!)
- **Trousseau sign (migratory thrombophlebitis):** Venous thrombosis in different places + hypercoagulability + pancreatic mass

- **Adenocarcinoma of the head of the pancreas:** Courvoisier sign + large, nontender gallbladder + itching + jaundice + migratory thrombophlebitis

Clinical Presentation: Patient (male > female) in the seventh–eighth decade of life with epigastric pain that radiates to the back and weight loss ± signs of biliary obstruction. Associated with superficial migratory thrombophlebitis. Metastasis occurs to Virchow node (left supraclavicular node) and periumbilical region (Sister Mary Joseph sign). Risk factors include smoking, chronic pancreatitis, hereditary pancreatitis, DM, diet high in saturated fat, obesity, and cirrhosis.

MoD: Adenocarcinoma has a high association with *K-ras* gene mutation and mutation of tumor suppressor genes p16 and p53. Most cases (65%) occur at the head of the pancreas.

Dx:

1. CT scan
2. FNA biopsy
3. CA19-9 tumor marker

Tx/Mgmt: Surgery (Whipple procedure aka pancreaticoduodenectomy), chemotherapy (gemcitabine) and RT

99 AR

Whipple procedure = resection of pancreas, duodenum, common bile duct and distal stomach

Signs, Symptoms and Ill-Defined Disorders

Upper Gastrointestinal Bleeding

Buzz Words: Bloody vomit, melena

Clinical Presentation: Melena, nausea, vomiting bright red blood, abdominal pain, and abdominal distention occurs. Upper GI bleeding is a potential source for massive blood loss and hemorrhagic shock.

MoD: Melena is dark, foul-smelling feces, which occur from protein denaturation after having hemoglobin exposed to gastric acid and pepsin. Source of hemorrhage is proximal to the ligament of Treitz. Major causes of upper GI bleed are esophageal varices, esophageal tear, peptic ulcer disease, AV malformations, and tumors.

Dx: Best initial test is EGD. The presence of rebound tenderness in a patient with upper gastrointestinal bleeding (GIB) should bring into consideration the possibility of bowel perforation.

Tx/Mgmt: NPO, provide supportive measures, replace lost intravascular volume, place nasogastric tube to decompress bowel, manage coagulopathies, and d/c any

QUICK TIPS
Any hemorrhage proximal to the ligament of Treitz is considered an upper GI bleed, while a distal hemorrhage is considered a lower GI bleed.

anticoagulants or antiplatelets. Provide blood transfusions to maintain adequate oxygen-carrying capacity (ideally hemoglobin >7.0 g/dL).

Lower Gastrointestinal Bleeding

Buzz Words: Hematochezia

Clinical Presentation: Blood per rectum: The color of the blood differs from depending on the source of hemorrhage. Blood from the left colon appears bright red once it comes out of the rectum. Blood from the right colon is partially digested by gut flora and has a brown color.

MoD: Source of hemorrhage is distal to the ligament of Treitz. Patients rarely develop hemorrhagic shock from a lower GI bleed.

Dx: Colonoscopy

Tx/Mgmt: Provide supportive measures, replace lost intravascular volume, manage coagulopathies, and discontinue any anticoagulants or antiplatelets.

Constipation

Clinical Presentation: Lack of defecation or flatus usually accompanied by abdominal distention and pain.

PPx: Drugs that most commonly cause constipation are calcium channel blockers (CCBs), opiates, tricyclic antidepressants, and calcium carbonate.

MoD: Decreased intestinal motility

Dx: Rule out hypothyroidism (i.e., serum thyroid stimulating hormone [TSH])

Tx/Mgmt: Patient education on most common causes for constipation, behavior modification, dietary modification, laxatives, and/or enema

Diarrhea

Clinical Presentation: Patient has high fecal output (i.e., >250 g of stool/day).

MoD: The three types of diarrhea are synthesized in Table 8.8.

Dx: Severe infectious diarrhea is a combination of blood in stool, volume depletion, abdominal pain/tenderness, and fever.

Tx/Mgmt: Initial treatment is based on severity, not etiology. Most antimotility agents can be used if there is no blood and no fever. Antibiotics are indicated in *severe* infectious diarrhea.

TABLE 8.8 Types of Diarrhea

	Osmotic	Secretory	Invasive
Characteristics	Osmotically active substance in the lumen High volume No inflammatory process	GI epithelial cells secrete ions to draw water along with them High volume	Invasion and damage of enterocytes Low volume Blood and leukocytes
Differential	>100 mOsm/kg	<50 mOsm/kg	Stool antigens, culture, and ova and parasites
Common causes	Giardiasis, osmotic laxatives, disacchari-dase deficiency	Enterotoxins, increased serotonin levels (carcinoid syndrome)	*Campylobacter, Shigella, Entamoeba histolytica*

Nausea and Vomiting

Buzz Words: Contraction alkalosis

Clinical Presentation: Nausea, vomiting, and rumination occur.

MoD: The physiologic causes of nausea can be synthesized into three different pathways:

- Gastrointestinal tract—$5HT_3$ receptors stimulated by mechanical and chemical irritants
- Chemoreceptor trigger zone (area postrema)—D_2 receptors stimulated by emetogenic substances in the cerebrospinal fluid (CSF)
- Vestibular system—H_1 and M_1 receptors stimulated by motion

Vomiting produces loss of volume and protons (for every H^+ there is a molecule of bicarbonate [HCO_3^-] generated in blood), which produces a metabolic alkalosis, commonly referred to as *contraction alkalosis*, which is responsive to infusion of saline.

Dx: Symptom referred by the patient

Tx/Mgmt: 5HT3 receptor antagonists ("setrons") are administered to aid in nausea produced from the GI tract, D_2 receptor antagonists (metoclopramide and domperidone) aid in nausea produced from the area postrema, antihistamines and antimuscarinics aid in nausea induced by motion sickness.

Disorders of the Salivary Glands and Esophagus

Disorders of the Salivary Glands

Stones

Buzz Words: Pain and swelling of the salivary glands

Clinical Presentation: Pain and swelling of the salivary glands caused by dehydration.

PPx: Avoidance of dehydration

MoD: Submandibular glands are the most commonly obstructed (80%–90%) by single stones within Wharton duct. Anticholinergic medications are associated with the development of stones.

Dx: Clinical diagnosis (e.g., palpation), high-resolution CT if too small

Tx/Mgmt:
1. Supportive (hydration, lozenges to stimulate saliva production); stones less than 2 mm will probably pass on their own.
2. NSAIDs

Sialadenitis

Buzz Words: Erythema and purulent drainage of salivary glands

Clinical Presentation: Elderly patient presents with pain, swelling, and tenderness of the oral cavity. May complain of mouth dryness. On exam erythema and purulent drainage may be identified.

PPx: Same as with stones; avoid dehydration

MoD: Infection of a salivary gland is usually preceded by the formation of a stone causing obstruction and stasis of secretions. Submandibular gland is most often involved. Chronic sialadenitis may cause gland atrophy and a significant decrease in volume of saliva produced.

Dx: Clinical diagnosis, can use CT

Tx/Mgmt: Dicloxacillin or cephalexin

Suppurative Parotitis

Buzz Words: Discharge of purulent material during examination of the buccal mucosa

Clinical Presentation: Elderly patient presents with pain and swelling at the angle of the mandible and periauricular region accompanied by fever and chills. During palpation of the parotid gland purulent discharge may be expressed from Stensen duct.

MoD: These infections are most commonly polymicrobial, and the pathogens most commonly isolated are S. aureus, S. viridans, and anaerobes.

Dx: Clinical diagnosis: Culture of secretions will most probably be contaminated by oral flora.

Tx/Mgmt: Fluid replacement and IV antibiotics (i.e., nafcillin, metronidazole, or vancomycin when methicillin-resistant S. aureus [MRSA] is suspected).

Esophagus

Achalasia

Buzz Words:

- **Achalasia**: Dysphagia + swallowing liquids harder than solids + Chagas disease + bird's-beak sign + patient sits straight to swallow liquids
- **Carcinoma of esophagus:** Dysphagia + swallowing solids harder than liquids
- **Plummer–Vinson** (increased esophageal cancer risk): Esophageal web + atrophic oral mucosa + spoon-shaped brittle nails (koilnychyia) + Fe-deficiency anemia

Clinical Presentation: Patient is usually younger than 50 y/o with nonprogressive difficulty swallowing both solids and liquids, weight loss, and heartburn unresponsive to PPI therapy. Can be noticed when there is difficulty passing scope into stomach during upper endoscopy.

MoD: Degeneration of the Auerbach ganglion cells resulting in failed relaxation of the lower esophageal sphincter (LES) and absence of peristalsis in the proximal part of the esophagus with food retention.

Dx:

1. Barium swallow shows *bird's-beak* narrowing in the lower third
2. Manometry (confirms Dx)
3. Chest x-ray (CXR) can show megaesophagus
4. Endoscopy to r/o Plummer–Vinson syndrome (would reveal fibrous web below cricopharyngeus muscle)

Tx/Mgmt:

1. CCBs + nitrates
2. Botox injections
3. Repeat dilatation
4. Heller myotomy versus fundoplication if GERD)

Dysphagia

Clinical Presentation: Patient has difficulty with swallowing. Accompanying symptoms may help aid in the further workup of the complaint.

MoD: Dysphagia may be classified into oropharyngeal versus esophageal or secondary to obstruction versus motility disorder.

Dx: Adequate interrogation should help pin down the probable cause of dysphagia. Oropharyngeal dysphagia is usually described as difficulty initiating a swallow and accompanied by coughing, nasopharyngeal regurgitation, choking, and aspiration. Esophageal dysphagia occurs a couple of seconds after initiating the swallow and is accompanied of sensation of food getting stuck in the esophagus.

Tx/Mgmt: Depends on the etiology

Zenker Diverticulum

Buzz Words: Mucosal outpouching in the hypopharynx + **halitosis** + elderly patient

Clinical Presentation: Male patient older than 60 y/o with oropharyngeal dysphagia, food regurgitation, and halitosis from decomposing food inside the diverticulum.

PPx: Avoid nasogastric tube due to high risk of perforation

MoD: Pseudodiverticulum (does not contain *muscularis* layer) within Killian triangle (posterior hypopharyngeal mucosa) secondary to weakness in cricopharyngeal muscles.

Dx: Barium swallow

Tx/Mgmt: Cricopharyngeal myotomy, diverticulectomy, flexible or rigid endoscopy

Esophagitis/Esophageal Reflux (GERD)

Buzz Words: Postprandial "heartburn" or chest discomfort/ epigastric pain + chronic cough + symptomatic relief with antacids

Clinical Presentation: The most common symptoms are postprandial retrosternal/epigastric pain, regurgitation, and chronic cough. Alarm symptoms that are concerning for malignancy are weight loss, dysphagia, bleeding, anemia, and recurrent vomiting. Can lead to Barrett esophagus.

PPx: Elevate head of bed, weight loss, smoking cessation; avoid caffeine, chocolate, spicy foods, fatty foods, carbonated beverages, and peppermint

MoD: Abnormally relaxed LES, which allows reflux of stomach contents to cause symptoms and complications. These contents can make way to the pharynx and larynx.

Dx: Clinical diagnosis: Electrocardiogram (ECG) to r/o myocardial infarction (MI)

Tx/Mgmt:
1. Lifestyle modification
2. PPI
3. If refractory to conservative treatment, surgery with Nissen fundoplication, resection, or endoscopic therapy

Esophagitis, Pill

Buzz Words: Epigastric pain s/p taking a pill → pill esophagitis

Clinical Presentation: Patient lies a lot on back, with complaints of dysphagia, odynophagia, or chest pain. Medications that most frequently produce esophagitis are aspirin, alprenolol, bisphosphonates, iron compounds, NSAIDs, potassium chloride, quinidine, and tetracycline.

PPx: Avoid these medications in patients prone to develop esophageal stasis.

MoD: Produced by prolonged mucosal contact with the contents of the medication. Any condition that prolongs or produces stasis of food in the esophagus is a direct risk for pill esophagitis.

Dx: EGD with biopsy to rule out other etiologies

Tx/Mgmt: Stop causative medication and use acid suppressants to avoid GERD, which might be exacerbating the injury.

Mallory–Weiss Syndrome

Buzz Words: Repeated painful emesis due to alcohol consumption + hematemesis + epigastric

Clinical Presentation: A Mallory–Weiss tear is a longitudinal tear of the mucosa at the gastroesophageal junction (GEJ) due to bouts of emesis from alcohol consumption. Patients typically present with epigastric pain and signs/symptoms of acute upper GI bleed.

MoD: Increased intra-abdominal pressure → longitudinal mucosal tear in the proximal stomach or distal esophagus from severe retching

Dx: EGD to document the tear

Tx/Mgmt: Most tears will heal with supportive therapy and acid suppression. Hypovolemia should be corrected aggressively. Hospitalization for observation is encouraged. Active bleeding at the time of EGD should be attended to (i.e., ligation or thermal coagulation).

Paraesophageal (Hiatal) Hernia

Buzz Words:
- **Hiatal hernia:** Retrocardiac air-fluid level + dysphagia + epigastric pain + GEJ displacement on imaging
- **Schatzki ring:** Patient greater than 65 years old + dysphagia + lower esophageal stricture + associated with hiatal hernia

Clinical Presentation: Most patients are asymptomatic or manifest only mild, intermittent symptoms. Those who do complain report epigastric or retrosternal pain, nausea, retching, and postprandial fullness.

MoD: Often the precise mechanism of development of the hernia is elusive. Paraesophageal hernias are classified depending on the abdominal organs protruding through the hiatus:

- Type I—sliding hernia, fundus remains in place while GEJ is displaced into the thorax, most common (90%).
- Type II—"true" paraesophageal hernia, GEJ remains in the place while the fundus is displaced into the thorax.
- Type III—both the GEJ and fundus are displaced through the hiatus.
- Type IV—wider defect where organs other than the stomach are displaced into the thorax.

Dx:

QUICK TIPS
Imaging studies would show retrocardiac air-fluid level within the esophagus.

- CXR
- Flexible endoscopy (r/o Schatzki ring, which is a thin circumferential scar in the lower esophagus due to trauma; tx with antireflux surgery)

Tx/Mgmt:

- Type 1 hiatal hernias → conservative
- Types 2–4 → surgical management

Diffuse Esophageal Spasm

Buzz Words:

QUICK TIPS
Dyspepsia = heartburn = post-prandial epigastric pain/fullness

- Mild inflammation of esophagus + prolonged high-amplitude contractions + high lower esophageal sphincter pressure + relaxation on swallowing
- Dysphagia worse with hot and cold liquids + chest pain that feels like MI + no regurgitation

Clinical Presentation: Diffuse esophageal spasm (DES) is a disorder of episodic chest pain and trouble swallowing that is exacerbated by hot and cold liquids.

MoD: Inflammation of esophagus → esophageal contractions

Dx:

1. Endoscopy
2. Manometry
3. Barium swallow (corkscrew esophagus)

Tx/Mgmt:

1. CCB + nitrates
2. Myotomy

Disorders of the Stomach, Small Intestine, Colon, Rectum, and Anus

Stomach

Important definitions to know:

Gastritis is inflammation of the gastric mucosa of any etiology, including from *H. pylori* and NSAIDs. Can present with dyspepsia and GI bleeding and is diagnosed with neutrophil infiltration of the glands through endoscope.

Gastroparesis is delayed gastric emptying that leads to bloating, constipation, nausea, and abdominal discomfort. It is often seen in conjunction with diabetes. Can be treated with dietary modifications (small frequent meals, low in fat and containing soluble fiber), prokinetic agents like metoclopramide or erythromycin (motilin receptor agonist), and antiemetics. If refractory to medical management, decompression (gastrostomy) and postpyloric feeding are considered.

Peptic Ulcer Disease

Buzz Words:

- **Gastric ulcer:** Epigastric/retrosternal pain **exacerbated** by eating
- **Duodenal ulcer:** Epigastric/retrosternal pain **improved** by eating

Clinical Presentation: Peptic ulcer disease (PUD) can occur in either the stomach or the duodenum. Food exacerbates the pain of the former but relieves the pain of the latter. In general PUD patients may experience epigastric pain provoked by eating as well as abdominal fullness, early satiety, and nausea. For gastric ulcers, patients with blood group A have a higher risk.

For duodenal ulcers, when perforation occurs, the gastroduodenal artery is the most commonly injured vessel; patient will manifest signs and symptoms of acute abdomen and upper GI bleed. Increased risk in patients with MEN1 syndrome.

PPx: Avoid NSAIDs and cigarettes

MoD: *H. pylori* (tennis racket–shaped organism) → impaired mucosal defense (gastric ulcer) or hyperacid secretion (duodenal ulcer)

Dx:

1. Urea breath test (increased CO_2 after urea ingestion because *H. pylori* converts urea to CO_2)
2. Blood antibodies to *H. pylori*

TABLE 8.9 Comparison Between Gastric and Duodenal Ulcers

	Gastric Ulcers	Duodenal Ulcers
Association with *Helicobacter pylori*	Duodenal > gastric	
Postprandial pain	Exacerbated	Relieved
Blood group commonly associated	Group A	Group O
Frequency of ulcer cases	25%	75%
Location	Lesser curvature of antrum	Anterior portion of first part of duodenum
Vessel involved when bleeding	Left gastric artery	Gastroduodenal artery
Diagnosis	EGD + biopsy	EGD alone
Carcinogenic risk	1%–4%	Almost none

EGD, Esophagogastroduodenoscopy.

3. *H. pylori* in feces
4. Direct biopsy (CLO test) to r/o cancer

Tx/Mgmt:
- If gastric ulcer, biopsy:
  - If complicated ulcer (e.g., bleeding/perf/obstruction) → surgery
  - If uncomplicated → *H. pylori* treatment and avoid NSAIDs
- If duodenal ulcer: *H. pylori* treatment. If atypical, test for serum gastrin; if gastrin is high, administer secretin stimulation test to r/o Zollinger-Ellison syndrome (ZES) (Table 8.9)

Peptic Ulcer Perforation

Buzz Words: "Washboard" abdomen, free air on CXR

Clinical Presentation: Sudden, severe, diffuse abdominal pain and abdominal rigidity, which may be accompanied by syncope. Exam is relevant for tachycardia, low temperature, weak pulse, and clammy skin.

PPx: Early diagnosis of peptic ulcer disease and adequate management

MoD: Most common sites of perforation are duodenal (60%), antral (20%), and body of the stomach (20%). Release of gastric acid into the peritoneal cavity produces an initial vasoplegic response.

Dx:
1. Upright CXR and abdominal films (± free air)
2. Abdominal CT

Tx/Mgmt: Nasogastric tube insertion, IV fluids, and PPI; if unstable, emergent operation

Small Intestine and Colon

Appendicitis

Buzz Words:
- **Appendicitis:** umbilical pain that migrates to the right lower quadrant (RLQ) + acute + leukocytosis + peritoneal signs + fever + **refusal to eat** + neutrophils w/ bands
- **Gastroenteritis: Intermittent** RLQ pain + anorexia + nausea:
  - The pain for appendicitis is NOT intermittent

Clinical Presentation: Patient presents with nausea and vomiting (N/V), aversion to food, and dull epigastric pain that migrates to McBurney point and can have positive Rovsing sign, Aaron sign, psoas test, and obturator sign. Diameter of appendix is greater than 6 mm in imaging studies. Children and elderly patients may have vague symptoms that make perforation and rupture more common than in adults. Very high yield for Surgery shelf. Easy to identify in question stem, so expect to be tested on mechanism, diagnostic steps, and management.

MoD: Obstruction of the lumen of the appendix is the most common cause of inflammation. Fecaliths, undigested seeds, pinworm infections, or lymphoid hyperplasia may be the culprits in obstruction. Once occluded, the epithelial lining continues to secrete mucus until the intraluminal pressure occludes venous outflow. Venous congestion and intraluminal stasis set the stage for bacterial overgrowth and progressive inflammation.

Dx:
1. CT to confirm acute appendicitis; if patient is pregnant or a child, ultrasound or MRI preferred
2. If reproductive-age female, hCG to r/o ectopic pregnancy, urinalysis (UA) to r/o urinary tract infection (UTI)

Tx/Mgmt:
1. Appendectomy
2. If cancer at base of appendix → right hemicolectomy

FOR THE WARDS

A normal-appearing appendix during surgical exploration should be removed regardless to avoid future complications.

 AR

Appendicitis—signs, symptoms, and causes

Angiodysplasia

Buzz Words: Lower GI bleed + small, dilated, thin-walled veins in GI tract + patient >50 y/o + aortic stenosis

Clinical Presentation: Patients usually don't notice occult blood loss, although signs and symptoms of lower GI bleed might manifest (i.e., hematochezia, melena, and sometimes hematemesis). It is the second leading cause of lower GI bleed in patients older than 60 y/o.

MoD: Ectatic, dilated, thin-walled vessels with tortuous submucosal veins; it is the most common abnormality of the GI tract. Lesions are commonly found in the cecum and ascending colon.

Dx:
1. CBC, iron studies
2. Fecal occult blood test (FOBT)
3. Colonoscopy and capsule endoscopy

Tx/Mgmt: Self-limited: If bleeding does not stop, epinephrine or coagulation from colonoscopy.

Diverticulosis and Diverticulitis

Buzz Words:
- **Acute diverticulitis:** Left lower quadrant (LLQ) acute abdomen + fever + leukocytosis + peritoneal pain
- **Diverticulosis:** LLQ chronic abdominal pain + no signs of acute infection ± signs of lower GI bleed

Clinical Presentation: Diverticula are sac-like protrusions from the colonic wall due to colonic muscular weakening. *Diverticulosis* refers to the presence of multiple diverticula in the colon. Diverticulitis refers to the inflammation and infection of these diverticula. The classic patient is older than 50 y/o with abdominal pain in the LLQ.

Diverticulitis would also present with fever, leukocytosis, and sudden manifestation of symptoms. Common complications of diverticulitis are perforation, abscess, fistula, and obstruction. The Hinchey classification allows for staging of colonic perforation in diverticular disease:
- Hinchey I—paracolonic abscess or phlegmon
- Hinchey II—pelvic or retroperitoneal abscess
- Hinchey III—purulent peritonitis
- Hinchey IV—feculent peritonitis

PPx: Vegetarian and high-fiber diets

MoD: Increased intraluminal pressure in the colon from constant strain (i.e., constipation) produces an outward bulge at points where blood vessels penetrate the bowel wall. Increasing age is a significant risk factor for the development of diverticula. Diverticulitis occurs when bacterial overgrowth happens within these protrusions.

Dx:
- **Diverticulosis:** Colonoscopy ± barium enema
- **Diverticulitis:** Abdominal CT (scope may cause perforation), which can distinguish between complicated and uncomplicated disease

Sigmoid Diverticulosis Video

Tx/Mgmt:

- **Diverticulosis:** High-fiber diet (most are asymptomatic); if persistent bleeding, angiographic/endoscopic treatment
- **Diverticulitis:** Antibiotic therapy (ciprofloxacin + metronidazole, TMP/SMX + metronidazole, or amoxicillin/clavulanate) and bowel rest
- Perforations should be immediately surgically managed.

Diverticula, diverticulosis, and diverticulitis

Hirschsprung Disease

Buzz Words: Neonate + to pass meconium + squirt sign

Clinical Presentation: Bilious emesis, abdominal distention, and failure to pass meconium within 48 hours of birth. May be complicated by enterocolitis, which carries a significant morbidity and mortality in newborns. Increased incidence occurs in Down syndrome, neurofibromatosis 1, MEN2 syndromes, and Waardenburg syndrome.

MoD: Incomplete migration of ganglion cells from their origin in the neural crest to the distal rectum.

Dx: Tight anal sphincter and squirt sign on digital rectal examination. Suction rectal biopsy (gold standard) taken 2 cm above dentate line shows absence of ganglion cells.

Tx/Mgmt: Surgical resection of the affected segment with preservation of the anal sphincter and primary anastomosis of the bowel

Hirschsprung disease (congenital aganglionic megacolon)

Paralytic Ileus

Clinical Presentation: Obstipation and oral intolerance occur usually lasting more than 3–5 days. Symptoms of prolonged ileus are distention, bloating, N/V, inability to pass flatus, and abdominal pain. Important risk factors for postoperative ileus are prolonged abdominal or pelvis surgery, open procedures, delayed initiation of enteral nutrition, intraabdominal inflammation.

PPx: Avoid medications known to impede peristalsis

MoD: Inflammatory process involving the intestinal smooth muscle cells, which disrupts normal peristaltic activity. Common causes are postoperative ileus, use of opiates or anticholinergics, severe illness, and hypothyroidism.

Dx: Exclude other causes of ileus (i.e., bowel obstruction, intra-abdominal infections, bowel perforation, etc.). Abdominal films show retained air in colon and rectum with no visible transition zone.

Tx/Mgmt: NG tube for decompression, fluid and electrolyte replacement, and pain management; serial abdominal examinations

Impaction

Buzz Words: Fecal loading in abdominal films

Clinical Presentation: Elderly patient who chronically suffers from constipation, with abdominal distention and prolonged failure to pass stool.

PPx: Eliminate potential causes of constipation + ensure dietary fiber intake of 20–25 g/day

MoD: Inability to sense and respond to the presence of stool in the bowel plays a role in the development of intestinal impaction.

Dx: Digital rectal exam would show copious amount of stool in the rectum. An abdominal film may aid in the diagnosis when proximal loops of bowel are involved in the absence of rectal impaction.

Tx/Mgmt:

1. Digital disimpaction may facilitate the passage of bowel through the anus.
2. Osmotic enemas may aid in the softening of the fecal matter.
3. Once disimpaction has been successfully performed, oral administration of polyethylene glycol can serve to prevent re-impaction.
4. Refractory cases can be managed with injection of local anesthetics to relax the pelvic floor along with abdominal massage or use of a colonoscope to fragment distal fecal matter.

Intestinal Obstruction/Stricture

Clinical Presentation: Intermittent abdominal pain, cramping, N/V, and distention occur. Exam will be noteworthy for signs of hypovolemia, increased peristalsis, and high-pitched bowel sounds (which will disappear as the bowel distends).

MoD: Normal flow of bowel contents is interrupted, leading to dilation, edema of the bowel wall, and proximal increase in intraluminal pressure. Excessive increase in pressure will obstruct blood flood and lead to bowel perforation. Postoperative adhesions are the most common cause of obstruction, followed by hernia, volvulus, intestinal inflammation, neoplasm, and prior irradiation.

Dx: Clinical diagnosis, which may be aided by abdominal CT scan to identify level and severity of obstruction.

Digital rectal examination should be performed to rule out impaction.

Tx/Mgmt: Decompression with nasogastric tube, volume replacement, and adequate management of pain. Prompt surgical exploration is required in complicated obstruction by ischemia, necrosis, or perforation. Patients with partial obstruction may be observed, with frequent reassessments in expectation of spontaneous resolution.

Irritable Colon/Irritable Bowel Syndrome

Buzz Words: Alternating diarrhea and constipation, pain decreased after bowel movement

Clinical Presentation: Nonspecific abdominal pain: Diarrhea, constipation, or patients alternating between these. It is associated with anxiety. Pain is relieved by a bowel movement and symptoms are less intense at night. Patients are rarely admitted to the hospital. Diagnosis made by Rome III criteria, which includes "recurrent abdominal pain or discomfort at least 3 days/month in the last 3 months associated" associated with ≥2 of change in frequency of stool, change in appearance of stool, and symptomatic improvement with defecation.

Rome III diagnostic criteria

PPx: Dietary modification, which consists in exclusion of gas-producing foods, low consumption of fermentable carbohydrates (FODMAPs—fermentable oligo-, di-, and monosaccharides and polyols), and lactose/gluten avoidance.

MoD: Pathophysiology remains uncertain; multiple theories and correlations have been postulated. Hypersensitization of visceral afferent nerves, mucosal immune system activation, and small bowel bacteria overgrowth to name a few.

Dx: Rome III criteria

Tx/Mgmt: Fiber and osmotic agents, antispasmodic agents, and tricyclic antidepressants (TCAs)

Ischemic Bowel

Buzz Words: Pneumatosis intestinalis, dead gut, abdominal pain out of proportion to the physical examination

Clinical Presentation: Commonly occurs in terminally ill patients receiving intensive care. It has a high mortality rate (60%–70%).

MoD: Reduced perfusion to the intestine from low cardiac output, arterial occlusion, venous congestion, or spasmodic vasoconstriction

Dx: Abdominal CT to identify signs of regional ischemia and intramural gas bubbles (pneumatosis intestinalis). Rising serum lactate is an early indicator of ischemic bowel. A high degree of clinical suspicion is required for patients who are being mechanically ventilated or continuously sedated; awaiting the appearance of gross abdominal manifestations might lead to a deadly delay in diagnosis.

Tx/Mgmt: Urgent exploratory laparotomy to resect injured segment of bowel. Provided that there are no contraindications, anticoagulants should be initiated in order to prevent further clot formation.

99 AR

Virtual colonoscopy of patient with sigmoid volvulus

Malnutrition

Buzz Words: Cachexia, sunken eyeballs, absent muscle mass, frailty

Clinical Presentation: Common in elderly, institutionalized, bedridden, homeless, or chronically alcoholic individuals

PPx: Most patients can be started on early postoperative enteral feeding (<48 hours).

MoD: Elderly patients usually consume less than half their recommended dietary allowance (RDA) owing to suppressed appetite, diminished sense of smell, depression, social isolation, and low income. Malnutrition sets the stage for impaired wound healing, increased risk of infection, and higher risk for perioperative mortality.

Dx: Visceral protein stores in organs (e.g., liver) are evaluated by measurement of serum albumin and transferrin. Somatic protein stores are evaluated by measuring the circumference of the arm. Low levels of albumin, prealbumin, transferrin, and retinol-binding protein correlate with malnutrition. Protein-energy malnutrition (PEM) can be classified by body mass index (BMI = weight [in kilograms]/height^2 [in meters]):
- Normal BMI = 18.5–24.9
- PEM grade I = 17–18.4
- PEM grade II = 16–16.9
- PEM grade III = <16

Tx/Mgmt: Any patient who is not able to consume at least 60% of his or her RDA requires adjunctive nutritional therapy through either the enteral or parenteral route. In selecting the route of access, duration of therapy should be taken into account. NGs and OGs should not be considered for patient who will require therapy for more than 4 weeks. Whenever possible, enteral nutrition is preferred over parenteral because it provides better glycemic control, avoids gut bacterial overgrowth, maintains the integrity of the mucosal barrier, and increases the variety of nutrients absorbed. Parenteral nutrition should be considered for patients who have not been able to tolerate/receive enteral feeds more than 7 days.

Malabsorption

Buzz Words: Oily, greasy, floating stool; patient with cystic fibrosis (CF) or chronic pancreatitis

Clinical Presentation: Patient presents with abdominal bloating and steatorrhea ± weight loss. Lipophilic vitamins (A, D, E, and K) and vitamin B_{12} will not be absorbed adequately (Table 8.10).

PPx: Adequately manage underlying condition.

MoD: Commonly due to defects in pancreatic secretion (i.e., chronic pancreatitis, CF), mucosal disorders (i.e., celiac disease, IBD), bacterial overgrowth (i.e., surgical alterations in GI anatomy, abnormal motility), or parasitic disease (*Giardia* most common).

Dx: Fecal fat test (Sudan III stain)

Tx/Mgmt: Supplement lipophilic vitamins. Pancreatic enzymes may be replaced orally for exocrine pancreatic insufficiency.

Dumping Syndrome

Buzz Words: Bloating + cramping + diarrhea + flushing + weakness/dizziness + palpitations + diaphoresis + recent GI surgery → dumping syndrome

TABLE 8.10 Common Vitamin Deficiencies in Malabsorption

Vitamin	Normal Function	Findings in Deficient States
A	Vision, epithelial tissue, growth in children	Nyctalopia, xerophtalmia, Bitot spots (conjunctival keratin spots), follicular hyperkeratosis, growth retardation
B_{12}	Red blood cell and neural development	Megaloblastic anemia, hypersegmented polymorphonuclear leukocytes, pancytopenia, posterior column and lateral corticospinal tract demyelination, glossitis
D	Bone mineralization and blood Ca^{2+} regulation	Pathologic fractures, tibial bowing, muscle spasms, tetany, rickets, osteomalacia
E	Antioxidant	Hemolytic anemia, peripheral neuropathy (posterior column degeneration), ataxia, peripheral edema, thrombocytosis
K	Clotting factor synthesis	Ecchymoses, gastrointestinal bleeding, prolonged prothrombin time/international normalized ratio and partial thromboplastin time

Clinical Presentation: After GI surgery (particularly postgastrectomy), patients may get dumping syndrome, which is a disorder characterized by carcinoid-like symptoms occurring after food ingestion. Early dumping syndrome occurs within 30 min due to rapid gastric emptying of hyperosmolar load. Late dumping syndrome occurs 1–3 hours after eating. This is a very high yield disorder on the Surgery shelf.

PPx: Avoid large amounts of sugar. Eat small meals frequently. Separate ingestion of solids and liquids.

MoD:
- Rapid influx of fluid + high osmotic gradient → small intestine from the gastric remnant of GI surgery (early dumping)
- Rapid influx of food + rapid rise in postprandial glucose → excessive release of insulin → vasomotor symptoms

Dx: Clinical diagnosis

Tx/Mgmt:
1. Change diet regimen
2. Octreotide
3. If refractory, surgical management

Lactose Intolerance

Buzz Words: Resolution after 1 day of avoiding milk products

Clinical Presentation: Abdominal distention, bloating, and diarrhea occur. It is rare in children younger than 6 y/o, rates increase with age.

PPx: Avoid dairy products

MoD: Lactase enzyme nonpersistence. Lactase normally hydrolyzes lactose into glucose and galactose, which can be absorbed by the intestinal epithelium. When lactose reaches the colon, bacteria convert it to short-chain fatty acids, hydrogen gas, and ketones. Could also be secondary to underlying disease (i.e., bacterial overgrowth, giardiasis, celiac disease, etc.).

Dx:
1. Clinical suspicion and improvement with dietary modifications
2. Stool osmotic gap greater than 125 mOsm/kg and pH less than 6.0 secondary to bacterial fermentation

Tx/Mgmt: Avoid dairy products or use lactase pills

Short-Bowel Syndrome

Buzz Words: Small bowel removed + enteral feeding + large amounts of liquid stool

Clinical Presentation: Patient who underwent extensive resection of intestines and manifests deficiency of macro- or micronutrients (see Table 8.11 for specific nutrient deficiencies) and diarrhea. It is associated with gastric hypersecretion, liver disease, and cholelithiasis.

MoD: Malabsorptive condition caused by absence of an essential segment of the bowel removed by surgical resection. The bowel becomes incapable of maintaining the patient's nutrient requirements on its own due to a reduction in absorptive surface area.

Dx: Clinical diagnosis

Tx/Mgmt: Replacement of fluids and electrolytes; resuming enteral feeding (intraluminal nutrients are the best stimulant for intestinal adaptation)

99 AR

Intestinal sites of nutrient absorption

Rectum and Anus

Abscess of Anal and Rectal Regions

Buzz Words: Palpable mass at the anal verge

Clinical Presentation: Patients present with pain in anorectal area ± fever. Four major variants exist, classified on their anatomic relation to the sphincters and muscles of the pelvic floor: intersphincteric, perianal, ischiorectal, and supraelevator. Most patients never seek medical attention.

MoD: Obstruction of the anorectal glands, located between the internal and external sphincters, leading to bacterial infection

Dx: Clinical diagnosis. MRI to see extent of infection

Tx/Mgmt: Incision and drainage (I&D), antibiotics if immunocompromised

TABLE 8.11 Commonly Tested Nutrient Deficiencies in Short-Bowel Syndrome

Segment missing	Nutrient deficiencies
Stomach	Vitamin B_{12} (lack of intrinsic factor)
Duodenum	Minerals: iron, calcium, and others
Ileum	Vitamin B_{12} (no absorption) and bile salts
Cecum	Potassium, short-chain fatty acids, and vitamin K

Anorectal Fistula

Buzz Words:
- Past anorectal abscess + perineal opening in skin + cord-like tract can be palpated + brownish purulent discharge + fecal streaks soiling underwear
- Operation for perianal fistula + area does not heal well + unhealing ulcers/fissures + purulent discharge + no palpable masses

Clinical Presentation: Patient has chronic drainage of pus or stool from a skin opening in the perirectal area ± mention of a prior perirectal abscess. It is associated with Crohn disease.

PPx: Treatment of Crohn disease, avoiding surgeries that weaken the muscular wall

MoD: Almost half of anorectal abscesses become fistulas that connect the rectal mucosa with the perirectal skin. Goodsall rule allows the examiner to predict the tract of the fistula by drawing an imaginary line between the ischial spines; all fistulas with external openings posterior to this line travel in a curvilinear fashion, while those with anterior openings travel in a radial fashion. Can occur due to prior surgeries, anorectal abscess or Crohn disease.

Dx: Fistulas are classified in relation to their anatomic tract (good for the wards but don't need to memorize for the shelf):
- Parks type 1—intersphincteric
- Parks type 2—transsphinteric
- Parks type 3—suprasphincteric
- Parks type 4—extrasphincteric

Tx/Mgmt:
1. Digital rectal examination (DRE), anoscope, proctosigmoidoscopy to r/o cancer
2. Biopsy to confirm Crohn disease if diagnosis not already made
3. Elective fistulotomy (marsupialization)
4. If Crohn, give patient metronidazole

FOR THE WARDS

Anorectal fistulas rarely heal spontaneously and require surgical management. The goal is to eradicate the fistula while preserving fecal continence.

Anal Fissure

Buzz Words: Exquisite pain with defecation + bright red blood per rectum (BRBPR) + fear of bowel movements + refuses physical examination (PE) because it's too painful to draw buttocks apart

Clinical Presentation: Severe, localized anorectal pain that increases with defecation, which is accompanied by streaks of blood on fecal matter. Most often it is located posteriorly.

PPx: Dietary modifications and medication interruption to avoid constipation, proper anal hygiene

MoD: Linear tears in the lining of the rectal canal below the level of the dentate line may be product of severe straining to defecate from constipation or a tight sphincter.

Dx:
1. Gentle traction of the buttocks (avoid DRE if painful)
2. If too painful, examine **under anesthesia** using DRE, anoscope, or proctosigmoidoscope to r/o cancer

Tx/Mgmt:
1. Stool softeners, sitz baths
2. Topical nitroglycerin
3. Botulinum toxin (relaxes sphincter)
4. Forceful dilation
5. Lateral internal sphincterotomy if refractory

Fecal Incontinence

Clinical Presentation: Involuntary loss of feces or flatus occur. Urge incontinence is characterized by an intense desire to defecate, with incontinence occurring despite efforts to retain stool. Passive incontinence consists in lack of awareness of need to defecate.

PPx: Avoid foods known to worsen symptoms

MoD: Incontinence can occur by alteration in any of the physiological components of defecation: sphincter function, stool volume/consistency, rectal compliance, cognitive function, anorectal awareness, and reflexes.

Dx: Flexible sigmoidoscopy to rule out malignancy or mucosal inflammation. Patients with sphincter defects should be evaluated with endoscopic ultrasound; those with intact sphincters should have rectal manometry performed.

Tx/Mgmt: Measures to reduced frequency and increase consistency of stool with bulking agents (i.e., methylcellulose) or antidiarrheal agents (i.e., loperamide)

Proctitis

Clinical Presentation: Rectal urgency, tenesmus, pain worsened by bowel movements, and mucous discharge occur. Risk factors for developing proctitis are previous radiation therapy, unprotected anal intercourse.

PPx: Use of condom during anal intercourse

MoD: *Chlamydia trachomatis* and *herpes simplex virus type 2* are common causes of proctitis in patients who engage in anal intercourse. Exposure to ionizing radiation is another possible etiology.

Dx: Clinical diagnosis: Sigmoidoscopy might show erythematous, friable, ulcerated rectal mucosa.

Tx/Mgmt: Aimed at relieving pain, usually with sitz baths, topical anesthetics, and oral analgesics. Those with chlamydial proctitis should receive tetracycline or doxycycline orally.

Hemorrhoids

Buzz Words:
- BRBPR + no pain → internal hemorrhoids
- BRBPR + pain + skin tags → external hemorrhoids
- Patient >50 y/o + hemorrhoids + BRBPR → colonoscopy to r/o cancer

Clinical Presentation: Hemorrhoids are swollen veins in the anus that can present as bright red blood coating fecal matter, anal pruritus, and pain. Risk factors for development of symptomatic hemorrhoids are age, portal hypertension, anal intercourse, pregnancy, straining, constipation, and anticoagulation/antiplatelet therapy.

Classified as either internal or external hemorrhoids:

Internal originate above the dentate line and are usually painless. External originate below the dentate line and produce pain when thrombosis occurs. Internal hemorrhoids are classified as follows:
- Grade I—do not prolapse
- Grade II—prolapse with defecation and return spontaneously into the anal canal
- Grade III—prolapse with defecation and require manual reduction
- Grade IV—not reducible

Treatment depends on the clinical degree. All patients should be started on prophylactic measures to avoid constipation and straining. Grade III can be managed with rubber-band ligation. Grade III–IV and mixed hemorrhoids may be offered surgical hemorrhoidectomy. Conventional procedures are the Ferguson (closed) hemorrhoidectomy and the Milligan–Morgan (open excision and ligation w/o mucosal closure) hemorrhoidectomy.

PPx: Fluids, fiber, prevention of constipation

MoD: Normal vascular structures of the anal canal that arise from three submucosal columns: right anterior, right posterior, or left lateral.

Dx:
1. DRE
2. Anoscopy
3. Flexible sigmoidoscope or proctosigmoidoscope to r/o anorectal cancer

Tx/Mgmt:
- Grade 1 → diet change
- Grade 2 → band ligation
- Grade 3 → band ligation, hemorrhoidectomy
- Grade 4 → Hemerrhoidectomy versus excisional thrombectomy for thrombosed external hemorrhoid not responding to medical therapy

Rectal Prolapse

Buzz Words: Elderly woman + multiple gestations + protruding rectal mass + rectal pain

Clinical Presentation: Thin, frail woman with history of multiple pregnancies who complains of mucosal mass protruding from rectal region, rectal pain, mild bleeding, fecal incontinence, and a wet anus. The mass may protrude after bowel movements and may be manually reducible. It is a type of procidentia, which just means an organ displacing downward from its anatomic position.

PPx: Dietary modifications and medication interruption to avoid constipation

MoD: Intussusception of a portion of rectum thorough the anal canal

Dx: Clinical diagnosis (physical exam would show a true prolapse rather than mucosal prolapse when radial folds or hemorrhoidal vessels can be identified)

Tx/Mgmt: Surgical resection of redundant sigmoid colon with fixation of the rectum (rectopexy) to the sacral fascia

Disorder of the Peritoneal Cavity

Ascites

Buzz Words: Abdominal fullness, fluid wave, flank dullness on percussion, shifting dullness

Clinical Presentation: Accumulation of fluid occurs in the peritoneal cavity. The most common cause is chronic liver failure, but other processes may induce it as well (e.g., nephrotic syndrome, malnutrition, protein-losing enteropathy, heart failure, carcinomatosis, etc.). Patients with abdominal hernias may suffer an exacerbation due to high pressure, with thinning of the overlying skin. Approximately 10% of patients will develop spontaneous bacterial peritonitis, which carries a mortality of 50% at 1 year.

PPx: Fluid and sodium restriction, avoid alcohol consumption

MoD: Transudation of fluid usually occurs from the intravascular space to the hepatic parenchyma, then leaking into the peritoneal cavity due to increased hydrostatic pressure (in the setting of portal hypertension) and decreased colloid oncotic pressure.

Dx: Abdominal exam reveals dullness to percussion and fluid wave on palpation. These signs become evident when accumulation is greater than 1.5 L. Ultrasound/CT can detect lower volumes of fluid in the peritoneal cavity. Diagnostic paracentesis aids in differential diagnosis (cell count, amylase level, triglyceride level, pH, and albumin). Anyone with ascites + fever must undergo paracentesis; spontaneous bacterial peritonitis is diagnosed with cells greater than 250/mm^3.

Tx/Mgmt: Fluid and Na$^+$ restriction (<2 g/day) and diuresis with spironolactone (to promote Na$^+$ excretion) ± furosemide. When respiration or mobility become severely limited, therapeutic paracentesis (8–10 L) is performed while administering IV albumin (8 g/L of fluid removed).

Disorders of the Liver and Biliary System, Noninfectious

Liver (*Table 8.12*)

Cirrhosis

Buzz Words: Micronodular pattern in hepatic surface + decreased LFTs

Clinical Presentation: Patient presents with signs and symptoms of hepatic failure, cholestasis, portal hypertension (HTN), hepatic encephalopathy, and decreased degradation of estrogens (i.e., gynecomastia, impotence, erectile dysfunction, and spider angiomas).

PPx: Depends on etiologic factor

MoD: Irreversible fibrosis of the liver parenchyma occurs. Regenerative nodules are formed as part of the reaction to injury and contain islands of healthy tissue surrounded by bands of fibrosis. Hydrostatic pressure in the portal system is increased by compression of nodules. See Box 8.1 for most common etiologic factors.

Dx: Palpation of RUQ is the best initial test with suspicion of cirrhosis. Liver biopsy confirms diagnosis.

Tx/Mgmt: Determination of etiology

TABLE 8.12 Simplified Meaning of Liver Function Tests

Test	Meaning
Albumin	Talks to the synthetic function of the liver and nutritional status of the patient
	May be low in malnutrition and nephritic syndrome
	Low albumin means little to no hepatic functional reserve
ALP	Biliary duct obstruction
	Caveat: bone can produce and leak the enzyme as well
ALT	Hepatocyte membrane damage and leak
	ALT > AST think viral hepatitis
AST	Hepatocyte membrane damage and leak
	AST > ALT think alcohol or drug toxicity
γGGT	Biliary duct obstruction
	Rises immediately after binge drinking
PT and INR	Talks to the synthetic function of the liver, most accurate marker

ALP, Alkaline phosphatate; *ALT,* alanine aminotransferase; *AST,* aspartate aminotransferase; *GGT,* γ-glutamyl tranferase; *INR,* international normalized ratio; *PT,* prothrombin time.

BOX 8.1 Most Common Causes of Cirrhosis

Alcoholic liver disease
Chronic viral hepatitis (i.e., hepatitis B virus and hepatitis C virus)
Hemochromatosis
Nonalcoholic fatty liver disease
Autoimmune disease (i.e., primary biliary cirrhosis and autoimmune
Wilson disease)
α_1-Antitrypsin deficiency

- Consider liver transplantation for end-stage dysfunction
- For cirrhosis + portal HTN → beta blockers to decrease portal pressure and transjugular intra-hepatic portosystemic shunt (TIPS)/lactulose for refractory portal HTN

Cirrhosis—definition and pathology

Dubin–Johnson Syndrome

Buzz Words: Black liver (dark pigment in hepatocytes) + episodes of self-resolving jaundice + direct (aka conjugated) bilirubinemia

Clinical Presentation: Usually asymptomatic, patient might present with mild jaundice w/o pruritus. Chronic conjugated hyperbilirubinemia is not associated with hemolysis. Condition may be exacerbated by illnesses, pregnancy, or use of oral contraceptives. It is associated with reduced prothrombin activity secondary to factor VII deficiency in 60% of cases.

MoD: Dysfunctional transport of conjugated bilirubin out of the liver. Autosomal recessive mutation in the *ABCC2* gene, which codes for MRP2 (multidrug resistance protein 2), used in the hepatocellular excretion of bilirubin glucoronides into bile canaliculi. Dense pigments composed of epinephrine metabolites accumulate in lysosomes, making the liver appear grossly black.

Dx:
1. Liver panel: Total bilirubin 2–5 mg/dL range, of which 50% is usually conjugated with normal LFTs.
2. UA: Bilirubinuria is common; may see urinary coproporhyrin I > coproporphyrin II.

Tx/Mgmt: No treatment required

Rotor Syndrome

Buzz Words: Normal-appearing liver (no black pigment) + episodes of self-resolving jaundice + direct (aka conjugated) bilirubinemia

Clinical Presentation: Patient presents with asymptomatic, chronic conjugated and unconjugated hyperbilirubinemia w/o evidence of hemolysis. There is normal liver histology (absent melanin pigments).

MoD: Defect in hepatic storage of conjugated bilirubin, which leaks into plasma; autosomal recessive inheritance

Dx: Similar labs to **Dubin-Johnson syndrome** (DJS). Urinary coproporphyrin excretion pattern allows to distinguish between DJS and rotor syndrome (Table 8.13).

Tx/Mgmt: No treatment required

Gilbert Syndrome

Buzz Words: Adult + jaundice in s/o stress (e.g., fasting, exertion) + unconjugated hyperbilirubinemia

TABLE 8.13 Interpretation of Urinary Coproporphyrin Excretion Patterns for Direct Bilirubinemia

	Healthy	Dubin-Johnson Syndrome	Rotor Syndrome
Total amount excreted	Normal	Normal	Elevated
Predominant type	Coproporphyrin III	Coproporphyrin I	Coproporphyrin I
Hepatocytes with dark pigment	No	Yes	No

Clinical Presentation: Recurrent episodes of jaundice are due to unconjugated hyperbilirubinemia. It is the most common inherited disorder of bilirubin glucoronidation.

MoD: Defect in the promoter of the gene that encodes UDP-glucoronosyltransferase 1A1.

Dx: Unconjugated (indirect) hyperbilirubinemia, total bilirubin is usually less than 3 mg/dL. Normal LFTs. Rifampin test: unconjugated bilirubin rises after administration of drug.

Tx/Mgmt: No treatment is required. Avoid irinotecan, it requires bilirubin-UGT–mediated glucronidation, and these patients are at increased risk for toxicity.

Crigler–Najjar Syndrome

Buzz Words:
- Indirect bilirubinemia + jaundice + kernicterus/bilirubin in basal ganglia + infant/child (does not live to adulthood) → type 1 Crigler-Najjar
- Indirect bilirubinemia + normal LFTs + adult (survives into adulthood) → type 2 Crigler Najjar

Clinical Presentation: Crigler-Najjar syndrome is an autosomal recessive disorder where metabolism of bilirubin is impaired, leading to a buildup of indirect bilirubin. Two subtypes exist: type 1 has severe hyperbilirubinemia (20–50 mg/dL) due to absent bilirubin UGT activity and leads to kernicterus, while type 2 has total bilirubin levels less than 20 mg/dL, has only reduced bilirubin UGT activity, and rarely leads to kernicterus. Type 1 patient dies before adulthood while type 2 lives into adulthood.

MoD: Autosomal recessive inheritance, decreased UGT activity → hyperunconjugated bilirubinemia

Dx: Liver panel (total bilirubin is higher than in Gilbert, normal LFTs)

Tx/Mgmt:
- If type 1 → phototherapy + plasmapheresis + liver transplant (only cure)
- If type 2 → no tx needed in many cases but phenobarbital and clofibrate if needed

End-Stage Liver Disease (Including Indications for Transplantation)

Buzz Words: Cirrhosis, cholestasis, portal HTN

Clinical Presentation: For the shelf, only know the Buzz Words for end-stage liver disease. For the wards, learn the Model for End-stage Liver Disease (MELD) score and indications for liver transplant.

QUICK TIPS

Crigler type 1 is worse than Crigler type 2

99 AR

Liver cholestasis—definition and pathology

Dx: The MELD score is a risk-stratification tool that uses bilirubin, creatinine, and the INR; it has been strongly correlated with 3-month survival. A MELD score of 30 correlates with a 50% 3-month survival. Patients awaiting liver transplantation are ranked according to MELD score and blood type by the United Network for Organ Sharing (UNOS).

Tx/Mgmt: Evaluation for transplantation should be obtained when MELD ≥10 and patient candidacy should be considered when MELD ≥15 (Table 8.14). Management should be directed to slowing the progression of disease, preventing further insults to the liver, preventing complications of cirrhosis, and adjusting dosing of medications according to preserved liver function.

Ischemic Hepatitis

Buzz Words: Liver shock, hypoxic hepatitis

Clinical Presentation: RUQ pain, nausea, vomiting, anorexia, and malaise occur. It is a rare phenomenon since the liver receives dual blood supply (proper hepatic artery and portal vein).

MoD: Diffuse hepatic infarction from acute hypoperfusion, severe hypoxemia, severe respiratory failure, or

TABLE 8.14 Indications for Liver Transplantation

Indication	Observations for Consideration
Acute liver failure (<26 weeks)	Receive highest priority for transplantation Severe liver injury + encephalopathy or impaired synthetic function (INR ≥1.5)
Cirrhosis	Complications of portal hypertension Manifestations of compromised liver function (i.e., hepatorenal syndrome)
Alcoholic liver damage	Patients required to have >6 months of abstinence, enrollment in rehabilitation, and adequate social support Transplantation offers a significant 5-year survival rate for these patients, and only 5%–7% return to excessive drinking
Neoplasms	Hepatocellular carcinoma (single lesion <5 cm), epithelioid hemangioendothelioma, and large hepatic adenomas
Metabolic disorders	Cystic fibrosis, α_1-antitrypsin deficiency, von Gierke disease, Andersen disease, hemochromatosis, Wilson disease, acute intermittent porphyria

associated with acute lower limb ischemia occur. There is an imbalance between oxygen demand and supply. Zone 3 of the hepatic acinus is the most susceptible to injury; furthest away from oxygenated blood supply.

Dx: ALT and AST may surpass the normal range by 50×.

Tx/Mgmt: Restoration of cardiac output. High mortality rates occur in patients who develop liver shock in the intensive care setting.

Hepatic Coma/Encephalopathy

Buzz Words: Flapping tremor, inability to sustain posture

Clinical Presentation: Irritability, confusion, altered mental state, asterixis (flapping of extended wrists), coma, and death.

PPx: The goal is to decrease the amount of available ammonia (NH_3) in the colon by decreasing the amount of amino acids for bacteria to metabolize (protein restricted diet), wiping out the gut flora (rifaximin), or converting ammonia into ammonium (NH_4), which cannot be absorbed by the colon.

MoD: Reversible metabolic disorder is due to increased serum NH_3 level. The urea cycle is defective in the setting of advanced liver dysfunction, allowing abnormally high levels of NH_3 to accumulate. Factors that may precipitate encephalopathy are:

- GI bleeds, which may precipitate encephalopathy due to increased nitrogen load in the lumen
- Portosystemic shunting
- Diuretics (thiazide/loop), which incite metabolic alkalosis, keeping ammonia in the NH_3 state

Identify any precipitating causes. Continue preventive measures to decrease gut absorption of NH3. Provide supportive therapy and nutritional support. Admit any patient with moderate-severe levels of confusion who might not be able to adhere to treatment.

Dx: Ammonia levels (hyperammonemia)

Tx/Mgmt: Lactulose to decrease NH_3 in blood; if confused, admit to hospital

Fatty Liver, Alcoholic Hepatitis

Buzz Words: Steatosis, steatohepatitis, ultrasound shows increased echogenicity, CT shows decreased hepatic attenuation, MRI shows increased fat signal. Yellow discoloration of the liver.

Clinical Presentation: Patients may be asymptomatic or manifest hepatomegaly and abdominal distention. Usually

10%–20% of patients will progress to develop cirrhosis if alcohol consumption is not interrupted.

PPx: Alcohol abstinence

MoD: Substrates of alcohol metabolism (i.e., glycerol 3-phosphate) are used to synthesize triglycerides (TGLs), which accumulate in the cytosol of hepatocytes. Alcohol also activates hormone-sensitive lipase, which increases TGL availability in blood and indirectly inhibits beta oxidation.

Dx:

1. Liver panel with GGT (to quantify alcohol consumption)
2. CT abdomen

Tx/Mgmt: Supportive: Treatment for alcohol substance use disorder (e.g., 12-step program, naltrexone, disulfiram)

Hepatorenal Syndrome

Buzz Words: History of liver dysfunction + acute kidney injury w/o renal organic dysfunction + poor response to fluid therapy (i.e., ascites resistant to diuretics)

Clinical Presentation: Presentation of kidney injury is usually insidious and labs will probably provide identification of disease process before any clinical manifestations become evident. Any patient with liver dysfunction and no known renal dysfunction who develops oliguria should be considered.

It is a diagnosis of exclusion with poor prognosis (mortality rate of 80%). Increased creatinine and blood urea nitrogen. Renal tubular function is preserved, therefore a random urine Na^+ should be less than 20 mEq/L, also proteinuria and hematuria should be absent. Biopsy would show normal renal parenchyma.

If possible, treat/cure cause of hepatic failure. Short-term return of liver function is the best management strategy. Supportive therapy, vasoactive (norepinephrine or vasopressin, midodrine) + albumin *gtt* (aka drip), and renal replacement therapy. Assess candidacy for liver transplant.

MoD: Loss of renal autoregulation as a complication of end-stage liver disease results in intense renal vasoconstriction and reversible ischemic injury (i.e., decreased glomerular filtration rate [GFR] in the absence of shock or renal dysfunction). Patient has poor response to fluid therapy. It is usually precipitated by hypovolemia (GI bleed) or a bacterial infection.

Dx:

1. Basic metabolic panel (BMP)

QUICK TIPS

Increased production of NADH accelerates conversion of DHAP to G3-P, which leads to formation of TGLs.

2. Liver panel
3. UA
4. BNP, echo to r/o heart failure

Tx/Mgmt:
1. Treat etiology of liver failure
2. Albumin
3. Supportive therapy
4. Dialysis
5. Liver transplant

Hepatopulmonary Syndrome

Buzz Words: Hypoxemia + history of liver disease

Clinical Presentation: Pulmonary dysfunction is due to primary liver dysfunction. Patient presents with symptoms of hypoxemia in the setting of liver disease and/or portal hypertension. Workup of the disease will show poor arterial hemoglobin saturation (<96%). Arterial oxygen tension (P_aO_2) while on room air determines severity of disease (mild, >80 mm Hg; moderate, 60–80 mm Hg; severe, <60 mm Hg). Evaluation for shunting is best done by getting a transthoracic contrast echocardiography. Chest imaging has nonspecific results. PFTs might indicated reduced diffusion capacity (low DLCO).

MoD: Pathogenesis is poorly understood. Intrapulmonary vascular dilations cause blood shunting, leading to an increased alveolar-arterial oxygen gradient (≥15 mm Hg). It is associated with increased levels of NO, endothelin-1.

Dx:
1. O_2 sat
2. Arterial line
3. CXR

Tx/Mgmt: Oxygen, liver transplant

Jaundice

Buzz Words: Icterus

Clinical Presentation: Yellow pigmentation occurs in skin and eyes. Unconjugated bilirubin (UGB) is lipophilic and can cross the blood-brain barrier (BBB), leading to kernicterus (accumulation in basal ganglia). Leakage of bile salts, bile acids, and cholesterol into the blood would manifest pruritus and xanthomas.

PPx: Depends on mechanism

MoD: There is accumulation of bilirubin, the end-product of heme degradation. Table 8.15 briefly depicts the distinct mechanisms in which jaundice may be produced.

TABLE 8.15 Mechanisms of Hyperbilirubinemia

Mechanism	Bilirubinemia	Causes
Increased bilirubin production	UCB > CB	Hemolytic anemia, Wilson disease, extravasation of blood
Decreased conjugation	UCB > CB	Physiologic jaundice of the newborn, breast milk jaundice, Gilbert syndrome, or Crigler-Najjar syndrome
Defective conjugation of UCB and secretion of CB	UCB ≈ CB	Viral hepatitis, pregnancy, or TPN
Decreased intrahepatic bile flow	CB > UCB	Primary biliary cirrhosis, drug-related (i.e., oral contraceptives and anabolic steroids), Dubin-Johnson syndrome, or Rotor syndrome
Decreased extrahepatic bile flow	CB > UCB	Gallstone, structural pancreatic anomalies (i.e., cancer, pancreas divisum, strictures), structural biliary anomalies (i.e., cholangiocarcinoma, primary sclerosing cholangitis), *Clonorchis sinensis* (Chinese liver fluke)

CB, Conjugated bilirubin; *TPN*, total parenteral nutrition; *UCB*, unconjugated bilirubin.

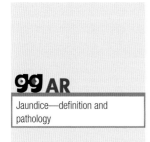

99 AR

Jaundice—definition and pathology

Dx: Adequate identification of risk factors for disease and interpretation of LFTs (see Table 8.12) are key to narrowing down the mechanism for the presentation.

Tx/Mgmt: Phototherapy is a safe method to treat severe unconjugated hyperbilirubinemia in newborns by increasing the solubility of UGB and allowing it to be excreted in urine. Administration of calcium carbonate modestly enhances the effect of phototherapy.

Nonalcoholic Fatty Liver Disease

Buzz Words: Yellow liver + liver fat signal on MRI + echogenicity on ultrasound

Clinical Presentation: Hepatic steatosis occurs in absence of causes for secondary fat accumulation (i.e., alcohol consumption, infection, medications, metabolic derangements). Patients are usually asymptomatic. Ultrasound shows increased echogenicity, CT shows decreased hepatic attenuation, MRI shows increased fat signal. Yellow discoloration of the liver is seen.

PPx: Avoid alcohol consumption

MoD: The primary pathophysiologic component is insulin resistance because it leads to increased TGL synthesis, hepatic uptake of free fatty acids, and lipolysis. Important regulators of hepatic insulin sensitivity are leptin, adiponectin, and resistin. Activation of stellate and hepatic progenitor cells leads to fibrosis of zone 3.

Dx:
1. LFTs
2. Ultrasound
3. MRI

Tx/Mgmt: Weight loss ± orlistat for patients who fail to lose weight through diet and exercise alone; avoid alcohol consumption

Portal Hypertension/Esophageal Varices

Buzz Words: Massive hematemesis, painless upper GI bleed, strange vascular markings around umbilicus

Clinical Presentation: It is usually asymptomatic until complications develop. Varices are seen at sites of portosystemic shunting (esophageal, umbilical, and hemorrhoidal), ascites, and congestive splenomegaly. Complications of portal hypertension include: variceal hemorrhage, ascites, and spontaneous bacterial peritonitis.

PPx: Treat the underlying cause to prevent progression and increased risk of variceal bleeds

MoD: Resistance to hepatic blood flow from intrasinusoidal HTN, which is secondary to regenerative nodule compression. Anastomosis from portal tributaries (i.e., esophageal, paraumbilical, and inferior rectal veins) to the cava system occur to shunt blood away. Resistance may also develop in the prehepatic (i.e., portal vein thrombosis) or posthepatic circulation (i.e., Budd–Chiari syndrome).

Dx:
1. Clinical diagnosis
2. U/S or CT
3. Measurement of hepatic venous pressure gradient with transjugular catheter (although rarely done)

Tx/Mgmt:
1. Management of ascites (fluid and Na^+ restriction + spironolactone, drain if breathing becomes impaired)
2. Prevention of variceal hemorrhage with nonselective beta blockers, ocreotide, and endoscopic ligation
3. Active hemorrhage may be managed with intraluminal compression (i.e., Sengstaken–Blakemore tube) or portocaval shunting (i.e., placement of transjugular intrahepatic portosystemic shunt)

Biliary System

Cholestasis

Buzz Words: "Bile lakes" inside hepatocytes

Clinical Presentation: Patient presents with jaundice with pruritus, malabsorption, cholesterol deposition in the skin (i.e., xanthomas), and light-colored stool (lack of stercobilin).

MoD: Hepatocellular cholestasis can be caused by drugs (i.e., OCCs or anabolic steroids), neonatal hepatitis, or pregnancy-induced (estrogen inhibits bile secretion). Obstructive cholestasis is usually due to blockage of the common bile duct (CBD): gallstone, primary sclerosing cholangitis, biliary atresia, or neoplasm at the head of the pancreas.

Dx: Hyperbilirubinemia, conjugated bilirubin greater than 50%, bilirubinuria, hypercholesterolemia, increased serum ALP and GGT, absent urobilinogen in the urine

Tx/Mgmt: Discontinue causative agent, remove source of obstruction, or treat medically according to inciting event.

99 AR

Liver cholestasis—definition and pathology

Ascending Cholangitis

Buzz Words:
- Charcot triad = fever + abdominal pain + jaundice
- Reynold pentad (suppurative cholangitis) = Charcot's triad + confusion + hypotension

Clinical Presentation: Fever, chills, RUQ abdominal pain, and jaundice occur. Elder or immunosuppressed patients may manifest hypotension only.

MoD: Infection of the biliary tract secondary to obstruction and stasis: Most common pathogens are *E. coli*, *Pseudomonas*, and *Enterobacter.*

Dx:
1. Elevated liver enzymes (especially ALP and GGT)
2. Imaging studies could show biliary dilation and a source of obstruction

Tx/Mgmt:
1. Antibiotic therapy and biliary drainage (endoscopic sphincterotomy with stone extraction ± stent placement). Preferred antibiotics are those with gram-negative and anaerobic coverage: pip/tazo, ampicillin/sulbactam, or ceftriaxone + metronidazole.
2. Urgent (open) biliary decompression is required in patients with failed ERCP or signs of acute suppurative cholangitis.

Cholelithiasis and Acute Cholecystitis

Buzz Words: Double-wall sign on ultrasound, Murphy sign

Clinical Presentation: RUQ pain (prolonged, steady, and severe), fever, nausea, vomiting, anorexia, and tenderness on palpation occur. Risk factors for stone formation are increasing age, obesity, excessive bile salt loss (terminal ileum disease), and female sex. Cholecystectomy is the preferred treatment for patients with symptomatic gallstones, porcelain gallbladder, cholecystitis, and asymptomatic gallstones in patients with SC disease. No surgery is needed for healthy asymptomatic patients. Antibiotic therapy should be initiated and continued until surgical removal with pip/tazo, ampicillin/sulbactam, or ceftriaxone + metronidazole. Patients refusing surgery or with high surgical risk can receive medical management with a bile acid supplement (ursodeoxycholic acid), which reduces biliary cholesterol secretion and increases biliary bile acid concentration. Medical management is associated with a high rate of recurrence.

PPx: (1) Weight loss; (2) avoid fibrates in patients with risk factors because they increase cholesterol content in bile therefore increasing the risk of stone formation; (3) ursodeoxycholic acid.

MoD: Cholesterol stones form in the setting of supersaturation of cholesterol in bile salts, which allows precipitation or gallbladder stasis. Pigmented stones are made of bilirubin and form when unconjugated bilirubin precipitates with calcium. Acute cholecystitis (inflammation of the gallbladder wall) occurs with stone impaction in the cystic duct, leading to gallbladder distention and bacterial overgrowth.

Dx:
1. Ultrasound (gallbladder wall >5 mm or edema), CT has lower sensitivity for small stones
2. Liver panel (normal bilirubin and LFTs)
3. Abdominal x-ray (AXR): pigmented gallstones can be visualized on abdominal films (cholesterol stones are radiolucent)

Tx/Mgmt:
1. Ursodeoxycholic acid
2. Antibiotics
3. Cholecystectomy

Choledocholithiasis

Buzz Words: CBD greater than 1 cm, stone in biliary tree

Clinical Presentation: RUQ or epigastric abdominal pain, jaundice, nausea, and vomiting

PPx: Weight loss and avoidance of fibrates in patients at risk for developing gallstones

MoD: Intermittent obstruction of the CBD occurs by a gallstone. Progression of obstruction can lead to acute cholangitis or acute pancreatitis.

QUICK TIPS
Clinical pearl: Pain from biliary colic is intermittent and resolves completely when the gallbladder relaxes, while pain from acute cholecystitis prevails for >4–6 h.

Gallstones (cholelithiasis)—definition and pathology

Acute cholecystitis—pathophysiology, symptoms, and diagnosis

Dx:
- Ultrasound identifies risk of having choledocholithiasis.
- Patients with prior cholecystectomy should undergo MRCP or endoscopic ultrasound to better assess possibility of choledocholithiasis.

Tx/Mgmt: Treatment is selected by risk of choledocholithiasis. Anytime that the abdomen is entered to perform a cholecystectomy, performance of a cholangiography or CBD exploration may be done to better assess risk:
- High-risk: ERCP with sphincterotomy + elective laparoscopic cholecystectomy
- Intermediate-risk: MRCP or elective laparoscopic cholecystectomy + intra-op evaluation of CBD
- Low-risk: direct cholecystectomy w/o additional imaging

Cholestasis Due to Parenteral Nutrition

Buzz Words:
N/A

Clinical Presentation: Hepatocellular and cholestatic injury that occurs after prolonged TPN (usually >2 weeks). Males > females and children > adults. Low birth weight, prematurity, duration of TPN, and intestinal stasis are significant risk factors.

PPx: Frequently assess the plausibility of reinitiating enteral nutrition to avoid prolonged periods of TPN.

MoD: Injury may vary widely between steatosis and mild hepatocellular damage to cirrhosis. Hepatic changes are related with prolonged rest of the enterohepatic circulation, changes in the nutritive composition, and the administration of nutrients from the hepatic artery rather than the portal vein.

Dx: Increase in serum conjugated bilirubin (>2 mg/dL), spike in liver enzymes, and exclusion other causes of hepatotoxic injury.

Tx/Mgmt: Cessation of TPN and treat small bowel bacterial overgrowth (metronidazole).

Gallstone Ileus

Buzz Words: Pneumobilia + intestinal obstruction

Clinical Presentation: Elderly woman with episodic subacute bowel obstruction. High rate of morbidity and mortality occurs.

PPx: Weight loss and avoidance of fibrates in patients at risk for developing gallstones

MoD: Mechanical bowel obstruction caused by impaction of a gallstone (usually >2 cm) at the ileocecal valve. These larger stone usually make their way to the bowel by way of a biliary-enteric fistula.

Dx: Abdominal CT is the preferred imaging study and would show intestinal obstruction with gallstone(s) in the ileum. Pneumobilia (air in the gallbladder) may be an associated finding secondary to the biliary-enteric fistula.

Tx/Mgmt: Surgical: Obstruction should be relieved with an enterotomy and stone removal. Patients with low-risk profiles should also have a concomitant cholecystectomy and closure of the biliary-enteric fistula.

Mirizzi Syndrome

Buzz Words: Obstructive jaundice, fever, RUQ pain

Clinical Presentation: Mirizzi syndrome occurs when a gallstone is lodged in the cystic duct. It has same risk factors as for cholecystolithiasis.

PPx: Weight loss and avoidance of fibrates

MoD: Hepatic duct obstruction occurs by extrinsic compression from an impacted stone in the cystic duct. It is associated with higher frequency of gallbladder cancer.

Dx: Elevated ALP + hyperbilirubinemia + RUQ ultrasound showing intrahepatic biliary dilatation and lith in the cystic duct

Tx/Mgmt: Laparoscopic cholecystectomy, during which the level of erosion and damage to the hepatic duct should be assessed to determine if repair is necessary.

Primary Biliary Cirrhosis

Buzz Words: Pruritus that does not improve with antihistamines

Clinical Presentation: Middle-aged woman of northern European descent who presents with pruritus, fatigue, and xanthelasma. Abdominal exam shows hepatomegaly and RUQ tenderness to palpation. May be associated with osteopenia, hyperlipidemia, and other autoimmune conditions (i.e., autoimmune hepatitis and Sjögren syndrome). It may progress to cirrhosis.

MoD: T-cell–mediated cholangiocyte damage, which allows bile leakage into the bloodstream. The etiology of pruritus is uncertain; it may be due to the increased production of endogenous opioids and retained bile salts.

Dx: Usually, ALP and GGT are elevated. Biopsy shows inflammation around bile ducts.

QUICK TIPS

Extrinsic compression of the HEPATIC duct, not the common bile duct.

AR

Primary biliary cholangitis—
causes, symptoms, diagnosis,
treatment, and pathology

Tx/Mgmt: Ursodeoxycholic acid is the best initial therapy. In patients with refractory disease, cholestyramine may reduce pruritus and slow down disease progression. Liver transplant in end-stage liver dysfunction.

Primary Sclerosing Cholangitis

Buzz Words: Beading of the bile ducts, "onion skin" fibrosis of the bile ducts

Clinical Presentation: Young adult male patient presents with jaundice, pruritus, and hepatosplenomegaly. It is associated with IBD in 70% of cases (ulcerative colitis > Crohn disease). May progress to portal hypertension, liver cirrhosis, and cholangiocarcinoma.

MoD: Obliterative, interrupted fibrosis of bile ducts (both intra- and extrahepatic). Association with HLA-DR52a (100% of the time), HLA-B8, HLA-Dr3, and HLA-Cw7 subtypes. These patients also have elevated IgM and p-ANCAs (80% of the time). Pruritus occurs due to bile salt deposition into the skin.

Dx:

1. Labs consistent with cholestasis; conjugated bilirubin greater than 50%, bilirubinuria, absent urine urobilinogen, increased ALP and GGT
2. ERCP would show narrowing and dilation of the bile ducts (*beading*)

Tx/Mgmt: Immunosuppressants (steroids, axathioprine, and MTX) and liver transplant

AR

Primary sclerosing cholangitis—
pathophysiology and symptoms

Disorders of the Pancreas

Acute Pancreatitis

Buzz Words:

- **Acute pancreatitis:** epigastric pain + acute abdomen (<24-hours pain) + radiating straight through back + N/V + amylase/lipase (lipase is more specific) + hypocalcemia
- Edematous pancreatitis: Alcohol + gallstones + panc + high hematocrit →
- **Hemorrhagic pancreatitis:** Edematous pancreatitis + **low** hematocrit + refractory to treatment
- **Pancreatic abscess** Persistent fever + leukocytosis 10 days s/p pancreatitis + pus collection
- **Pancreatic pseudocyst:** Mass in pancreas + 5 **weeks s/p pancreatitis** + upper abdominal trauma + early satiety/vague discomfort due to fluid around pancreas

Clinical Presentation: Acute and severe epigastric abdominal pain that irradiates posteriorly, N/V. Tenderness is felt on palpation. Might also manifest signs of volume depletion. Classically described signs are Grey–Turner (flank hemorrhage) and Cullen (periumbilical hemorrhage).

Increased serum amylase and lipase; lipase more specific. Imaging studies (CT/ultrasound) are necessary to determine if a stone is the culprit and if removal is needed. Magnetic resonance cholangiopancreatography (MRCP) gives the best image of the ductal structure of both pancreas and biliary systems. In the setting of necrosis, sampling by aspiration is warranted to rule out superinfection.

Replete intravascular volume! Dehydration is the most common cause of mortality. Rest the pancreas (NPO) and provide pain management. ERCP allows for removal and dilation of strictures. Surgical debridement is indicated in the setting of infected necrosis that does not improve with broad-spectrum antibiotics.

PPx: Avoidance of alcohol

MoD: Many causes of pancreatitis (Box 8.2): Identication of the cause allows for adequacy in management. There must be activation of enzymes within the pancreatic ductal system to produce pancreatitis (i.e., obstruction, activation by calcium, drug toxicity, etc.). This event will initiate a systemic inflammatory response, which may set the setting for disseminated intravascular coagulopathy (DIC), shock, and sepsis. A significant amount of peripancreatic fluid accumulates (*third space*) as the pancreas digests itself. Splenic vein thrombosis may occur, since most of

---

FOR THE WARDS

Know the Ranson criteria

QUICK TIPS

In pancreatitis, serum amylase is normal if (1) there is hyperlipidemia (interferes with amylase production), (2) increased urinary excretion of amylase, (3) near destruction of pancreatic parenchyma.

BOX 8.2 Common Causes of Acute Pancreatitis

Gallstone obstruction
Alcohol
Drugs: azathioprine, furosemide, thiazides, trimethoprim-sulfamethoxazole, valproate
Hypertriglyceridemia
Hypercalcemia
Structural pancreatic anomalies: cancer, pancreas divisum, strictures
Recent endoscopic retrograde cholangiopancreatography, gastric, or biliary surgery
Infection: Coxsackie virus, mumps, *Mycoplasma pneumoniae*
Trauma (i.e., seat belt injury)

the pancreatic venous drainage goes to the splenic vein (classic finding: antral varices w/o esophageal varices).

Dx:

1. Lipase/amylase
2. CT
3. Ultrasound to find out cause (e.g., gallstones)

Tx/Mgmt:

1. NPO, NG suction, IV fluids
2. Drain if pancreatic abscess

Chronic Pancreatitis

Buzz Words: Radiographic dyes show a "chain of lakes" appearance in the major duct + dystrophic calcifications + repeated episodes of past pancreatitis + steatorrhea + hypocalcemia + diabetes + constant epigastric pain

Clinical Presentation: Patient (men > women) presents with debilitating abdominal pain and history of repeated episodes of pancreatitis. Patient may manifest deficiency in any of the following vitamins: A, B_{12}, D, E, or K (see Table 8.10 for manifestations). Amylase and lipase will probably be within normal range (no enzymes left to release). Dystrophic calcifications may be seen on abdominal films or CT scans. Most accurate test is the secretin stimulation test (given IV). The bentiromide test assesses the ability of chymotrypsin to cleave orally administered bentiromide to para-aminobenzoic acid (measured in urine). Oral supplementation of pancreatic enzymes and fat-soluble vitamins are taken. Simple analgesics or NSAIDs are used. Refractory pain management may be mediated with ganglion block with injection guided by endoscopic ultrasound. It has a poor prognosis; 50% mortality within 10 years. Can lead to splenic vein thrombosis.

PPx: Treatment of acute pancreatitis, avoidance of alcohol

MoD: Repeated attack of acute pancreatitis produce duct obstruction. Calcification and dilation of the major ducts occur. Type 1 DM may develop in 70% of cases of chronic pancreatitis.

Dx: CT and/or ERCP

Tx/Mgmt:

1. Insulin for diabetes
2. Pancreatic enzymes for steatorrhea
3. Pain control
4. Surgery to drain pancreatic duct

Hereditary Pancreatitis

Buzz Words: Pancreatitis in child, family history of similar episodes

Clinical Presentation: Pancreatitis occurs before 20 years of age. One-third of patients develops pancreatic insufficiency and are at a greater risk for pancreatic cancer.

PPx: Avoid alcohol, smoking, limit dietary fat intake, and supplement with daily multivitamins and antioxidants

MoD: Mutations in the serine protease 1 gene (*PRSS1*) may promote premature activation of trypsinogen or interfere with the inactivation of trypsin. Other genes that may be implicated are *SPINK1, CFTR, CPA1*, and *CLDN2*. Autosomal dominant inheritance.

Dx: Genetic testing should be done for young patients in whom a discernible cause is not identified.

Tx/Mgmt: Management is identical to previously discussed for acute pancreatitis. Pancreatectomy with islet auto-transplantation may be considered for patients with opioid addiction due to chronic pancreatitis.

Pancreatic Cyst/Pseudocyst

Buzz Words: Persistent increase in serum amylase more than 10 days, walled-off pancreatic necrosis, hemosuccus pancreaticus

Clinical Presentation: Development of a fluid-filled abdominal mass in a patient recovering from acute pancreatitis (20% of cases) associated with amylase levels, which have remained elevated for a prolonged period of time. Amylase should return to normal levels in 2–4 days. These cysts can suffer spontaneous infection. Involvement of adjacent vessels could result in a pseudoaneurysm, which may rupture and produce GI bleed (hemosuccus pancreaticus).

MoD: The amount of amylase in the fluid surpasses the renal clearance of amylase.

Dx: Abdominal CT scan

Tx/Mgmt:
- Less than 5 cm f/u with more scans, will most likely resolve on its own.
- Greater than 5 cm or symptomatic lesion, requires guided drainage (endoscopic-ultrasound or CT).

Pancreatic Insufficiency

Clinical Presentation: Mild insufficiency might manifest abdominal discomfort and bloating while severe insufficiency would manifest malabsorption with steatorrhea, fat-soluble vitamin deficiency, and vitamin B_{12} deficiency.

MoD: Chronic pancreatitis, cystic fibrosis, hemochromatosis, and Shwachman-Diamond syndrome. Malabsorption occurs when greater than 90% of the exocrine function has been destroyed.

Dx: Decreased fecal elastase-1

Tx/Mgmt: Similar management as described for chronic pancreatitis

Traumatic and Mechanical Disorders

Post–Gastric Surgery Syndromes

Blind Loop Syndrome

Clinical Presentation: Patient who had a gastrectomy (Billroth II or Roux-en-Y procedure) in the past who presents with foul-smelling diarrhea, weight loss, and weakness. Patients may present with megaloblastic anemia (secondary to folate and B_{12} deficiency), peripheral neuropathy (B_{12} deficiency), and steatorrhea (from deconjugation of bile salts).

MoD: Bacterial overgrowth in the segment of bowel that is excluded from the pass of chyme. These bacteria can interfere with folate absorption, vitamin B_{12} absorption, and/or enterohepatic circulation.

Dx: B12 levels

Tx/Mgmt: Broad-spectrum antibiotics are used to halt bacteria overgrowth. Definitive treatment requires a second procedure to avoid having a blind loop of bowel present.

Adhesions

Clinical Presentation: It is most commonly asymptomatic. Symptomatic patients may present with signs and symptoms of bowel obstruction, multiple miscarriages, or failure to conceive.

PPx: Meticulous surgical technique with minimal manipulation of peritoneal surfaces. Solid or liquid barriers can be used to prevent adhesion formation after abdominal surgery.

MoD: Adhesions form after any sort of manipulation of the intra-abdominal organs during surgery. They are considered to be the normal peritoneal response to surgical injury. It is a common cause of bowel obstruction.

Dx: Clinical suspicion + confirmation on surgical exploration

Tx/Mgmt: Surgical lysis of adhesions is indicated in patients who manifest bowel obstruction or with the purpose of aiding in conception and improvement of fertility.

Hernias

Direct Inguinal Hernia

Buzz Words: The defect in the abdominal wall is inside the Hesselbach triangle (i.e., medial to the inferior epigastric vessels).

Clinical Presentation: Older male patient presents with bulge in groin, which protrudes during abdominal straining. These hernias rarely occur in women or children.

PPx: Dietary habits that prevent constipation and the excessive straining

MoD: These lesions tend to be acquired over time as a result of excessive pressure and tension on the abdominal wall.

Dx: Clinical diagnosis

Tx/Mgmt: Surgical repair of the defect. Patients with signs of incarceration or bowel obstruction should be taken to the OR urgently. The operative technique depends on the surgeon's level of expertise and comfort. Table 8.16 mentions some of the techniques that can be performed.

Indirect Inguinal Hernia

Buzz Words: Defect in the abdominal wall is outside Hesselbach triangle, through the inguinal canal and lateral to the inferior epigastric vessels.

Inguinal hernia

QUICK TIPS

Hesselbach triangle = inguinal ligament + rectus abdominis + inferior epigastric vessels

TABLE 8.16 Repair of Inguinal Hernias (For the Wards Only!)

Repair Type	Procedure
Classic tissue repairs	Halstead repair
	Bassini repair
	McVay repair
	Marcy repair
	Shouldice repair
Anterior mesh repairs	Lichtenstein repair
	Mesh-plug repair
	Prolene hernia system
Preperitoneal repairs	Stoppa repair
	Kuggel repair
Laparoscopic repairs	Totally extraperitoneal repair
	Transabdominal preperitoneal repair

Clinical Presentation: Young patient presents with a bulge in the groin that protrudes during abdominal straining. These hernias occur more commonly on the right side. It is the most common groin hernia in men and women.

PPx:

Dietary habits that prevent constipation and excessive straining

MoD: Congenital defect in which the processus vaginalis remains patent. Intraabdominal organs protrude through both the internal and external inguinal rings.

Dx: Clinical diagnosis

Tx/Mgmt: Patients with signs of incarceration or bowel obstruction should be taken to the OR urgently. (See Table 8.16.)

Femoral Hernia

Buzz Words: Reducible bulge in the groin

Clinical Presentation: Bulge in the groin (usually lower than inguinal hernias), which protrudes during abdominal straining. These hernias occur most commonly in women. Femoral hernias are highly susceptible to incarceration due to the rigid structures that surround the femoral canal.

MoD: Similar to direct inguinal hernias, these are acquired defects secondary to laxity in the abdominal wall. The defect usually occurs near the attachment of the transversus abdominis muscle onto Cooper ligament (i.e., through the femoral ring), with abdominal organs going into the femoral canal.

Dx: The defect in the abdominal wall is inferior to the inguinal ligament.

Tx/Mgmt: Surgical repair: The femoral hernia can be repaired from different approaches (i.e., inguinal, thigh, laparoscopic, or abdominal) as long as the femoral canal is occluded.

Umbilical Hernia

Buzz Words: Periumbilical bulge that protrudes with straining

Clinical Presentation: Periumbilical bulge that protrudes with straining. Rare hernias in adults, most commonly present in newborns. Females > males. It is associated with obesity, ascites, and pregnancy. Incarceration is common in men.

PPx: Dietary habits that prevent constipation and the excessive straining

MoD: Dilation of the umbilical ring and protrusion of omentum (most commonly) into the hernial sac. Ascites in

---

MNEMONIC

Remember the contents of the femoral triangle from lateral to medial with the mnemonic **NAVEL**: femoral **N**erve, **A**rtery, **V**ein, **E**mpty space (where femoral hernias occur), and **L**ymph nodes the setting of preexisting umbilical hernia produces thinning of the skin and increases risk of spontaneous rupture.

Dx: Clinical diagnosis

Tx/Mgmt: Asymptomatic hernias do not require repair. Small symptomatic hernias can be repaired quickly through an open approach, while larger defects are better handled via a laparoscopic approach.

Penetrating Wounds, Abdominal

Buzz Words: Hemodynamic instability s/p abdominal trauma (knife or gunshot)

Clinical Presentation: It is an emergent condition that requires immediate laparotomy. Depending on the awareness and neurologic status of the patient, obtaining a description of the mechanisms of injury may be a possibility.

MoD: Penetrating abdominal trauma

Dx: FAST (focused abdominal sonography for trauma) can be done at the bedside to evaluate for presence of hemoperitoneum. Multidetector CT is another quick imaging technique that might help to show whether the integrity of the abdominal wall is compromised. On initial physical examination it is crucial to identify if the abdominal cavity was penetrated.

Tx/Mgmt: Adequate fluid resuscitation, initiate broad-spectrum antibiotics, provide adequate pain management, and perform emergent laparotomy if indicated (Box 8.3). Reporting of abdominal stab wounds to local authorities might be warranted.

Perforation of Hollow Viscus and Blunt Trauma

Buzz Words: Free abdominal air, pneumoperitoneum, mesenteric air, fecal matter in peritoneal cavity

Clinical Presentation: It is an emergent condition that requires immediate laparotomy. History of abdominal trauma

---

BOX 8.3 Indications for Emergent Exploratory Laparotomy

Evisceration of intra-abdominal organs
Signs of gastrointestinal hemorrhage
Hemodynamic instability
Signs of peritonitis
Impalement

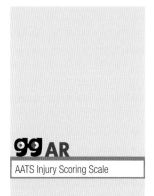

AATS Injury Scoring Scale

(penetrating or blunt) + signs and symptoms of acute abdomen.

MoD: Trauma

Dx: Abdominal CT scans should be performed only in stable patients, would show discontinuity in the wall of hollow viscus, mesenteric hematoma, free intraabdominal fluid, signs of active bleeding, or extravasation of intravenous contrast.

Tx/Mgmt: Emergent exploratory laparotomy: Mesenteric and intramural hematomas can resolve without the need for surgery.

Perforation/Rupture of Esophagus (Boerhaave Syndrome)

Buzz Words: Pneumomediastinum + L pneumothorax in the patient who was vomiting earlier that day.

Clinical Presentation: Acute, intense retrosternal pain that begins during vomiting and is aggravated by swallowing. May be accompanied by hoarseness, back pain, subcutaneous emphysema, and dyspnea. It is often associated with alcohol intoxication or bulimia in young patients. Can also occur during endoscopic examinations.

MoD: Spontaneous full-thickness rupture of the esophagus after forceful retching. Results in contamination of the mediastinal cavity.

Dx: CXR may show left-sided pneumothorax, pneumomediastinum, or esophageal thickening. Barium should not be used as a contrast medium for fluoroscopy.

Tx/Mgmt:
1. NPO, nutritional support, broad-spectrum antibiotics, and IV PPI are the mainstays of medical management
2. Surgical repair within 24 hours for patients with perforation

Congenital Disorders

Intussusception

Buzz Words: Colicky abdominal pain + patients have to squat to relieve pain + 6–12 month old + vague mass on right side of abdomen + empty RLQ + currant jelly stools + preceded by viral infection + bull's-eye sign on ultrasound → intussusception

Clinical Presentation: Child presents with intermittent abdominal pain, distention, cramping, vomiting, and bloody stools. Some cases have been associated with the

rotavirus live-attenuated vaccine. Can also have association with recent viral infection.

MoD: Three-quarters of cases are idiopathic, while the
other quarter have an underlying condition that creates
a nidus for intussusception. Meckel diverticulum is a
common cause of intussusception. The overlying bowel
loop entraps the mesentery, occluding blood flow to the
inner loop.

Dx:
1. Abdominal ultrasound may detect layers of intestine
   within another loop of bowel, often described as
   coiled-spring lesion or *bull's-eye* sign
2. Barium or air enema

Tx/Mgmt:
1. Barium or air enema
2. Surgery if reduction not achieved

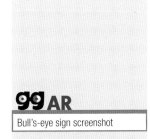
Bull's-eye sign screenshot

Necrotizing Enterocolitis

Buzz Words:
- Premature infants + first feed + feeding intolerance + abdominal distention + **bleeding stools** +
  rapidly dropping platelet count (a sign of sepsis in
  babies)
- A 5-day-old former 33-week preemie develops
  bloody diarrhea
- AXR with air in bowel wall and portal veins + preemie + vomiting + leukocytosis
- Nonpreemie + heart condition (e.g., DiGeorge) + any
  condition that predisposes to hypoperfusion + poor
  feeding + bloody stools

Clinical Presentation: Necrotizing enterocolitis (NEC) is the
destruction of colon by infection. Occurs in **premature**
infant who develops abdominal distention, tenderness,
vomiting, rectal bleeding, and diarrhea. It is associated
with pneumatosis intestinalis on AXR.

MoD: Ischemic necrosis of the mucosa, which allows bacterial invasion (e.g., *Staphylococcus epidermidis*), with
subsequent dissection of gas into the muscularis and
portal system. Immaturity of GI tract appears to be a
significant risk factor.

Dx: Clinical diagnosis: Abdominal films show pneumatosis
intestinalis; labs show thrombocytopenia, metabolic
acidosis, and blood in stool samples.

Pneumatosis intestinalis AXR:

Tx/Mgmt:
1. NPO
2. broad-spectrum Abx, IV fluids/nutrition (i.e., TPN)

3. If abdominal wall erythema, air in biliary tree, pneumatosis intestinalis or pneumoperitoneum → surgery

Volvulus

Buzz Words:
- *Coffee bean*–shaped bowel on abdominal film, *whirl* sign (twisting of mesentery), loss of haustral markings
- Elderly patient + tympanic air-fluid levels + distended colon/abdomen + tenderness + air-filled loop in RUQ that tapers down toward the LLQ with a parrot's beak

Clinical Presentation: Elderly patient with slowly progressive abdominal pain who finally develops signs and symptoms of bowel obstruction (discussed previously) and significant abdominal distention. It has significant mortality risk (20%–25%).

MoD: Bowel twists around its own mesentery. Common causes are chronic constipation, laxative abuse, fiber-rich diet, and Chagas disease.

Dx:
1. AXR (air-filled coffee-bean shape RUQ)
2. CT abdomen
3. Proctosigmoidscopy

Tx/Mgmt:
1. Rectal tube
2. Proctosigmoidoscopic exam
3. Flexible sigmoidoscopy in attempt to untwist the segment of bowel, followed by rectal tube placement
4. Exploratory laparotomy reserved for failed endoscopic correction

99 AR

Abdominal film of patient with sigmoid volvulus

Annular Pancreas

Buzz Words: Pancreas around the duodenum on imaging

Clinical Presentation: Most patients are asymptomatic but some infants may manifest abdominal distention, vomiting, and feeding intolerance. This malformation predisposes to pancreatitis and duodenal obstruction from subsequent fibrosis. It is associated with Down syndrome, esophageal/duodenal atresia, polyhydramnios, and Meckel diverticulum.

MoD: Failure of the ventral bud to rotate around the duodenum, forming a ring around the second portion of the duodenum

Dx: AXR, ultrasound

Tx/Mgmt: Correction is done by surgically bypassing the annulus (i.e., duodenoduodenostomy in children and duodenojejunostomy or gastrojejunostomy in adults). Modification of the structural configuration of the pancreas is strongly discouraged.

Biliary Atresia

Buzz Words: Neonatal conjugated hyperbilirubinemia

Clinical Presentation: Jaundice in newborn is accompanied by acholic stools and dark-colored urine. Abdominal exam is notable for splenomegaly and a firm liver. It is associated with lateralization anomalies (i.e., situs inversus and asplenia).

MoD: Inflammatory process that causes obstruction or absence of bile duct. Mutations of the *CFC1* gene (regulates L-R distribution in embryonic development) have been associated with biliary atresia.

Dx: Conjugated hyperbilirubinemia: Cholangiogram is gold standard for confirmation.

Tx/Mgmt: Kasai procedure (hepatoportoenterostomy) may confer palliation of obstruction initially. Nonetheless, most patients (60%–80%) will eventually require liver transplantation.

99 AR
Biliary atresia—definition and pathophysiology

Cleft Lip and/or Palate

Buzz Words: Complicated breastfeeding, nasal speech and communication between nasal and oral cavities

Clinical Presentation: Incidence is 1:800 live births. Cleft lip and palate is the most common presentation, occurring in 50% of cases. Cleft lip alone occurs in 25% of cases and is more common in males. Cleft palate alone occurs in 25% of cases and is more common in females.

Complications from cleft lip/palate include inadequate suction during breastfeeding, malocclusion, speech problems, and eustachian tube dysfunction (i.e., chronic otitits media).

PPx: Avoid smoking and drugs known to cause this malformation during pregnancy.

MoD: Failure in fusion of facial processes. Associated with teratogenic drug exposure during pregnancy (e.g., phenytoin, valproic acid, thalidomide). Defect is present in 60%–80% of patients with Patau syndrome (trisomy 13), Potter sequence (think oligohydramnios), and CATCH-22.

Dx: Physical exam

Tx/Mgmt: Surgical closure of the defect is the preferred modality of treatment. Cleft lip is usually closed at 3 months of age; cleft palate closure follows usually before 1 year of age. Missing teeth should be replaced by prosthesis. Sometimes palatal function is not restored completely and speech therapy is required.

Esophageal Atresia

Buzz Words: Polyhydramnios, drooling, and cyanosis with feeds

Clinical Presentation: Newborn presents with excessive drooling. Breastfeeding attempt produces coughing, perioral cyanosis, and a drop in hemoglobin saturation. Commonly this will present in association to a tracheoesophageal fistula (85% of cases). Tracheal esophageal fistula/esophageal atresia (TEF/EA) form part of the VACTERL association.

MoD: Polyhydramnios develops due to inability of the fetus to swallow amniotic fluid.

Dx: X-ray showing nasogastric tube in the atretic esophageal pouch after an attempt to pass the tube into the stomach

Tx/Mgmt: Primary anastomosis when the distance between the proximal and distal esophageal segments allows

MNEMONIC

VACTERL association: Vertebral anomalies, Anal atresia, Cardiac defects, Tracheoesophageal fistula, Esophageal atresia, Renal anomalies, and Limb defects

Malrotation Without Volvulus

Buzz Words: Bands of peritoneum attaching the cecum to the lateral abdominal wall, duodenum with a *corkscrew* appearance, incomplete rotation around the superior mesenteric artery (SMA)

Clinical Presentation: Vomiting, abdominal distention, and tenderness occur. Usually occurs in patients with other congenital anomalies.

MoD: Incomplete rotation of the cecocolic limb around the SMA, which means that the cecum ends in the mid-upper abdomen and is attached to the R lateral abdominal wall by bands of peritoneum (Ladd bands). These bands cross the duodenum causing intrinsic obstruction and compression. In malrotation, the third portion of the duodenum does not pass between the abdominal aorta and the SMA.

Dx: Contrast enema shows a high, medially directed cecum.

Tx/Mgmt: Ladd procedure consists in division of Ladd bands + widening of the mediastinum + appendectomy + fixation of the cecum and colon in their correct anatomical location.

Meckel Diverticulum

Buzz Words: Failed obliteration, blind pouch connected to ileum, pancreatic acini in mucosa, ectopic gastric mucosa, fecal matter in umbilical area at birth

Clinical Presentation: Painless melena and iron deficiency anemia occur during the first years of life. Another presentation could be bowel obstruction secondary to small bowel intussusception (diverticulum functions as nidus). It is the most common congenital anomaly of the small bowel. A ligament between the terminal ileum and umbilicus may be identified during surgical exploration of the abdomen.

MoD: Omphalomesenteric (vitelline) duct remnant, which usually obliterates by the seventh week of embryonic development. Pouch may contain retained gastric (most common), pancreatic, colonic, jejunal, duodenal, or endometrial tissues. Ectopic gastric acid produces mucosal ulceration and bleeding.

Dx: ^{99m}Tc nuclear scan to identify gastric mucosa.

Tx/Mgmt: Segmental bowel resection in all symptomatic patients or young patients due to potential for complications.

QUICK TIPS

The rule of 2's: 2 inches long, 2 feet from ileocecal valve, 2% of population, 2% are symptomatic

Pyloric Stenosis

Buzz Words: Projectile vomiting, palpable "olive-like" RUQ abdominal mass

Clinical Presentation: Baby (3–5 weeks of age) w/ forceful nonbilious vomiting that occurs after feeding. Abdominal exam is notable for hyperperistalsis and palpable pyloric sphincter in 70% of cases. Males > females.

MoD: Hypertrophy of the pyloric sphincter, usually not present at birth but develops over the first 3–5 weeks of life. NO synthase deficiency precipitates the disease.

Dx: Abdominal ultrasound shows increased pyloric muscle thickness length and diameter.

Tx/Mgmt:
1. Laparoscopic pyloromyotomy
2. Correction of electrolyte abnormalities and fluid repletion

3. Early reinitiation of feeding

Gastric Outlet Obstruction

Buzz Words: Enlarged gastric bubble in abdominal film

Clinical Presentation: Epigastric abdominal pain, nausea, and vomiting occur after eating. Also related to early satiety, weight loss, and abdominal distention.

MoD: Mechanical obstruction of the stomach and duodenum. Common causes of compression are pancreatic cancer, gastric lymphoma, Crohn disease, peptic ulcer disease, fibrosis after caustic injury, gastric bezoars, and percutaneous endoscopic gastrostomy tube migration.

Dx: Metabolic derangements from excessive vomiting are hypokalemia and hypochloremic metabolic alkalosis. Abdominal CT will most likely point out the cause of compression.

Tx/Mgmt: Medical management consists of NPO + nasogastric tube, address electrolyte and metabolic imbalances, fluid replacement, and IV PPI. Nonsurgical candidates (patient-determined or disease-determined) can have a self-expanding metal stent placed endoscopically.

Tracheoesophageal Fistula

Buzz Words: Cyanosis during breastfeeding

Clinical Presentation: Coughing and cyanosis occur after feeding in newborn. If the defect is not corrected, aspiration pneumonia will ensue.

MoD: Cyanosis is secondary to laryngospasm to protect airway after aspiration of milk/formula.

Dx: Fistula can normally be identified in a lateral chest film. Fluoroscopic imaging studies are performed with water-soluble contrast agents (DO NOT USE BARIUM) to avoid chemical pneumonitis.

Tx/Mgmt: Surgical ligation of the fistula through a cervical approach when the fistula is isolated. In cases with EA, resection and primary anastomosis of the esophageal segments is preferred.

Wilson Disease

Buzz Words: Hepatic dysfunction between 8 and 16 years + young child + Kayser–Fleischer ring + wing-beating tremors + seizures + ataxia + dysarthria + tremor + dystonia + Parkinsonism + tics

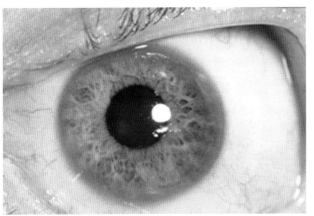

FIG. 8.1 Kayser-Fleischer ring. (From OpenStax: http://cnx.org/content/m15007/latest. Used under Creative Commons Attribution 4.0 License.)

Clinical Presentation: Wilson disease is a disorder of copper regulation, whereby a mutation on chromosome 13 leads to accumulation of copper in hepatocytes, cornea, basal ganglia, and kidneys. This leads to many unique signs and symptoms, such as Kayser-Fleischer ring and wing-beating tremor (Fig. 8.1). The diagnostic lab results are also classically tested. Make sure to know that Wilson disease is present when ceruloplasmin is low and urine copper is high. Also be sure to memorize treatment options, since this disease is so frequently tested.

PPx: Low-copper diet

MoD: AR mutation in *ATP7B* gene (chromosome 13) → copper accumulates in hepatocytes, then cornea, basal ganglia and kidneys

Dx:
1. Serum ceruloplasmin (low)
2. Urine copper (high)
3. Liver biopsy

Tx/Mgm:
1. Chelation with penicillamine, trientene, and zinc
2. Low-copper diet
3. Liver transplant in advanced disease

Adverse Drug Effects

Drug-Induced Changes in Motility

Chronic Laxative Abuse

Buzz Words: Factitious diarrhea, contracting alkalosis

Clinical Presentation: Woman who works in health care with profuse watery diarrhea associated with cramping abdominal pain. Signs of dehydration may be present.

MoD: Voluntary abuse of osmotic laxatives (i.e., magnesium, sorbitol, lactulose, polyethylene glycol)

Dx: Hypokalemia and metabolic (contraction) alkalosis. Those abusing magnesium cathartics will have hypermagnesemia. Stool osmotic gap usually exceeds 75 mOsm/kg. Diagnosis of exclusion after ruling out organic causes of diarrhea.

Tx/Mgmt: Electrolyte and fluid replacement, referral to psychiatric evaluation

Opioids

Buzz Words: N/A

Clinical Presentation: Patient with chronic pain managed with opioids or substance abuse disorder who complains of abdominal distention, failure to pass flatus, and diffuse abdominal pain.

PPx: Prophylactic laxative therapy for patients requiring chronic pain management

MoD: Opioids inhibit bowel motility through direct and anticholinergic mechanisms. Longer transit times allow for excessive reabsorption of fluids from feces, creating rock-solid fecal matter and impaction. In the setting of chronic opioid abuse, tolerance does not develop to constipation (or miosis either).

Dx: Clinical diagnosis

Tx/Mgmt: Cathartic, stool softener, or osmotic laxatives to rehydrate fecal matter and allow for uneventful passing.

Drug-Induced Gastritis, Duodenitis, and Peptic Ulcer (NSAIDs)

Buzz Words: N/A

Clinical Presentation: Same presentation as that described previously for gastritis, duodenitis, and peptic ulcer disease.

PPx: Use of selective cyclo-oxygenase-2 (COX-2) inhibitors (i.e., celexocib)

MoD: The arachidonic acid degradation pathway allows the formation of proinflammatory and physiologically active molecules that aid in platelet aggregation, vasoconstriction, and protection of gastric mucosa. Nonselective inhibition of COX from NSAIDs reduces the stimulus to maintain mucous production, mucosal perfusion, and increases gastric acid production.

Dx: Clinical suspicion and signs of improvement when the drug is discontinued.

Tx/Mgmt: Avoiding nonselective COX inhibitors

Drug-Induced Hepatitis

Buzz Words: Symptoms or abnormal labs that appear to have a time relationship with initiation of a drug.

Clinical Presentation: Most patients are asymptomatic, within those who do manifest symptoms the most common would be nausea, vomiting, RUQ pain, jaundice, malaise, low-grade fever, acholic stools, and choluria.

PPx: Awareness of marginal liver function and avoidance of hepatotoxic drugs in these patients.

MoD: Drug-induced injury may be classified in several ways, perhaps the most useful is by clinical presentation: hepatocellular, cholestatic, or mixed injury. Table 8.17 presents the most common causative agents by method injury.

Dx: Hepatocellular injury will be characterized by elevation in ALT and AST more than 3× the upper limit of normal (ULN). Cholestatic injury will be characterized by elevation of alkaline phosphatase (ALP) more than 2× ULN. Hyperbilirubinemia will be present in both injuries.

Tx/Mgmt: Withdrawal of drug thought to have caused the injury.

Drug-Induced Pancreatitis (e.g., Thiazides)

Buzz Words: Elevated serum amylase and lipase after initiating a new drug

Clinical Presentation: It is similar to presentation mentioned earlier for acute pancreatitis. Patients have excellent prognosis with a low risk of mortality once the drug is stopped.

TABLE 8.17 Causative Agents of Drug-Induced Hepatitis by Injury

Injury	Agents
Hepatocellular	Acetaminophen, isoniazid, halothane, methyldopa
Cholestasis	Amoxicillin-clavulanate, amiodarone, oral contraceptives, anabolic steroids, rifampin
Mixed	Captopril, ibuprofen, phenytoin

PPx: Awareness of drug prescription in patients with marginal pancreatic function

MoD: Pathogenesis of drug-related insult is poorly understood. Some drugs that can cause pancreatitis are azithromycin, furosemide, thiazides, TMP-SMX, and valproate.

Dx: Clinical suspicion, there are no distinguishing clinical features from other causes of pancreatitis. Preventable or modifiable causes of pancreatitis should be excluded.

Tx/Mgmt: Management of acute pancreatitis (describe earlier) + cessation of drug use.

GUNNER PRACTICE

1. A 19-year-old female comes to you complaining of low-grade fever, severe fatigue, nausea and jaundice for the past 3 days. She is sexually active, with multiple partners, and uses condoms inconsistently. Her temperature is 38.6°C and her liver is palpable 4 cm below the costal margin. Which of the following is the best serologic marker for this patient's condition?
   A. Anti-HBs
   B. Anti-HBe
   C. Anti-HCV
   D. IgM Anti-HBc
   E. IgG Anti-HBc

2. A 50-year-old male who has a history of prolonged alcohol abuse is brought to you by his daughter for increasing confusion. A couple of weeks ago, he began feeling drowsy and had a hard time falling asleep. He has progressively become confused and disoriented. He can still recognize his daughter and neighbors but cannot sustain a simple conversation. He denies abdominal pain, fever, or chills. Last year he was admitted to the hospital for upper gastrointestinal bleeding, which was due to ruptured esophageal varices. He suffers from hypertension, which has been managed by enalapril, spironolactone, and propranolol. On examination, he is lethargic and disheveled. His vital signs are blood pressure 119/74 mm Hg, pulse 72/min, respirations 18/min, and temperature 36.8°C. His liver feels firm on palpation with a span of 7 cm at the midclavicular line. There is no shifting dullness, and the spleen is not palpable. He cannot recall the date, reason for his visit, or his home

address. Neurologic exam reveals asterixis. Which of the following is the most appropriate management at this time?

A. Neomycin
B. Restriction of protein intake
C. Lactulose
D. Oral branched chain amino acid supplements
E. Stop spironolactone

3. A 25-year-old male who has returned from a trip to India presents with severe watery diarrhea, which has been present for the past 2 days. He denies any blood or mucus in his stool and has had 10 episodes of diarrhea so far. On interrogation he accepts that he feels slightly lightheaded. He denies nausea, vomiting, fever, or chills. He mentions eating fresh fruit during his trip. Which is the most likely pathogen causing this patient's presentation?

A. *Clostridium difficile*
B. *Bacillus cereus*
C. Enteroinvasive *E. coli*
D. *Rotavirus*
E. Enterotoxic *E. coli*
F. *Shigella*

ANSWERS: What Would Gunner Jess/Jim Do?

1. WWGJD? A 19-year-old woman comes to you complaining of low-grade fever lasting a couple of weeks, severe fatigue, nausea, and jaundice for the past 3 days. She has been using ibuprofen to control her fever for the past weeks. Her medical history is unremarkable and takes no medications. She is sexually active, with multiple partners, and uses condoms inconsistently. Her father is a diabetic and her mother died of breast cancer at age 59. Her temperature is 38.6° C and her liver is palpable 4 cm below her costal margin. Which of the following is the best serologic marker for this patient's condition?

Answer: D, IgM Anti-HBc.

Explanation: The correct answer is IgM Anti-HBc (option D). This individual is engaging in risky sexual behaviors that constitute an important risk factor for hepatitis B infection. Her clinical presentation is consistent with acute hepatitis. Serologic markers of acute disease are HBsAg and anti-HBc IgM type. Also IgM anti-HBc is the only positive marker during the *window* period of hepatitis B infection.

A. Anti-HBs → Incorrect. Anti-HBs follows the disappearance of HBsAg and would not be elevated during the acute phase of infection.

B. Anti-HBe → Incorrect. Anti-HBe is the earliest marker of the recovery phase and would not be elevated during the acute phase of infection.

C. Anti-HCV → Incorrect. Anti-HCV would be found in patients with hepatitis C infection. Commonly tested risk factors for HCV infection are IV drug abuse with needle sharing rather than risky sexual behaviors.

D. IgG Anti-HBc → Incorrect. IgG Anti-HBc usually appears weeks after the acute phase and is associated with decreasing levels of IgM type. These remain elevated for life.

2. WWGJD? A 50-year-old male who has a history of prolonged alcohol abuse is brought to you by his daughter for increasing confusion. A couple of weeks ago, he began feeling drowsy and had a hard time falling asleep. He has progressively become confused and disoriented. He can still recognize his daughter and neighbors but cannot sustain a simple conversation. He denies abdominal pain, fever, or chills. Last year he was admitted to the hospital for upper gastrointestinal

bleeding, which was due to **ruptured esophageal varices.** He suffers from hypertension, which has been managed by enalapril, spironolactone, and propranolol. On examination, he is lethargic and disheveled. His vital signs are blood pressure 119/74 mm Hg, pulse 72/min, respirations 18/min, and temperature 36.8°C. His liver feels firm on palpation with a span of 7 cm at the midclavicular line. There is no shifting dullness, and the spleen is not palpable. He cannot recall the date, reason for his visit, or his home address. Neurologic exam reveals asterixis. Which of the following is the most appropriate management at this time?

Answer: C, lactulose.

Explanation: This patient is suffering from hepatic encephalopathy. Lactulose is the first-line of therapy to treat hyperammonemia by lowering the intraluminal pH and driving the conversion of ammonium (NH_4) to ammonia (NH_3), which is not well absorbed by the gut. In addition, this drop in pH inhibits bacterial overgrowth.

A. Neomycin → Incorrect. Neomycin is an aminoglycoside commonly used to eradicate gut flora but is less efficacious than lactulose. It is considered a second-line drug.

B. Restriction of protein intake → Incorrect. Restriction of protein intake is part of the prophylactic measures that can be taken to prevent hepatic encephalopathy by decreasing the nitrogen load in the gut. Patients should be encouraged to consume less than 70 g of protein each day.

D. Oral branched chain amino acid supplements → Incorrect. Oral branched chain amino acid supplements have an unclear role in the treatment of encephalopathy.

E. Stop spironolactone → Incorrect. As a K-sparing diuretic, spironolactone aids in the prevention of ascites in this patient with end-stage liver disease.

3. WWGJD? A 25-year-old male who has returned from a trip to India presents with severe watery diarrhea, which has been present for the past 2 days. He denies any blood or mucus in his stool and has had 10 episodes of diarrhea so far. On interrogation he accepts that he feels slightly lightheaded. He denies nausea, vomiting, fever, or chills. He mentions eating fresh fruit during his trip. Which is the most likely pathogen causing this patient's presentation?

Answer: E, enterotoxic *E. coli.*

The pathogen most likely linked to this traveler's diarrhea is ETEC. This secretory diarrhea is brought upon by the enterotoxins (LT and ST toxins), which mediate passive diffusion of chloride ions from the epithelial cells into the gut lumen.

A. *Clostridium difficile* → Incorrect. *C. difficile* is usually secondary to antibiotic exposure and development of pseudomembranous colitis.

B. *Bacillus cereus* → Incorrect. *B. cereus* is usually associated with food poisoning, in which preformed bacterial toxins induce nausea and vomiting a couple of hours after eating re-heated rice or other starchy foods.

C. Enteroinvasive *E. coli* → Incorrect. Enteroinvasive *E. coli* is associated with eating undercooked red meat and presents with bloody diarrhea. *E. coli* O157:H7 produces verotoxin (shiga-like toxin), which may progress to hemolytic uremic syndrome.

D. *Rotavirus* → Incorrect. *Rotavirus* causes watery diarrhea in children.

F. *Shigella* → Incorrect. *Shigella* usually causes dysentery (blood and mucus).

Gynecologic Disorders

Drake Lebrun, Hao-Hua Wu, Leo Wang, Rebecca Gao, and Wanda Ronner

9

Introduction

Gynecologic disorders seen on the Medicine shelf exam include conditions affecting the breast and the female genital tract. There is substantial overlap between material tested on the Medicine shelf exam, Surgery shelf exam, and Ob-Gyn shelf exam; however, the content on the Medicine shelf is more limited in scope and focuses on the work-up and treatment of disorders that are medically treated.

In addition to understanding the clinical aspects of these conditions, you are also expected to be able to narrow down a differential diagnosis for relevant chief complaints, such as nipple discharge, breast mass, or ovarian mass. This is relatively straightforward as long as you master the important differentiating factors between similar disorders. For example, if you are answering a question related to nipple discharge, you need to know that different colors of discharge are associated with specific conditions: straw-colored discharge that varies cyclically is likely due to fibrocystic change, purulent discharge is likely due to a breast abscess, and bloody discharge is either due to intraductal papilloma or papillary cancer. Lastly, examiners expect you to know the underlying pathogenesis of common gynecologic neoplasms, such as cervical cancer arising from HPV-induced dysplasia or endometrial cancer arising from unopposed estrogen exposure.

This chapter is divided into three primary sections: (1) Breast Disorders; (2) Disorders of the Cervix, Ovary, Uterus, Vagina, and Vulva; and (3) Gunner Practice. Breast disorders are further subdivided into infectious and inflammatory conditions, benign neoplasms, and malignant neoplasms. Disorders of the cervix, ovary, uterus, vagina, and vulva are subdivided into benign conditions and malignant neoplasms.

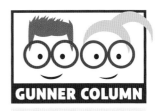

GUNNER COLUMN

Breast Disorders

Infectious, Immunologic, and Inflammatory Disorders

Mastitis

Buzz Words: Focal breast pain + breast erythema + nipple cracking + variations in temperature from one part of

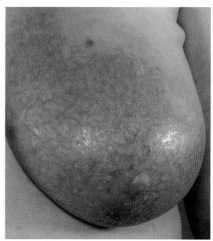

FIG. 9.1 Mastitis. Photo demonstrating localized breast erythema. (From Mayo Clinic. http://www.mayoclinic.org/diseases conditions/mastitis/multimedia/mastitis/img-20008120 By permission of Mayo Foundation for Medical Education and Research. All rights reserved.)

breast to another + infectious symptoms (fever, malaise, myalgias)

Clinical Presentation: See Fig. 9.1:

- Age/gender: Breastfeeding females
- Chief complaint: Painful breast ± nipple discharge

MoD: Bacteria (most often *Staphylococcus aureus*) enter the breast via small cracks in the skin caused by breastfeeding, causing a superficial infection of breast tissue.

Dx:

1. Physical exam revealing a tender erythematous breast.
2. Elevated white blood cell (WBC) count.

Tx/Mgmt:

1. Oral antibiotics, anti-staphylococcal antibiotics; dicloxacillin or cephalexin are first line. Trimethoprim-sulfamethoxazole is indicated if the patient is at risk for methicillin-resistant *S. aureus.*
2. If unresponsive to oral antibiotics, use intravenous (IV) antibiotics.
3. If unresponsive to IV antibiotics, suspect abscess, which requires surgical treatment.

Breast Abscess

Buzz Words: Painful palpable fluctuant breast mass + purulent nipple discharge + skin erythema + infectious symptoms (fever, malaise, myalgias)

Clinical Presentation:

- Age/gender: Breastfeeding females

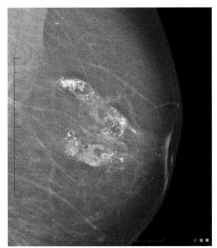

FIG. 9.2 Fat necrosis. Mammogram demonstrating spiculated calcifications that are highly consistent with fat necrosis, especially after a known history of trauma to the breast. (From Radiopaedia. https://radiopaedia.org/images/1884198.)

- Chief complaint: Painful breast mass ± purulent nipple discharge
- PMH: History of preceding mastitis

PPx: Can be prevented by timely and appropriate treatment of mastitis and the mother should be encouraged to continue breastfeeding with affected breast.

Mechanism of Disease (MoD): Progression of a superficial infection of breast tissue leading to a localized collection of pus and associated tissue destruction.

Dx:
1. Physical exam reveals a warm, tender fluctuant breast mass with associated purulent nipple discharge.
2. Elevated WBC.
3. Ultrasound to localize mass.

Tx/Mgmt:
1. Ultrasound-guided needle aspiration of abscess until no collection remains.
2. Incision and drainage may be used if the overlying skin is destroyed or if the abscess is unresponsive to aspiration.

Inflammatory Disease of Breast (Fat Necrosis)

Buzz Words: Pain and/or tenderness following trauma to breast + skin retraction + spiculated calcifications on mammography (Fig. 9.2)

Clinical Presentation:
- Age/gender: Adult females (40s and 50s)
- Chief complaint: Usually asymptomatic and found incidentally. Patients may complain of a breast lump.

- Risk factors include pendulous breasts and **recent history of breast surgery**.

MoD: Trauma disrupts fatty breast tissue → fat cells undergo necrosis → release of cytokines incites a localized inflammatory response. Eventually reparative fibrosis walls off and replaces the area of necrosed fat.

Dx:

1. History or implied history of trauma
2. Mammography (ill-defined, irregular spiculated calcifications)

Tx/Mgmt:

1. Reassurance and observation: Excision is unnecessary as there is no increased risk of breast cancer.

Benign and Undefined Disorders

Solitary Breast Cyst

Buzz Words: Small rounded or oval fluid-filled sac + non-tender + smooth borders

Clinical Presentation:

- Age/gender: Adult premenopausal and perimenopausal females
- Chief complaint: Usually asymptomatic and found incidentally. Patients may complain of a breast lump.

MoD: Lobule in the terminal grows into a fluid-filled mass.

Dx:

1. Ultrasound to visualize mass
2. Aspiration of fluid
3. Mammogram

Tx/Mgmt: Reassurance and observation because most cysts will resolve spontaneously. Drainage of fluid can be performed if the cyst enlarges or becomes painful.

Fibrocystic Change

Buzz Words: Multiple painful bilateral breast masses + straw-colored nipple discharge + fluctuation in size and severity with menstrual cycle

Clinical Presentation:

- Age/gender: Premenopausal females
- Chief complaint: Cyclic breast swelling, pain, and tenderness

MoD: Exaggerated response of breast tissue to physiologic hormonal changes during menstrual cycle.

Dx:

1. Fine-needle aspiration (FNA) of fluid

Tx/Mgmt:

1. Oral contraceptive pills (OCPs)
2. Danazol (androgen agonist), bromocriptine (dopamine agonist), and tamoxifen (selective estrogen antagonist

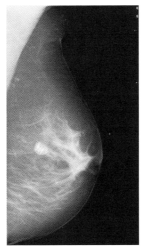

FIG. 9.3 Fibroadenoma. Mammogram demonstrating a small well-circumscribed solid lesion. (Case courtesy of Dr. Giorgio M. Baratelli, Radiopaedia.org, rID: 29466.)

in the breast) may be used in severe cases if OCPs are ineffective.
3. Nonsteroidal anti-inflammatory drugs (NSAIDs) for pain.

Fibroadenoma

Buzz Words: Firm, rubbery, nontender round mass + freely moveable + well-circumscribed + often solitary and unilateral + *no* fluctuation in size with menstrual cycle + slow or no growth (vs. phyllodes tumors, which grow rapidly)

Clinical Presentation:
- Age/gender: Young adult females (late teens and 20s)
- Chief complaint: Usually asymptomatic and found incidentally. Patients may complain of a breast lump.

MoD: Benign proliferation of breast epithelium and stroma.

Dx:
1. Mammogram to visualize lesion (Fig. 9.3)
2. Ultrasound to differentiate solid versus cystic components
3. FNA

Tx/Mgmt:
1. If asymptomatic: Observation and reassurance because most fibroadenomas will be reabsorbed.
2. If mass enlarges or is persistent for more than 3 months: Excisional biopsy.

3. If mass is very large (>5 cm): FNA to rule out cystosarcoma phyllodes.

Phyllodes Tumor (Cystosarcoma Phyllodes)

Buzz Words: **Very large** (>6 cm) nontender mass + warm erythematous skin overlying mass + freely moveable + well-circumscribed + **rapid growth**

Clinical Presentation:
- Age/gender: Adult females (40s and 50s)
- Chief complaint: Breast lump

MoD:
1. Benign proliferation of breast epithelium and stroma that may contain malignant cells.

Dx:
1. Mammogram to visualize lesion
2. Ultrasound to differentiate solid versus cystic components
3. Core-needle biopsy to rule out underlying aggressive malignancy

Tx/Mgmt: Wide local excision due to (1) high rate of local recurrence with simple excision, and (2) 10% of phyllodes tumors contain malignant cells.

Intraductal Papilloma

Buzz Words: Bloody or serosanguinous nipple discharge + no concurrent breast mass

Clinical Presentation:
- Age/gender: Adult females (20s–40s)
- Chief complaint: Bloody nipple discharge

MoD: Benign growth of epithelial lining (papilloma) arises within the lactiferous ducts (intraductal).
- Papilloma intermittently blocks the duct → nonbloody discharge.
- Large papillomas can twist around their stalk → infarction → bloody discharge.

Dx:
1. Cytology of discharge to rule out invasive papillary cancer.
2. Mammogram to rule out other lesions: Mammogram will not show papilloma due to its small size.

Tx/Mgmt:
1. Surgical excision of involved duct.

Malignant Neoplasms

Breast Cancer

Buzz Words: Irregular fixed breast mass + spiculated mass on imaging + asymmetric + architectural distortion + retraction of overlying skin and/or nipple + "orange peel" skin

Invasive ductal carcinoma   **Invasive lobular carcinoma**

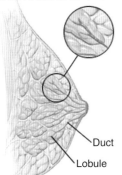 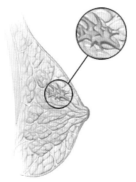

Duct

Lobule

FIG. 9.4 Anatomic origins of invasive breast neoplasms. Normal ducts and lobules are seen as well as tumors arising from those structures. (From www.drugs.com.)

texture (peau d'orange) + eczematous lesion of nipple/areola + palpable axillary lymph nodes

Clinical Presentation:
- Age/gender: Older females
- Chief complaint: Breast lump with associated skin changes. Often asymptomatic and found on screening mammography.
- Risk factors:
  - History of ductal carcinoma in situ (DCIS) or lobular carcinoma in situ (LCIS) (Fig. 9.4)
  - Increased lifetime estrogen exposure due to younger age at menarche, nulliparity, older age of first live birth, older age at menopause, obesity, and long-term (>5 years) use of hormone-replacement therapy
  - Prior exposure to ionizing radiation (e.g., treatment of Hodgkin lymphoma during childhood)
  - Family history of gynecologic malignancies
  - First-degree relatives with breast cancer: Risk increases with number of first-degree relatives and early age at time of Dx
  - BRCA1/BRCA2 genes are associated with bilateral pre-menopausal breast cancer and ovarian cancer

PPx:
- USPSTF: Biennial mammograms from age 50 to 74
- American Cancer Society: Annual mammograms from age 45 to 54, then annual or biennial for as long as woman is in good health

Dx:
1. Screening mammography
2. Needle biopsy or FNA
3. Staging workup for metastatic disease

TABLE 9.1 Breast Neoplasms

	Description	Classic Presentation	Treatment
Lobular carcinoma in situ (LCIS)	**Non-invasive** proliferation of malignant epithelial cells in breast lobules	Asymptomatic Incidental finding on biopsy for an unrelated indication	Observe Selective estrogen-receptor modifiers
Ductal carcinoma in situ (DCIS)	**Non-invasive** proliferation of malignant epithelial cells in breast ducts	Asymptomatic Found on screening mammography showing clustered microcalcifications	Lumpectomy + radiation therapy Simple mastectomy for extensive multicentric lesions
Invasive cancer		Ill-defined fixed breast mass, irregular asymmetric mass with spiculations mass and architectural distortion on imaging	Lumpectomy + radiation therapy Simple mastectomy for larger lesions Radical mastectomy for disease with axillary node involvement
Lobular carcinoma	Invasive proliferation of malignant epithelial cells in breast **lobules**	Less common than ductal carcinoma Frequently bilateral	
Ductal carcinoma	Invasive proliferation of malignant epithelial cells in breast **ducts**	More common than lobular carcinoma	

Tx/Mgmt: Depends on stage (Table 9.1):
- Lumpectomy with sentinel lymph node biopsy
- Simple mastectomy
- Radical mastectomy

Paget Disease of the Breast

Buzz Words: Eczema (scaling, crusting, ulceration) of the nipple/areolar complex (Fig. 9.5) + unilateral + malignant intraepithelial cells (Paget cells) +/− concurrent underlying breast cancer (~90% of cases)

Clinical Presentation:
- Age/gender: Adult females (50s and 60s)
- Chief complaint: Pain and/or itching of nipple

MoD: Malignant cells invade into epidermis of the nipple → inflammation of the nipple → spread to areola → eczematous changes of the nipple/areolar complex

Dx:
1. Diagnostic biopsy of skin demonstrating presence of intraepithelial adenocarcinoma cells (Paget cells) within the nipple
2. Mammography to identify an associated mass

Tx/Mgmt: Surgical resection of the lesion: Exact means of resection (breast-conserving vs. simple mastectomy

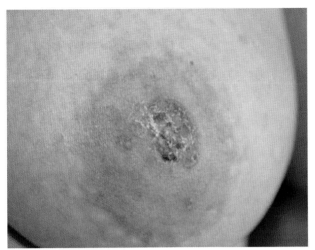

FIG. 9.5 Paget disease of the breast. Photo demonstrating classic physical exam findings such as scaling, crusting, and ulceration near the nipple/areolar complex. (From Lage D, Volpini Cde A, Sasseron Mda G, Daldon P, Arruda L: Paget's disease: the importance of the specialist. *An Bras Dermatol* 85(3):365–369, 2010.)

vs. radical mastectomy) and need for adjuvant therapy depend on the indicated treatment for the concurrent underlying breast cancer.

Disorders of the Cervix, Ovary, Uterus, Vagina, and Vulva

Benign Neoplasms and Cysts

Endocervical and Endometrial Polyps

Buzz Words: Intrauterine heavy bleeding + irregular bleeding + post-coital bleeding

Clinical Presentation:
- Age/gender: Adult females (40s and 50s)
- Chief complaint: Often asymptomatic, postmenopausal bleeding
- Tamoxifen (selective estrogen receptor modulator) is a risk factor

MoD: Benign proliferation of endometrial glands and stroma within the uterus or endocervical canal: Polyps can has a stalk (pedunculated) or may be flat.

Dx:
1. Ultrasound to non-invasively visualize lesion
2. Hysteroscopy to visualize lesion with option for immediate removal

Tx/Mgmt:
- If woman is premenopausal: Symptomatic polyps should be removed via hysteroscopy. Asymptomatic

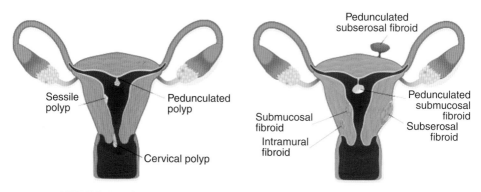

UTERINE POLYPS   UTERINE FIBROIDS

FIG. 9.6 Figure demonstrating differences between locations of polyps and fibroids. Polyps are benign proliferations of **endometrium**, while fibroids are benign proliferations of **myometrium**. (From www. fibroids.com.)

polyps can be observed unless patient is at risk for infertility, endometrial hyperplasia, or endometrial carcinoma.
- If woman is postmenopausal: All polyps should be removed via hysteroscopy because (1) polyps can mask bleeding from other concerning sources; and (2) polyps can be premalignant or malignant.

Leiomyomata Uteri (Uterine Fibroids)

Buzz Words: Firm irregular palpable uterine mass(es) (Fig. 9.6) + heavy bleeding + painful menses + fluctuates in size with menstrual cycle

Clinical Presentation:
- Age/gender: Adult premenopausal and perimenopausal females (30s to 50s).
- Chief complaint: Often asymptomatic: Patients may complain of heavy bleeding, painful menses, irregular bleeding, and abdominal pain.
- African-American women are at highest risk.

MoD: Benign proliferation of smooth muscle cells within the uterus: Fibroids are stimulated by estrogen → fluctuate in size with menstrual cycle. Fibroids regress after menopause.

Dx:
1. Physical exam may detect a nontender **irregularly** enlarged "lumpy" uterus
2. Pelvic ultrasound
3. Tissue biopsy to confirm diagnosis

Tx/Mgmt:
- If asymptomatic or mild symptoms: reassurance and observation

- If moderate symptoms: OCPs, gonadotropin-releasing hormone (GnRH) agonists (e.g., leuprolide)
- If severe symptoms in a woman who has completed childbearing: Hysterectomy or uterine artery embolization
- If severe symptoms in a young woman who wants to preserve fertility: Myomectomy (uterus-preserving resection of one or more fibroids)

Benign Ovarian Cysts and Neoplasms

Buzz Words: Adnexal mass on ultrasound + usually asymptomatic

Clinical Presentation:
- Age/gender: Adult females
- Chief complaint: Often asymptomatic: Patients may complain of pelvic pain or dyspareunia.

MoD: There are several types of benign ovarian cysts and masses:
- **Follicular cysts**: Follicle fails to rupture during follicular maturation. Unilateral.
- **Corpus luteum cysts**: Corpus luteum fails to regress → continues to secrete progesterone → delays menstruation. Can become hemorrhagic → rupture → acute abdominal pain and hemoperitoneum. Unilateral.
- **Theca lutein cysts**: Excess human chorionic gonadotropin (hCG) → growth of large bilateral ovarian cysts. Causes of excess hCG include molar pregnancy and choriocarcinoma.
- **Endometriomas**: Ectopic endometrial growth within ovary. "Chocolate cysts."
- **Dermoid cysts (mature termatomas):** Proliferations of multiple germ cell layers (ectoderm, endoderm). May contain multiple tissue types including hair, teeth, skin, etc.
- **Cystadenomas**: Proliferations of epithelial cells.
- **Fibromas**: Proliferations of stromal cells producing collagen and extracellular matrix.

Dx:
1. Transvaginal ultrasound
2. Excise any mass with worrisome features (e.g., multiloculated, irregular, solid and cystic aspects) for definitive pathologic diagnosis

Tx/Mgmt:
- Follicular cysts and corpus luteum cysts: Observe. Most benign cysts will resolve on their own. Oral contraceptives may be used to suppress future cysts
- Dermoid cysts: Cystectomy (or oophorectomy if very large) for pathologic Dx and to rule out malignancy.

TABLE 9.2 Pap Smear Screening Guidelines

Woman's Age	How Often Should a Woman Have a Pap Test?
Under 21 years old	No testing needed
21–30 years old	Pap test every 3 years
30–65 years old	Pap test every 3 years or Pap and HPV every 5 years
65 years old or older	No testing needed

From http://www.health.ny.gov/diseases/cancer/cervical/campaign/

QUICK TIPS

Large ovarian masses can occasionally rupture, leading to acute abdominal pain and rebound tenderness.

QUICK TIPS

Large ovarian cysts can also twist upon their pedicle, leading to ovarian torsion (a surgical emergency). Torsed ovaries present with nausea, vomiting, and waxing and waning pain.

99 AR

USPSTF cervical cancer screening guidelines

QUICK TIPS

High-risk HPV serotypes (16, 18, 31, 45) use specific proteins (E6 and E7) to inactivate key tumor suppressor genes (p53 and Rb, respectively). This promotes cervical dysplasia and ultimately progression to cervical squamous cell carcinoma. This same process is also seen in squamous cell carcinomas arising in the head, neck, and anus. The most important risk factor for HPV infection is multiple sexual partners.

- Cystadenomas: Oophorectomy
- Fibromas: Cystectomy (or oophorectomy if very large)

Precancerous and Malignant Neoplasms

Cervical Cancer

Buzz Words: Postcoital bleeding + HPV infection

Clinical Presentation:

- Age/gender: Adult females
- Chief complaint: Usually asymptomatic: Post-coital bleeding is the most common symptom.
- Risk factors:
  - HPV infection (high-risk serotypes 16, 18, 31, 45) and its associated risk factors (e.g., multiple partners)
  - HIV
  - Cigarette smoking
  - Systemic immunosuppression (e.g., chronic steroid use, chemotherapy). Diethylstilbestrol (DES) is a risk factor for clear cell subtype

PPx: Pap smear screening (Table 9.2)

MoD: High-risk HPV serotypes can inactivate key tumor suppressor genes (p53 and Rb), promoting cervical dysplasia, and ultimately progression to cervical squamous cell carcinoma.

Dx:

1. Speculum exam may demonstrate friable mass on cervix
2. Pap smear
3. Colposcopic biopsy for definitive histologic Dx

Tx/Mgmt:

- If the lesion is confined to the cervix: Cold-knife conization (removal of a wedge-shaped portion of affected cervix and endocervical canal).
- If the lesion is confined to the upper vagina and parametrium: Radical hysterectomy or radiation therapy.
- If the lesion extends beyond the upper vagina or parametrium: Chemoradiation.

- **Colposcopic biopsy**: Abnormal areas on the cervical surface are visualized by applying acetic acid to the surface. Biopsies are taken of any abnormal areas.
- **Conization**: A cone-shaped portion of the cervix is removed via electrosurgical excision or surgical scalpel.

QUICK TIPS

Following a positive Pap smear and/or HPV test, additional diagnostic tests are ordered to confirm or rule out a diagnosis of cervical dysplasia. These tests include: colposcopic biopsy and conization

Endometrial Hyperplasia
Buzz Words: Uterine bleeding in postmenopausal woman + thickened endometrial stripe
Clinical Presentation:
- Age/gender: Perimenopausal and post-menopausal females
- Chief complaint: Heavy uterine bleeding and/or post-menopausal bleeding
- Risk factors:
  - Increased lifetime estrogen exposure due to younger age at menarche, nulliparity, older age of first live birth, older age at menopause, obesity, long-term (>5 years) use of hormone-replacement therapy
  - Chronic anovulation (e.g., polycystic ovarian syndrome), estrogen-secreting ovarian tumors, tamoxifen use, hereditary non-polyposis colon cancer (HNPCC) syndrome
  - Hypertension, diabetes mellitus
PPx: Avoid exposure to unopposed estrogen
MoD: Excess estrogen stimulation without progesterone → unopposed proliferation of endometrial glands and stroma → endometrial hyperplasia
Dx:
1. Pelvic ultrasound to visualize thickened endometrial stripe
2. Endometrial biopsy to confirm diagnosis, rule out carcinoma, and assess the severity of cellular atypia and architectural changes
Tx/Mgmt:
- If cells do not demonstrate atypia: Progesterone therapy
- If cells are atypical: Dilation and curettage
- Hysterectomy may be appropriate in postmenopausal women who have completed childbearing.

Endometrial/Uterine Cancer
Buzz Words: Uterine bleeding in postmenopausal woman + thickened endometrial stripe
Clinical Presentation:
- Age/gender: Perimenopausal and postmenopausal females

- Chief complaint: Heavy, irregular, or postmenopausal bleeding
- Risk factor: Endometrial hyperplasia—risk factors are the same as those for endometrial hyperplasia

PPx: Avoid exposure to unopposed estrogen

MoD:

- Type I: Estrogen-dependent progression of endometrial hyperplasia
- Type II: Non-estrogen-dependent carcinogenesis, occurring in the setting of tumor suppressor mutations (e.g., p53) or atrophic endometrium

Dx:

1. Pelvic ultrasound can demonstrate a thickened endometrial stripe, but tissue diagnosis is still required.
2. Endometrial biopsy is definitive.
3. CA-125 can be used to assess spread and treatment effectiveness.

Tx/Mgmt:

- Stage I and II: Total abdominal hysterectomy + bilateral salpingoophorectomy
- Stage III and IV: Total abdominal hysterectomy + bilateral salpingoophorectomy + pelvic and para-aortic lymph node dissection + radiation therapy

Ovarian Cancer

Buzz Words: Ascites + abdominal distension + abdominal pain + early satiety + constipation + elevated CA-125

Clinical Presentation:

- Age/gender: Post-menopausal females
- Chief complaint: Non-specific (ascites, early satiety, constipation)
- Risk factors: Family history of ovarian or breast cancer. Increased estrogen exposure due to infertility, nulliparity. Age. BRCA1/BRCA2. Genetic syndromes including HNPCC, Turner syndrome. OCPs are protective because they decrease the number of ovulatory cycles.

PPx: Screening for ovarian cancer is not indicated except in select high-risk subgroups (e.g., patients with known BRCA1/2 mutations).

MoD: The ovary consists of three primary tissue types: epithelial cells, germ cells, and stromal tissue. Malignant neoplasms can arise from each of these.

Dx:

1. Transvaginal ultrasound to visualize a mass
2. **Elevated CA-125** (elevated in epithelial-derived neoplasms)
3. Biopsy

gg AR

APGO (Association of Professors of Gynecology and Obstetrics) ovarian cancer video

Tx/Mgmt:
1. Surgical resection including total abdominal hysterectomy, bilateral salpingo-oophorectomy, and removal of pelvic and para-aortic lymph nodes
2. Chemotherapy
3. Radiation therapy for palliation or persistent disease

Vulvar Dysplasia and Cancer

Buzz Words: Solitary raised crusted nodule, plaque, ulcer, or mass on the labia majora + vulvar itching

Clinical Presentation:
- Age/gender: Post-menopausal females in 50s and 60s
- Chief complaint: Vulvar mass and/or pruritis
- Risk factors: Smoking, HPV infection, vulvar dystrophy (e.g., lichen sclerosus), history of cervical cancer

PPx: HPV vaccination, treatment of vulvar dystrophy if present

MoD: Two mechanisms of vulvar carcinogenesis:
- HPV-induced cellular dysplasia progresses to squamous cell carcinoma
- Chronic inflammation progresses to cellular dysplasia and eventually neoplasia

Dx: Vulvar biopsy

Tx/Mgmt: Surgical excision

Gestational Trophoblastic Disease

Buzz Words: hCG production + "snowstorm" uterus on imaging + grape-like intrauterine vesicles ± bilateral theca lutein ovarian cysts

Clinical Presentation:
- Age/gender: Pregnant or post-partum females
- Chief complaint: Irregular and/or heavy vaginal bleeding during early pregnancy
- Risk factors: Asian ethnicity

MoD: Proliferation of placental tissue is due to abnormal fertilization. Multiple subtypes of gestational trophoblastic disease (GTD) include:
- Molar pregnancy (benign with malignant potential):
  - Complete: 46XX (all paternally derived) implants in uterine wall. Non-viable without associated embryo. Presents as irregular and/or heavy vaginal bleeding with enlarged uterus.
  - Incomplete: 69XXX/XXY (paternally and maternally derived) embryo implants in uterine wall. Presents as a missed abortion.
- Invasive moles (malignant): Persistent molar pregnancy after evacuation. Presents as rising hCG after dilation and curettage.

99 AR

Gestational trophoblastic disease video

- Choriocarcinoma (malignant): Necrotizing malignant cancer arising late post-partum, up to years after pregnancy.

Dx:

1. High serum hCG (>100,000 mIU/mL).
2. Pelvic ultrasound may demonstrate snowstorm pattern in uterus in the case of a complete mole and/or large bilateral multiloculated ovarian cysts (theca lutein cysts).

Tx/Mgmt: Specific treatment depends on GTD subtype (see below). Follow all patients with serial hCG measurements until hCG level reaches 0. Provide reliable contraception to ensure hCG measurements are accurate.

- Molar pregnancy: Dilation and curettage
- Invasive mole: Chemotherapy
- Choriocarcinoma: Chemotherapy

GUNNER PRACTICE

1. A 42-year-old female presents to her gynecologist for a lump in her left breast. She states that she first noticed the lump 2 months ago. The lump has grown rapidly in size since she first noticed it, which prompted her to visit her gynecologist. The lump is firm, non-tender, and not associated with nipple discharge. She denies fever, chills, chest wall tenderness, shortness of breath, myalgias, or muscle weakness. She has a history of asthma, which is well controlled with intermittent albuterol. Her family history is notable for hypertension and diabetes mellitus. She has no family history of breast or ovarian cancer. Menarche occurred at age 12 and her periods have been regular since then. She has never been pregnant. Examination reveals a large, firm, freely moveable mass in the upper outer quadrant of the patient's left breast. The skin overlying the mass appears shiny and somewhat stretched. A mammogram demonstrates a large 6-cm, well-circumscribed mass with smooth margins. Which of the following is the most appropriate next best step in the management of this patient?
   A. FNA
   B. Magnetic resonance imaging (MRI)
   C. Reassurance and observation
   D. Lumpectomy followed by adjuvant radiation therapy
   E. Core needle biopsy

2. A 61-year-old woman presents to her gynecologist for a red rash on her left breast. She reports that the rash started 6 months ago and has been associated with persistent itchiness and crusting despite multiple treatments with over-the-counter moisturizing creams. She denies nipple discharge or breast pain. She denies fever, chills, weight loss, or change in appetite. She has a history of hypertension and hyperlipidemia, which are well controlled with lisinopril and atorvastatin, respectively. Physical exam is notable for a red crusty ulcerative lesion, approximately 3 cm in diameter, overlying the left nipple and areola. In addition to performing a skin biopsy of the lesion, what other step is most appropriate in the management of this patient?
   A. Leuprolide
   B. Breast ultrasound
   C. Mammogram
   D. Topical steroid
   E. Wide local excision of the nipple/areolar complex

3. A 31-year-old African-American female presents to her gynecologist for heavy menstrual bleeding and pelvic pain. Menarche occurred at age 13 and menses had been regular up to 8 months ago when her menses became heavy and painful. Her last menstrual period was 10 days ago. She has never had children, but is actively trying to get pregnant and would like to have children within the next few years. She is otherwise healthy and takes no medications. She has never smoked and drinks occasionally. Her mother died of a heart attack at age 75. On bimanual exam, she has a palpable, firm, irregularly enlarged mass on her uterus. Pelvic ultrasound reveals a large homogeneous hypoechoic mass arising from the myometrium. Which of the following is the next best step in the management of this patient's condition?
   A. Leuprolide
   B. Computed tomography (CT) of the abdomen and pelvis
   C. Hysterectomy
   D. Myomectomy
   E. Dilation and curettage

ANSWERS: What Would Gunner Jess/Jim Do?

1. WWGJD? A 42-year-old female presents to her gynecologist for a lump in her left breast. She states that she first noticed the lump 2 months ago. The lump has grown rapidly in size since she first noticed it, which prompted her to visit her gynecologist. The lump is firm, nontender, and not associated with nipple discharge. She denies fever, chills, chest wall tenderness, shortness of breath, myalgias, or muscle weakness. She has a history of asthma that is well-controlled with intermittent albuterol. Her family history is notable for hypertension and diabetes mellitus. She has no family history of breast or ovarian cancer. Menarche occurred at age 12 and her periods have been regular since then. She has never been pregnant. Examination reveals a large, firm, freely moveable mass in the upper outer quadrant of the patient's left breast. The skin overlying the mass appears shiny and somewhat stretched. A mammogram demonstrates a large 6 cm, well-circumscribed mass with smooth margins. Which of the following is the most appropriate next best step in the management of this patient?

Answer: E, Core needle biopsy

Explanation: This patient in her early 40s presents with a rapidly growing freely movable well-circumscribed breast mass. This is most consistent with **cystosarcoma phyllodes (phyllodes tumor).** Phyllodes tumors are proliferations of epithelial and stromal breast tissue, similar to fibroadenomas. However, unlike fibroadenomas, phyllodes tumors often occur in women in their 30s and 40s, are larger, grow more rapidly, and may harbor malignant cells. Core needle biopsy is the preferred method of definitive pathologic diagnosis for cystosarcoma phyllodes after initial imaging.

A. FNA → incorrect. FNA has a high false-negative rate and is not appropriate for biopsy of potential phyllodes tumors. Core needle biopsy is the preferred method for making a pathologic diagnosis.

B. MRI → Incorrect. Although more advanced imaging modalities, such as MRI, may better characterize this mass, a pathologic diagnosis is required.

C. Reassurance and observation → Incorrect. Reassurance and observation are not indicated if there is suspicion for cystosarcoma phyllodes. Cystosarcoma phyllodes may harbor malignant cells; thus, tissue biopsy is required to confirm the diagnosis and rule out malignancy. Moreover, the standard of care for cystosarcoma phyllodes is wide local excision. Reassurance and observation would be appropriate if this mass were a smaller and less locally aggressive fibroadenoma.

D. Lumpectomy followed by adjuvant radiation therapy → Incorrect. A definitive tissue diagnosis is required before any surgery is performed.

2. WWGJD? A 61-year-old woman presents to her gynecologist for a red rash on her left breast. She reports that the rash started 6 months ago and has been associated with persistent itchiness and crusting despite multiple treatments with over-the-counter moisturizing creams. She denies nipple discharge or breast pain. She denies fever, chills, weight loss, or change in appetite. She has a history of hypertension and hyperlipidemia, which are well controlled with lisinopril and atorvastatin, respectively. Physical exam is notable for a red crusty ulcerative lesion, approximately 3 cm in diameter, overlying the left nipple and areola. In addition to performing a skin biopsy of the lesion, what other step is most appropriate in the management of this patient?

Answer: C, Mammogram

Explanation. This postmenopausal female presents with an eczematous lesion affecting the nipple. This is most consistent with Paget disease of the breast. Paget disease of the breast is frequently associated with a concurrent underlying breast neoplasm. In addition to skin biopsy to confirm the diagnosis of Paget disease, this patient should also undergo a mammogram to identify any potential underlying neoplasms.

A. Leuprolide → Incorrect. Leuprolide is a GnRH analog that decreases levels of estrogen and testosterone. It is used to treat uterine fibroids and certain types of breast cancer. It is not used to treat Paget disease of the breast.

B. Breast ultrasound → Incorrect. Breast ultrasound may help to identify an underlying breast neoplasm; however, a mammogram is more sensitive than ultrasound alone.

D. Topical steroid → Incorrect. Topical steroid is not an appropriate treatment for Paget disease of the breast.

E. Wide local excision of the nipple/areolar complex → Incorrect. A definitive tissue diagnosis is required before any surgery is performed.

3. WWGJD? A 31-year-old African-American female presents to her gynecologist for heavy menstrual bleeding and pelvic pain. Menarche occurred at age 13 and menses had been regular up to 8 months ago when her menses became heavy and painful. Her last menstrual period was 10 days ago. She has never had children but is actively trying to get pregnant and would like to have children within the next few years. She is otherwise healthy and takes no medications. She has never smoked and drinks occasionally. Her mother died of a heart attack at age 75. On bimanual exam, she has a palpable, firm, irregularly enlarged mass on her uterus. Pelvic ultrasound reveals a large homogenous hypoechoic mass arising from the myometrium. Which of the following is the next best step in the management of this patient's condition?

Answer: D, Myomectomy

Explanation: This African-American female has menorrhagia, cyclic pelvic pain, an irregularly enlarged uterus, and a myometrial mass on imaging. This is most consistent with a **fibroid.** In a young female who has not completed childbearing, the most appropriate treatment option is a uterus-preserving myomectomy.

A. Leuprolide → Incorrect. Leuprolide is a GnRH agonist that is used to treat fibroids. However, leuprolide inhibits gonadotropin secretion and thus prevents pregnancy. In a patient actively seeking to have children, leuprolide is not an appropriate first-line treatment option.

B. CT of the abdomen and pelvis → Incorrect. Advanced imaging modalities such as CT or MRI are not typically indicated for most fibroids.

C. Hysterectomy → Incorrect. Hysterectomy would permanently prevent this patient from getting pregnant and is thus not an appropriate treatment option. Hysterectomy is appropriate for patients who have completed childbearing.

E. Dilation and curettage → Dilation and curettage is an appropriate treatment for symptomatic uterine polyps. Dilation and curettage is not an appropriate treatment for fibroids.

Renal, Urinary, and Male Reproductive System

Kumar Nadhan, Hao-Hua Wu, Leo Wang, Rebecca Gao, and Sean Harbison

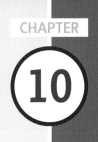

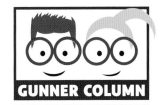

GUNNER COLUMN

Introduction

The renal, urinary, and male reproductive system comprises a series of tubes that conduct unidirectional flow, much like slides in a water park. Questions about this water park are high yield on the Surgery shelf because they allow examiners to test anatomy, principles of basic physics (yes, it has come back to haunt you), and your understanding of how one monkey wrench can ruin an entire organ and the whole body. For example, a ureteral kidney stone can cause fluid backup, leading to kidney damage, subsequent retention of blood urea nitrogen (BUN), and finally brain dysfunction.

Luckily for you, most pathology in this system can be conquered with a thorough understanding of the anatomy combined with the knowledge that any disruption in flow will affect all proximal parts of the organ system. Thus, take time to learn the anatomy from urine/semen production site to excretion. All flow in this system is excretory (leaving the body) liquid. This chapter will first attack the renal and urinary system from top down anatomically.

Infectious Disorders

Upper Urinary Tract

The upper urinary tract encompasses the kidney down to but not including the bladder. Problems in the upper urinary tract follow a general sequence of events. First, the urinary tract is obstructed, most often by kidney stones. Then a bacterial infection develops proximal to the obstruction, which presents as fever and pyuria on urinalysis (>10 WBCs per high-power field). Ultimately, the ascending infection results in progressive damage to proximal structures. The most common bacteria that cause infection in the urinary tract are gram-negative bacteria, most notably *Escherichia coli* and *Proteus*.

Xanthogranulomatous Pyelonephritis
Buzz Words: Chronic kidney stones + flank pain + *Proteus Mirabilis* + kidney mass + lipid-laden macrophages

Clinical Presentation: A 40-year-old woman with recurrent kidney stones and urinary tract infections (UTIs) presents with fever and chronic flank pain.

MoD: Chronic obstruction (usually by kidney stones) → infection → massive destruction of kidney induced by lipid-laden macrophages

Dx:
1. Urinalysis shows pyuria, WBC casts, and macrophages. Lipid-laden macrophages are pathognomonic.
2. Urine culture can show *E. coli* or *Proteus.*
3. Computed tomography (CT) or x-ray shows a mass in the kidney, often mistaken for cancer.

Tx/Mgmt: Surgery is definitive but can be supplemented with antibiotics.

Renal and Perinephric Abscess

Buzz Words: Suspected pyelonephritis refractory to treatment + >14 days + abdominal pain + past UTI

Clinical Presentation: An adult patient with diabetes presents with vague flank pain and fever that has lasted for more than 14 days despite adequate antibiotic treatment for pyelonephritis.

MoD:
- Wound/pulmonary infection→ hematogenous spread (*Staphylococcus aureus*)
- UTI → ascending infection
- Secondary complication of pyelonephritis

Dx: CT scan shows mass inside (renal) or outside (perinephric) renal capsule.

Tx/Mgmt:
1. Percutaneous
2. Antibiotics can be used to prevent spread of infection.

(Acute) Pyelonephritis

Buzz Words: Unilateral costovertebral angle (CVA) tenderness + >103°F fever + anorexia + vesicoureteral reflux (VUR)

Clinical Presentation: A 30-year-old woman with recurrent UTIs presents with CVA tenderness, high fever, and nausea/vomiting.

MoD: Obstruction → UTI → Ascending bacteria → infection of renal parenchyma

Dx:
1. Urinalysis (UA) (pyuria and WBC casts)
2. Urine culture (WBCs >100,000/mL)

Tx/Mgmt:
1. Oral antibiotics based on culture; fluoroquinolones and trimethoprim-sulfamethoxazole (TMP-SMX) are most common.

2. Severe pyelonephritis or high-risk patients (pregnant, elderly) → IV antibiotics, most commonly ceftriaxone, and hospitalization

Pyonephrosis

Buzz Words: Pyelonephritis + pus in renal pelvis + hydronephrosis

Clinical Presentation: This is a rarely tested complication of pyelonephritis but worth noting so you are not surprised if you come across hydronephrosis within the kidney.

Prophylaxis (PPx): Treat urinary tract obstruction promptly.

Mechanism of Disease (MoD): Urinary tract obstruction → ascending infection → pyelonephritis → pus accumulates in collecting system → distention of renal pelvis → abscess can form, which may progress condition to sepsis or kidney failure.

Diagnostic Steps (Dx):
1. Kidney ultrasound
2. Abdominal CT scan

Treatment and Management Steps (Tx/Mgmt): Drainage via image-guided retrograde or percutaneous ureteral stent placement

Genitourinary Tuberculosis

Buzz Words: Immigrant + prisoner + positive purified protein derivative (PPD) + pyuria + microscopic hematuria + chest x-ray (CXR) showing upper lobe cavitation

Clinical Presentation: A recent immigrant from Southeast Asia with human immunodeficiency virus (HIV) infection presents with microscopic hematuria. CXR shows an upper lobe cavitation.

MoD: Direct infection or miliary disease

Dx:
1. PPD
2. CXR (3) tuberculosis (TB) organisms in urine (urinary acid-fast bacilli [AFB] may be negative, since TB seeps into urine only intermittently).

Tx/Mgmt: Treat underlying TB (e.g., pyrazinamide, rifampin, isoniazid, and ethambutol)

Lower Urinary Tract and Urinary Tract Infections of Unspecified Location

The lower urinary tract involves the bladder down to the urethral opening. Pathology of the lower tract is more common but less severe than that of the upper tract, so management will lean away from surgical intervention. Common lower urinary tract symptoms consist of urinary urgency, frequency, burning, and hematuria.

UTI/Cystitis

Buzz Words: Young female + pelvic pressure (discomfort or fullness) + lower urinary tract symptoms + indwelling catheter + recent honeymoon

Clinical Presentation: A 20-year-old female presents with pelvic discomfort, dysuria, and frequent urination.

PPx: Adequate hydration and frequent diuresis

MoD: Urethral infection → ascending UTI → inflammation of bladder

Dx:
1. Dipstick (positive leukocyte esterase, WBC count, or increased nitrites)
2. Urine culture (bacteria >100,000/mL)

Tx/Mgmt: Antibiotics—TMP-SMX, fluoroquinolone, nitrofurantoin

gg AR

UTI In-Depth Video

Urethritis

Buzz Words: Young male + mucopurulent urethral discharge + dysuria + absent systemic signs + unprotected sexual activity

Clinical Presentation: A 20-year-old sexually active male with a history of UTIs presents with urethral discharge and dysuria.

PPx: Protection during sexual activity, decrease number of partners

MoD: Sexually transmitted disease of *Neisseria gonorrhoeae* (50%–80% cases), *Chlamydia trachomatis, Ureaplasma, Trichomonas vaginalis*

Dx: Mucopurulent discharge can be enough to diagnose. Can confirm with urine dipstick showing leukocyte esterase and WBCs.

Tx/Mgmt: Oral antibiotic therapy covering gonorrhea and chlamydia

Chlamydia

Buzz Words: Teenage sexually active female + yellow discharge + dysuria + dyspareunia

Clinical Presentation: An 18-year-old sexually active female presents with dysuria. She has multiple sexual partners.

PPx: Screening

MoD: Sexual intercourse → infection of urethra

Dx: Urinary nucleic acid amplification test (NAAT) for *C. trachomatis*. Supplement pregnancy test to avoid teratogenic antibiotics (e.g., doxycycline).

Tx/Mgmt:
1. Antibiotics covering both chlamydia and gonorrhea
2. Treat sexual partners to avoid reinfection

Immunologic and Inflammatory Disorders

Upper Urinary Tract

Inflammatory pathology of the upper urinary tract mainly consists of disease of the kidney glomerulus. Glomerular disease can be broadly divided into two categories, nephritic and nephrotic syndromes.

Nephritic syndrome involves glomerular inflammation and presents as hematuria, hypertension, oliguria, RBC casts, increased BUN and creatinine.

Nephrotic syndrome results from podocyte disruption and presents as more than 3.5 g/day proteinuria (frothy urine), hypoalbuminemia, hyperlipidemia, edema, and hypercoagulability. Definitive diagnosis of nephrotic syndrome is both more than 50 mg/kg per day urinary protein excretion and hypoalbuminemia. It is sometimes referred to as the "Oh Shit" syndrome = nephrOtic, prOtein, hypO-albuminemia, edema from lOw plasma Oncotic pressure. Understand that diseases may have features of both nephritic and nephrotic syndrome, but we categorize them generally into one of the two. We start with the nephritic syndromes, continue with nephrotic, and then cover additional upper tract inflammatory conditions.

Alport Syndrome

Buzz Words: Nephritic and nephrotic syndromes + cataracts + deafness + males in the family

Clinical Presentation: A 16-year-old male presents with hematuria and deafness. On further questioning, other males in the family also have a history of hematuria, deafness, and renal insufficiency.

MoD: Inherited collagen 4 defect → poor basement membrane structure in kidneys, ears, and eyes

Dx:
1. UA
2. Basic metabolic panel (BMP)
3. Electron microscopy shows split, "basket weave" thinning and thickening, glomerular basement membrane

Tx/Mgmt: Angiotensin converting enzyme (ACE) inhibitors/angiotensin type 1 receptor blockers (ARBs) to decrease proteinuria

Membranoproliferative Glomerulonephritis (Glomerular Disease Due to Hepatitis C)

Buzz Words: Chronic hepatitis C + new onset nephrotic or nephritic syndrome + cryoglobulinemia + "tram track" on glomerular basement membrane (GBM)

Clinical Presentation: A patient with chronic hepatitis C has microscopic hematuria found on a UA done for UTI evaluation.

PPx: Treat underlying disease

MoD: Chronic Hep C infection → immune complex (Ag-antibody) deposits in glomerular subendothelium → immune complement pathways activated → disrupts glomerular structure

Dx:
1. UA
2. BMP
3. Electron microscopy shows tram-track GBM

Tx/Mgmt: Treat underlying disease

Membranous Glomerulosclerosis (Glomerular Disease Due to Hepatitis B)

Buzz Words: Hepatitis B + nephrotic syndrome + massive proteinuria + foamy urine + "spike-and-dome"

Clinical Presentation: An 8-year-old child with hepatitis B from rural China has bubbles in his urine.

PPx: Treat underlying disease

MoD: Chronic Hep B infection → immune complex (antigen-antibody) deposits in glomeruli subepithelium → podocytes disrupted in hepatitis B virus (HBV) (membranous nephropathy)

Dx:
1. UA
2. BMP
3. Hepatitis B serology
4. Electron microscopy shows spike-and-dome GBM

Tx/Mgmt: Spontaneous resolution in children, manage HBV in adults

Poststreptococcal Glomerulonephritis (PSGN)

Buzz Words: Child + 2 weeks post-URI or skin infection + edema + cola-colored urine + hypertension + "lumpy bumpy" GBM + antigen–antibody complexes with subendothelial immunoglobulin (Ig)G and IgM deposition + elevated antistreptolysin-O (ASO) + decreased complement

Clinical Presentation: A 5-year-old girl has brown-colored urine and hypertension after a URI.

MoD: Group A strep (GAS) infection of skin or pharynx → type 3 hypersensitivity (HS) reaction 2 weeks later → subepithelial immune complex deposition → GBM disruption

Dx:
1. UA shows RBC casts (nephritis)
2. BMP
3. Positive strep antigen serology
4. Immunofluorescence (IF) shows lumpy-bumpy GBM

Tx/Mgmt: Supportive: spontaneous resolution in 2–3 weeks. Loop diuretics as needed for hypertension.

Immunoglobulin A Nephropathy (Berger Disease)

Buzz Words: Episodic hematuria + renal insufficiency + recent URI or gastroenteritis + nephritic syndrome + Henoch-Schönlein purpura + mesangial deposits on light microscopy (LM) + IgA stain on IF

Clinical Presentation: 12-year-old boy has hematuria and petechiae after a URI.

MoD: → increased synthesis of IgA → deposits in glomerular mesangium (next to capillaries) → GBM disruption

Dx:
1. Urinalysis shows RBC casts.
2. BMP
3. Confirmation with kidney biopsy, but clinical diagnosis is often sufficient. IgA may be elevated but is NOT diagnostic.

Tx/Mgmt: ACE inhibitors/ARBs to manage hypertension and proteinuria

Lupus Nephritis

Buzz Words: Lupus symptoms (fatigue, fever, butterfly rash, arthritis) + nephrotic and/or nephritic syndrome + wire loops on light microscopy (LM) + subendothelial deposits on electron microscopy (EM) + full house on IF

Clinical Presentation: A woman who has a history of lupus presents with hematuria.

PPx: Early detection by evaluating renal function in SLE patients with or without renal disease symptoms

MoD: Chronic lupus → deposited anti-dsDNA immune complexes and autoantibodies attack GBM antigens → GBM disruption

Dx:
1. UA
2. BMP
3. Renal biopsy

Tx/Mgmt:
1. Corticosteroids
2. ACEIs/ARBs
3. Dietary restriction of fat for hyperlipidemia

QUICK TIPS

Most common nephrotic syndrome in children

Minimal Change Disease (Lipoid Nephrosis)

Buzz Words: Child + facial edema + recent immunization or bee sting + normal light microscopy + foot process effacement

Clinical Presentation: A 4-year-old child with a recent URI presents with facial edema.

MoD: Infection/immunization → GBM loses podocytes → GBM loses negative charge → negatively charged albumin lost

Dx: Clinical diagnosis: EM shows podocyte effacement.

Tx/Mgmt: Corticosteroids produce full resolution.

Thin Basement Membrane Disease/Nephropathy

Buzz Words: Asymptomatic + persistent, benign microscopic hematuria + incidentally found on UA + family history of hematuria + no hypertension + normal on LM + thin basement membrane on EM

Clinical Presentation: This is also known as benign familial hematuria. Incidental UA finding of microscopic hematuria.

MoD: Hereditary genetic defect → thin GBM → intermittent asymptomatic hematuria

Dx: Clinical diagnosis

Tx/Mgmt: Spontaneous resolution (Table 10.1)

Acute Interstitial Nephritis (Tubulointerstitial Nephritis)

Buzz Words: Recent penicillin/gentamicin/NSAID/IV contrast use + allergic rash + fever + hematuria + WBC casts + eosinophils

Clinical Presentation: A patient recently on penicillin presents with fever and a new rash.

MoD: Medication (e.g., gentamicin) → hypersensitivity reaction → inflammation of interstitium surrounding kidney tubules → decreased renal function → creatinine clearance

Dx:
1. BMP
2. UA (eosinophils in urine)
3. Renal biopsy (rarely performed)

Tx/Mgmt: Remove offending medication

Acute Tubular Necrosis

Buzz Words: Crush injury + contrast + hypotension + muddy-brown casts + oliguria + normal BUN/CR but increased on BMP due to oliguria

Clinical Presentation: Acute tubular necrosis is, as the name suggests, the rapid death of renal tubular cells. At this

TABLE 10.1 Glomerular Disease

Disease	Buzz Words	Syndrome	Dx	Tx
Alport syndrome	Cataracts, deafness, males in family	Nephritic	EM: Basket-weave split GBM	ACEIs/ARBs
Hepatitis C	Cryoglobulinemia	Nephritic/nephrotic	EM: Tram-track GBM	Manage Hep C
Hepatitis B	Immigrant, foamy urine, massive proteinuria	Nephrotic	EM: Spike-and-dome GBM	Supportive
Poststreptococcal glomerulonephritis	URI, skin infection, cola-colored urine	Nephritic	Streptococcal antigen serology	Supportive
IgA nephropathy	URI, gastroenteritis	Nephritic	Clinical	ACEIs/ARBs
Lupus nephritis	Rash, arthritis	Nephritic/nephrotic	Renal biopsy	Supportive; corticosteroids, ACEIs/ARBs
Minimal change disease	Facial edema, URI, immunization, bee sting	Nephrotic	Clinical	Corticosteroids
Thin basement membrane disease	Asymptomatic, familial hematuria	Nephrotic	Clinical	Supportive

point, there is irreversible kidney damage. It is the most common cause of acute kidney injury (AKI). Acute tubular necrosis (ATN) most commonly affects hospitalized patients and is made up of three phases. First is the *inciting event* or *injury*, most often ischemia. Next is the *maintenance phase*, characterized by oliguria and hyperkalemia, which lasts up to 3 weeks. Last, the *recovery phase*, characterized by polyuria and possible hypokalemia. A typical patient presents with oliguria after volume depletion (diarrhea, vomiting), long time spent down, or a scan or procedure requiring contrast dye.

PPx: Adequate fluid administration

MoD: Ischemia or nephrotoxic substances (e.g., contrast, myoglobinuria, hemoglobinuria) → tubular cells die and slough off

Dx:

1. BMP
2. UA shows muddy-brown casts
3. Positive response to fluid repletion

Tx/Mgmt: IV fluid repletion→ spontaneous resolution

QUICK TIPS

PCT and TAL = Hardest-working cells of renal tubule = need most blood = die first during ischemia

Papillary Necrosis

Buzz Words: Hematuria + proteinuria + sickle cell + NSAIDs + diabetic with acute pyelonephritis

Clinical Presentation:
- Chief complaint: flank pain
- Past medical history (PMH): Chronic analgesic use, diabetes, sickle cell

MoD: Pyelonephritis in diabetes, chronic analgesic abuse, or sickle cell sickling causes ischemia and death of papillae.

Dx:
1. BMP
2. UA

Tx/Mgt: Supportive

HIV Nephropathy

Buzz Words: African American + HIV + hematuria + nephrotic syndrome

Clinical Presentation: Hematuria and/or proteinuria occur in an HIV patient.

PPx: Proper management of HIV

MoD: HIV progresses → infects kidney epithelial cells → inflammation

Dx:
1. BMP
2. UA
3. Kidney biopsy shows focal segmental glomerulosclerosis (FSGS).

Tx/Mgmt: Antiretroviral therapy

Lower Urinary Tract

Interstitial Cystitis/Bladder Pain Syndrome

Buzz Words: Chronic (>6 weeks) suprapubic pain + lower urinary tract symptoms + NO evidence of infection + gross hematuria + radiation exposure or malignancy

Clinical Presentation: Interstitial cystitis is a complex condition that serves as a last-resort diagnosis for chronic suprapubic pain. There is no evidence of inflammation; rather, it is a chronic pain syndrome much like fibromyalgia. This is rarely tested but should be considered if the questions make clear that all etiologies have been thoroughly explored with unsuccessful outcomes.

Dx:
1. CBC
2. UA and urine culture (UCx)
3. Kidney ultrasound

4. Cystogram if sclerotherapy
5. Vesicoureterogram. (6) Cystoscopy
Tx/Mgmt: Relieve symptoms to maintain quality of life

Neoplasms

Benign Neoplasms and Cysts

Renal Oncocytoma

Buzz Words: Painless hematuria + flank pain + well-circumscribed mass + central scar

Clinical Presentation: Renal oncocytoma is the most common benign neoplasm of the kidney. Incidental imaging finding or painless hematuria, flank pain, abdominal mass.

MoD: Collecting duct cell proliferation

Dx:
1. BMP
2. UA
3. CT or MRI
4. Biopsy (eosinophilic cells filled with mitochondria)

Tx/Mgmt: Surgical resection if mass >1 cm

Renal Cyst

Buzz Words: Incidental renal mass + asymptomatic + hypoechoic center

Clinical Presentation: Renal cysts, the most common renal masses, are often asymptomatic and found incidentally. Simple cysts are benign, requiring no treatment. Complex cysts (explained further on) require more attention, as they carry risk for malignancy. Incidental finding on imaging.

Dx: Ultrasound shows anechoic (dark) center in simple cysts or septation and/or solid components in complex cysts.

Tx/Mgmt: No treatment if simple cyst. Surgical removal if complex cyst.

Malignant Neoplasms

Wilms Tumor/Nephroblastoma

Buzz Words: Toddler + palpable abdominal mass + hematuria + hemihypertrophy + aniridia + mental retardation

Clinical Presentation: Wilms tumors are the most common and should be your go-to answer for early childhood renal masses. Wilms is one condition of both the Beckwith-Wiedemann syndrome and WAGR (Wilms tumor, aniridia, genitourinary malformation, mental retardation) complex, most recognized by hemihypertrophy and aniridia, respectively.

Affected children may have a palpable unilateral abdominal mass.

MoD: WT1/WT2 mutation → loss of function of tumor suppressor genes → embryonic glomerulus proliferates

Dx:
1. Kidney ultrasound
2. CT

Tx/Mgmt: Nephrectomy with possible supplementary chemotherapy and radiation

Renal Cell Carcinoma

Buzz Words: Older male + smoker + palpable mass + flank pain + hematuria + weight loss

Clinical Presentation: RCC is a silent assassin because it is often already metastatic at presentation. The most common renal malignancy in adults, it is often associated with paraneoplastic syndromes (i.e., ACTH, EPO). RCC is also seen in von Hippel-Lindau syndrome (think RCC with hypertension) and tuberous sclerosis (think RCC with CNS, cardiac, and skin pathology).

PPx: Quit smoking

MoD: PCT cell proliferation

Dx:
1. BMP
2. UA/UCx
3. Abdominal ultrasound or CT

Tx/Mgmt:
1. Surgically resect if tumor is localized.
2. Chemotherapy if tumor has metastasized.

Transitional Cell Carcinoma

Buzz Words: Painless hematuria + cyclophosphamide + smoking + aniline dyes + phenacetin

Clinical Presentation: This is a test favorite as it is the most commonly seen malignancy of the urinary system, located in the bladder, ureter, and/or renal pelvis. A 50-year-old Caucasian man with a significant smoking history and a history of working in a cloth-dying factory presents with painless hematuria.

PPx: Smoking cessation

MoD: Chemical carcinogens

Dx:
1. BMP
2. UA/UCx
3. Cystoscopy

Tx/Mgmt: Transurethral resection

TABLE 10.2 Acute Kidney Injury

Type	Problem	Causes	Common BUN/Cr
Prerenal (MC)	Hypoperfusion	Hypotension, volume loss, cardiac failure	>20
Intrinsic	Renal cell dysfunction	Nephrotoxins (rhabdomyolysis) or irreversible ischemia	<15
Postrenal	Output obstruction	Obstruction: BPH, nephrolithiasis	15–20

Metabolic and Regulatory Disorders

The following sections discuss the spectrum of renal insufficiency, or loss of function. Renal insufficiency may occur due to acute or chronic pathologies, all of which result in predictable sequelae: hyperkalemia, acidemia, electrolyte imbalance, acidosis, and azotemia/uremia. Azotemia is the state of elevated BUN and Cr in the blood. Uremic syndrome, the symptoms resulting from BUN buildup, has toxic effects on all organs in the body, most notably causing inflammation of the cardiac sac and mental status changes. These effects are more often seen with chronic renal insufficiency when BUN is greater than 50 mg/dL.

Acute

Acute Kidney Injury (Table 10.2)
Buzz Words:
- **AKI:** Hospitalized patient + sudden oliguria + hypotension + elevated Cr levels + heart failure + rhabdomyolysis + diuretics
- **Prerenal failure:** Elevated urine osmolarity + decreased urine Na + low FeNa (<1%) + elevated BUN:Cr (>20:1) + hyaline cast on UA
- **Intrinsic failure:** Glomerulonephritis + AKI
- **Postrenal failure:** Complete obstruction of the urinary tract + renal failure + low urine osmolarity (<35) + elevated urine Na (>40) + elevated FeNa (>1%) + BUN:Cr >15:1

Clinical Presentation: AKI is a SUDDEN drop in kidney function that may be superimposed on chronic kidney damage. It is on the same spectrum as renal failure, since renal tubular cells are damaged, but the kidney maintains the ability to recover functionality. The tubular cell damage may be reversible or irreversible depending on the cause and extent of the damage.

Damage can be done by various mechanisms neatly classified based on location: prerenal, intrarenal, and postrenal. AKI must be treated immediately to avoid potentially fatal sequelae.

- BUN = normally reabsorbed by kidney
- Azotemia = rise in BUN in an asymptomatic patient
- Uremia = rise in BUN in a symptomatic patient

PPx: Hydration for potentially hypovolemic patients

MoD:

- Prerenal—reversible ischemia (hypotension, volume loss, cardiac failure)
- Intrinsic AKI—nephrotoxins (rhabdo) or irreversible ischemia
- Postrenal—Obstruction (benign prostatic hyperplasia [BPH], nephrolithiasis)

Dx:

1. BMP
2. Urinalysis
3. Kidney ultrasound if postrenal suspected

Tx/Mgmt: Manage the resultant electrolyte and fluid abnormalities (IV fluids) while figuring out the cause (prerenal, intrinsic, or postrenal) → kidney function will return to normal:

- **Prerenal:** Avoid NSAIDs, ACEi, maximize renal perfusion by treating underlying cause
- **Intrinsic:** Eliminate offending agents, trial of furosemide
- **Posterenal:** Bladder catheterization

Chronic Kidney Disease

Chronic kidney disease (CKD) is formally identified as GFR less than 60 mL/min for more than 3 months. By this point, the kidneys have essentially shriveled up (can be seen on ultrasound), continuing to lose function until they eventually enter end-stage renal disease (ESRD) and ultimately renal failure (RF). The following conditions are variations of CKD, most of which lack a definitive cure and must be managed symptomatically.

End-Stage Renal Disease

Buzz Words: Diabetes + HTN + glomerulonephritis + uremic syndrome + electrolyte abnormalities + anemia

Clinical Presentation: In ESRD, the kidney is on its last breath! Also be mindful that ESRD is the only condition for which patients are eligible for Medicare despite not meeting age requirements.

Dx:

1. BMP → GFR—may estimate via Cr
2. Urinalysis

Tx/Mgmt: There is no cure short of transplantation, so manage complications as they come, concentrating on electrolytes (e.g., hyperkalemia), volume overload, and infection. Patients are often on hemodialysis.

Cystinuria

Buzz Words: Familial renal colic + cyanide nitroprusside–positive urine + hexagonal/benzene crystals + radiopaque staghorn calculi + rotten-egg smell

Clinical Presentation:
- Age: Less than 20 years
- Chief complaint: Renal colic
- PMH: Kidney stones during childhood, family history of stones in males

MoD: Autosomal recessive positively charged amino acid transporter deficiency → cysteines bond → hexagonal cystine crystals accumulate, forming stones → staghorn calculi

Dx:
1. UA shows hexagonal crystals
2. Urinary cyanide nitroprusside

Tx/Mgmt:
1. Hydration
2. Acetazolamide (alkalinization of urine increases cystine solubility)

Fanconi Syndrome

Buzz Words: Polyuria/polydypsia + metabolic acidosis + rickets/osteomalacia + family history

Clinical Presentation:
- Age: Less than 10 years
- Chief complaint: Polyuria and polydipsia
- PMH: Renal tubular acidosis or rickets in family

MoD: Proximal tubule resorption defect caused by any damage to the kidney: cystinuria (main cause in children), Wilson disease, nephrotoxic drugs such as cisplatin

Dx:
1. BMP
2. Urinalysis (excess amino acids, glucose, bicarbonate, potassium)

Tx/Mgmt:
1. Correct resultant nutritional deficiencies and metabolic acidosis. This is a type 2 renal tubular acidosis (RTA II); hypokalemic hyperchloremic normal gap acidosis.
2. Kidney transplant if severe.

MNEMONIC

AEIOU = indications for dialysis: Acidosis (pH < 7.1), Electrolytes (potassium > 6.5), Intoxicants (lithium, ethylene glycol, methanol, salicylates), Overload (volume), Uremia with systemic effects (mental status changes, pericarditis)

Hypertensive Renal Disease (Hypertensive Nephrosclerosis)

Buzz Words: Long-standing HTN + increase in BP + papilledema + sudden decline in renal function + African American

Clinical Presentation: Long-term systemic hypertension may eventually lead to progressive renal failure. This can take on a benign or malignant form. You will most often be tested on the latter, as presented here.

- Age: Greater than 60 years
- Gender: Men > women
- Chief complaint: Blood pressure spike (diastolic >115)

PPx: Control HTN

MoD: Increased systemic blood pressure → increased renal capillary pressure → compensatory thickening or sclerosis of afferent arterioles → narrower arteriolar lumen → ischemia → decreased renal function → exacerbation of HTN → heart failure or stroke

Dx:

1. BMP
2. UA (increased Cr excretion with possible proteinuria/hematuria)

Tx/Mgmt: Decrease BP

Nephrolithiasis (Renal and Ureteral Calculi)

Buzz Words:

- **Nephrolithiasis:** Colicky flank pain + radiates to groin + dehydrated + hematuria + loop diuretics
- **Uric acid stone:** Radiolucent + flat square plates
- **Calcium oxalate:** Radiodense + bipyramidal ovals + biconcave ovals
- **Struvite stones:** Radiodense + staghorn calculi + rectangular prisms
- **Cysteine stones:** Radiolucent "stop sign" stones

Clinical Presentation:

- Age: 20–50 years
- Gender: Men > women
- Chief complaint: Flank pain
- Medications: Chemotherapy, loop diuretics, acetazolamide

PPx: Hydration

MoD: Low fluid consumption or substance accumulation in urine → supersaturation of calcium (MC), oxalate, and/or uric acid in the urine → formation of stones

- Hypercalciuria from increased intestinal absorption or renal excretion

- Hyperuricemia from gout or chemotherapy
- Struvite stones from bacteria producing ammonia (e.g., *Proteus, Klebsiella*)

Dx:
1. UA
2. Kidneys, ureters, bladder (KUB)
3. Spiral CT without contrast

Tx/Mgmt: IV fluids and analgesia as needed for all patients, further measures depend on size of stone and severity of pain:
- <0.5 cm spontaneous passage; hydrate and analgesics as needed.
- >0.7 cm removal:
  1. Shock-wave lithotripsy
  2. Stent
  3. Nephrostomy

Renal Tubular Acidosis

Buzz Words:
- **RTA:** Hyperchloremic + unexplained normal gap metabolic acidosis
- **Type 1 (distal):** RTA + fluid contraction + hypokalemia + nephrolithiasis + rickets
- **Type 2 (proximal):** RTA + hypokalemia + hypophosphatemic rickets + alkaline urine
- **Type 4:** RTA + hyperkalemic hyperchlroemic non–anion gap metabolic acidosis + alkaline urine

Clinical Presentation: Renal tubular acidosis (RTA) is a metabolic acidosis characterized by hyperchloremia and a normal anion gap. There are three major types of RTA, resulting from injury to different parts of the renal tubule. The glomerulus is spared in all three.

MoD: Renal tubule cell defect → insufficient urinary acid excretion → metabolic acidosis:
- Type 1 → Distal tubule defect → Decreased hydrogen excretion
- Type 2 → Proximal tubule defect → Increased bicarbonate excretion
- Type 4 → Aldosterone-related defect → Decreased hydrogen and potassium excretion, hyperkalemia is a distinguishing feature of RTA 4

Dx: NAG metabolic acidosis → rule out other causes → urinary pH

Tx/Mgmt: Treat underlying cause:
- Type 1 → sodium bicarbonate to correct metabolic acidosis
- Type 2 → Sodium restriction to stimulate bicarbonate resorption

Vascular Disorders

The kidney is highly susceptible to ischemia, as its blood supply lacks extensive branching. Thus, disruption of blood flow cannot be easily combated by anastomosis or collateral circulation.

Renal Artery Stenosis

Renal artery stenosis (RAS) is a narrowing of the renal artery. It has numerous etiologies, most notably atherosclerosis, fibromuscular dysplasia, and nephrosclerosis (discussed earlier). All forms of RAS entail renovascular hypertension through the renin-angiotensin system. Naturally RAS also results in renal insufficiency as a result of ischemic tubular cell damage.

QUICK TIPS
RAS = MCC secondary to arterial hypertension

Atherosclerosis

Buzz Words: Elderly male + abdominal bruit + headache + unexplained severe HTN + high renin levels + renal insufficiency

Clinical Presentation:
- Age: Greater than 50 years
- Gender: Men > women
- Chief complaint: Headache
- PMH: Atherosclerosis, smoking, diabetes, hyperlipidemia

PPx: Control metabolic syndrome

MoD: Metabolic syndrome → arterial insult → atherosclerotic plaque formation → narrowing of renal artery → decreased renal perfusion → (1) increased renin-angiotensin (2) tubular cell ischemic atrophy

Dx:
- Renal arteriogram—cannot be used in renal failure
- Magnetic resonance angiography (MRA)—safe in renal failure

Tx/Mgmt:
1. Control HTN
2. Revascularization if (a) greater than 80% stenosis, (b) ACE inhibitors raise Cr levels, (c) greater than 50% with positive scintigraphy

Fibromuscular Dysplasia

Buzz Words: Young female + abdominal bruit + severe HTN (>200/100) + ACE inhibitors exacerbate HTN + high renin levels

Clinical Presentation: Along with narrowing of the renal arteries, fibromuscular dysplasia may affect the carotid and vertebral arteries. Compromise of either artery

leading to the brain can lead to ischemic or hemorrhagic stroke:
- Age: Less than 40 years
- Gender: Women > men
- Chief complaint: Headache

Dx:
1. Renal arteriogram
2. MRA

Tx/Mgmt:
1. Revascularization by stenting if severe
2. Manage HTN
3. Aspirin prophylaxis if carotid or vertebral artery affected

Acute Arterial Event

Renal Vein Thrombosis

Buzz Words: Nephrotic syndrome + renal cell carcinoma + sudden renal insufficiency + sudden flank pain

Clinical Presentation: Flank pain is present in a hypercoagulable patient (OCPs, cancer, nephrotic syndrome).

MoD: Hypercoagulable state → thrombosis → decreased renal perfusion

Dx:
1. BMP
2. UA/UCx
3. Renal venography
4. Intravenous pyelogram (IVP)

Tx/Mgmt:
1. Treat underlying cause
2. Anticoagulation; prophylaxis for pulmonary embolism

Renal Infarction

Buzz Words: Sudden flank pain + cardiac arrhythmia + valvular disease + recent angiogram

Clinical Presentation:
- Age: Greater than 50 years
- Gender: Women > men
- Chief complaint: Sudden flank pain
- PMH: Heart failure, myocardial infarction (MI), valvular disease

MoD:
- Cardiac arrhythmia → thromboemboli → renal artery occlusion
- Angiogram → cholesterol crystals dislodged from arterial atherosclerotic plaque → embolization

Dx:
1. BMP
2. UA/UCx

3. ECG for MI
4. CT with contrast to view infarction
5. Arteriogram to locate occlusion

Tx/Mgmt:
- Cardiac origin:
  1. Anticoagulation
  2. Revascularization
- Cholesterol emboli—supportive treatment only

Traumatic and Mechanical Disorders

Bladder Rupture

Buzz Words: Pelvic fracture + hematuria + suprapubic pain + unstable pelvis

Clinical Presentation: Chief complaint: Suprapubic pain

PPx: Urinate before driving

MoD: Distended bladder → pelvic trauma → bladder rupture: Extraperitoneal rupture is most common.

Dx: Retrograde cystogram with pre- and postvoid imaging

Tx/Mgmt:
- Extraperitoneal rupture: Foley
- Intraperitoneal rupture: Surgical repair with suprapubic cystostomy

Neurogenic Bladder

Buzz Words: Overflow incontinence + urgency/frequency + stroke + spinal cord damage

Clinical Presentation: Hyperactive or hypoactive bladder occurs in a patient with a history of stroke or spinal cord damage.

MoD: Stroke, Parkinson disease, spinal lesion → neurologic dysfunction → sympathetic and parasympathetic nervous system imbalance → bladder dysfunction

Dx:
1. BMP
2. UA/UCx
3. Postvoid residual volume

Tx/Mgmt:
- Hyperactive—anticholinergics
- Hypoactive—intermittent self-catheterization

Urinary Tract Obstruction

Buzz Words: BPH + renal colic + low urine flow + hydronephrosis

Clinical Presentation: Urinary tract obstruction has numerous etiologies and variations; however it can be defined by a general principle. Proximal to the blockage, there is urine buildup within and eventual dilation of the urinary tract structures. BPH is the most commonly encountered obstruction. Other causes include kidney stones, cancer, trauma, and urethral stricture.

- Age: Greater than 50 years
- Gender: Men > women
- Chief complaint: Renal colic
- PMH: BPH, prostate cancer, UTI, kidney stones

MoD: Blockage of the urinary tract → fluid backup → hydronephrosis

Dx:

1. BMP
2. UA
3. Renal ultrasound shows distention of structures proximal to obstruction.

Tx/Mgmt:

- BPH—prostatectomy
- Urethral obstruction—Foley catheterization, stent placement

Posterior Urethral Valves

Buzz Words: Antenatal ultrasound + newborn male + no urination in first day

Clinical Presentation:

- Age: Neonate
- Gender: Male only
- Chief complaint: Hydronephrosis on antenatal ultrasound

MoD: Congenital defect due to embryogenic malformation

Dx:

- Antenatal ultrasound during gestation
- Voiding cystourethrogram for newborn

Tx/Mgmt:

1. Foley catheter—relieves obstruction.
2. Endoscopic resection is curative.

Renal Laceration

Buzz Words: Abdominal trauma + rib fracture + gross hematuria + flank pain

Clinical Presentation: Gross hematuria after trauma

MoD: Penetrating or blunt abdominal trauma

Dx: CT scan

Tx/Mgmt:

- Exploratory laparotomy if penetrating trauma per protocol
- Expectant management if blunt trauma

Ureteral Laceration/Avulsion/Disruption

Buzz Words: Motor vehicle accident (MVA) + pelvic trauma + abdominal or ob/gyn surgery + flank pain

Clinical Presentation: Flank pain and bruising after trauma or surgery

MoD: External trauma or iatrogenic during abdominal surgery

Dx: CT with contrast

Tx/Mgmt: Surgical repair or stent placement

Urethral Diverticulum

Buzz Words: Lower urinary tract symptoms + anterior vaginal wall mass + recurrent UTI

Clinical Presentation:
- Chief complaint: Lower urinary symptoms
- PMH: Recurrent UTI

MoD: Outpouching of urethral mucosa toward the vaginal canal → urine pools in the pouch → UTI

Dx: Voiding cystourethrography

Tx/Mgmt: Surgical repair

Urinary Incontinence

Buzz Words: Retirement home + inability to control urination with coughing/laughing + diabetes + BPH + cannot reach toilet in time

MoD:
- **Stress incontinence**: Pelvic floor weakness increased abdominal pressure (cough, sneeze) exceeds resistance → urinary leakage
- **Urge incontinence**: Detrusor muscle hyperactivity → increased frequency of bladder emptying
- **Functional incontinence**: Unable to get to the bathroom in time despite normal urinary tract
- Physiology—for example, delirium, depression, immobility
- **Overflow incontinence**: Bladder hypoactivity (diabetic neuropathy) or distal obstruction (BPH) → urinary retention → frequent voiding but low volume

Dx
1. BMP
2. UA/UCx

Tx/Mgmt:
- **Stress**—(1) Pelvic floor exercises. (2) Surgical repair of pelvic floor.
- **Urge**—Anticholinergics decrease detrusor activity.
- **Functional**—Decrease volume of intake and treat underlying cause.
- **Overflow**—Cholinergics to increase detrusor activity.

Vesicoureteral Reflux

Buzz Words: Child with UTI + high fever + flank pain

Clinical Presentation:
- Age: Less than 10 years
- Chief complaint: Burning on urination
- PMH: Recurrent UTI

MoD: Congenital malformation of ureter at vesicoureteral junction → unable to prevent retrograde urine flow → carries bacteria up to kidney

Dx:
1. BMP
2. Urine culture for infection
3. Voiding cystourethrogram to confirm VUR

Tx/Mgmt:
1. Empiric antibiotics for infection → update after culture.
2. Antibiotic prophylaxis until spontaneous resolution. Use typical UTI-associated medication; for example, TMP-SMX and nitrofurantoin.

Congenital Disorders

Double Ureter

Buzz Words: Child with UTI + VUR ruled out

Clinical Presentation: Congenital ureter anomalies—duplicate ureters and collecting systems—are most often detected by prenatal imaging, which shows hydronephrosis. However, you are more likely to be tested on the late presentation form, which is a cause of UTI in children.
- Age: Less than 10 years, especially less than 3 months
- Chief complaint: Painful urination
- PMH: Recurrent UTI

MoD: Congenital defect from error in embryogenesis

Dx: Kidney ultrasound

Tx/Mgmt:
1. Antibiotics for UTI
2. Surgery, if needed, after child is 1 year old.

Horseshoe Kidney

Buzz Words: Child with UTI + Turner syndrome + ureteropelvic junction obstruction (UPJ) + kidney stones + kidney fused at midline

Clinical Presentation:
- Age: Less than 10 years
- Chief complaint: Painful urination or renal colic

MoD: Lower kidney poles fuse at midline during embryogenesis → altered anatomy predisposes to stones and infection

- Altered anatomy may include UPJ
- Associated with Turner syndrome

Dx:
1. IVP
2. CT

Tx/Mgmt: Kidney function is preserved; treat complications as needed.

Renal Hypodysplasia and Agenesis

Buzz Words: Small or absent kidney + small birth size + poor growth

Clinical Presentation: A 9-month-old infant has an absent kidney, found incidentally on ultrasound. His mother has hypertension and took lisinopril during pregnancy.

MoD: Genetic or teratogenic (ACEIs/ARBs during pregnancy)

Dx: Renal ultrasound

Tx/Mgmt: Supportive

GUNNER PRACTICE

1. An 18-year-old Caucasian woman comes into clinic complaining of severe headaches that have gotten progressively worse over the last 6 days. She has been under increased stress lately and believes this to be the cause of her headaches. She has taken NSAIDs daily for the headaches but states that this does not help. She has no prior medical history, does not smoke, no family history of headaches, and exercises regularly. She plays volleyball for her school and was hit in the head by a stray ball during practice last week. She fell down but did not lose consciousness. She has a BMI of 21 kg/m^2. On physical exam, her pulse is 70/min, respirations 15/min, and blood pressure is 200/120 mm Hg. Cardiopulmonary and neurologic examinations show no abnormalities. Lab results show elevated renin levels. What is the most likely cause of her headache?
   A. Head injury
   B. NSAID abuse
   C. Fibromuscular dysplasia
   D. Stress
   E. Migraine

2. A 3-year-old boy is brought into the hospital by his parents after they saw blood stains on his underwear. They had seen the blood spots once before a week ago but haven't seen any blood in the toilet. The boy has not been irritable but had a cold 1 month ago. He is pleasant

upon exam, is of normal height and weight for his age, and makes good eye contact but ignores commands. Physical exam is normal. The father mentions that the boy has had trouble walking in the last 6 months and occasionally bumps into objects. What is the next step?

A. Reassure the parents that their son is developing normally

B. Kidney biopsy

C. Urinalysis

D. Begin lowest dose of ACE inhibitor therapy

E. Pelvic CT

3. EMS rushes into the trauma bay with a 36-year-old woman who was pulled from a car accident. She was the driver in a head-on collision with another car, going about 60 mph at the time of collision. She is fully responsive and complaining of pain around her belly button. She says she feels like something is trying to claw its way out of her stomach. Primary exam shows patent airway, symmetrical breathing, and full pulses bilaterally. She has minor lacerations on her legs and forehead that have begun to clot. Upon moving the patient's left leg, she screams in pain, as her leg feels loose or disconnected from her hip. Pulse is 80, respiratory rate 16, and blood pressure 130/80 mm Hg. What is the next step in management?

A. Immediate surgery

B. Retrograde cystogram

C. X-ray of the abdomen/pelvis

D. MRI of the abdomen/pelvis

E. CT of the abdomen/pelvis

ANSWERS: What Would Gunner Jess/Jim Do?

1. WWGJD? An 18-year-old Caucasian woman comes into clinic complaining of severe headaches that have gotten progressively worse over the last 6 days. She has been under increased stress lately due to college applications and believes this to be the cause of her headaches. She has taken advil daily for the headaches, but states they do not help. She has no prior medical history, does not smoke, no family history of headaches, and exercises regularly. She plays volleyball for her school and was hit in the head by a stray ball during practice last week. She fell down, but did not lose consciousness. She has a BMI of 21kg/m². On physical exam, her pulse is 70/min, respirations 15/min, and blood pressure is 200/120 mm Hg. Cardiopulmonary and neurologic examination shows no abnormalities. Lab results show elevated renin levels. What is the most likely cause of her headache?

Answer: C, Fibromuscular dysplasia

Explanation: Pt is a young female with no past medical history with severely elevated blood pressure. This high blood pressure at such a young age and no other explanation should immediately raise flags for fibromuscular dysplasia. The headache is most likely a direct result of the elevated blood pressure.

A. Head injury → Incorrect. A blow to the head with a volleyball is unlikely to cause a severe head injury. This is supported by the fact that the patient did not lose consciousness.

B. NSAID abuse → Incorrect. Four days of NSAID use is unlikely to cause rebound headache, and this does not explain the elevated blood pressure.

D. Stress → Incorrect. Cannot explain elevated blood pressure.

E. Migraine → Incorrect. Cannot explain elevated blood pressure.

2. WWGJD? A 3-year-old boy is brought into the hospital by his concerned parents afterthey saw blood stains in his underwear. They have seen the blood spots once before a week ago, but haven't seen any blood in the toilet. The boy has not been irritable in the last two weeks, but had a cold 1 month ago. The boy is pleasant upon exam, playing with his toy airplane. He is of normal height and weight for his age, makes good eye contact, but ignores commands. Physical exam is normal. The father mentions the boy has had some trouble

walking in the last 6 months. He occasionally bumps into objects. What is the next step?

Answer: C, Urinalysis

Explanation: The boy has suspected Alport syndrome with glomerulonephritis, deafness, and altered vision. Urinalysis will identify the glomerulonephritis, mainly showing proteinuria.

A. Reassure the parents that their son is developing normally → Incorrect. The Pt has clear developmental delays.

B. Kidney biopsy → Incorrect. Although electron microscopic examination of a kidney specimen will show the typical split GBM in Alport, this is invasive and should not be done as the first step.

D. Begin lowest dose of ACE inhibitor therapy → Incorrect. Diagnosis should be confirmed and the extent of the disease should be evaluated before initiating treatment.

E. Pelvic CT → Incorrect. CT can eventually be used if no other etiologies are found, but it is not the correct first step for a patient suspected of having Alport syndrome.

3. WWGJD? EMS rushes into the trauma bay with a 36-year-old woman who was pulled from a car accident. She was the driver in a head on collision with another car, going about 60mph at the time of collision. She is fully responsive and complaining of pain around her belly button. She says she feels like something is trying to claw its way out of her stomach. Primary exam shows patent airway, symmetrical breathing, and full pulses bilaterally. She has minor lacerations on her legs and forehead that have begun to clot. Upon moving the patient's left leg, she screams in pain as her leg feels loose or disconnected from her hip. Pulse is 80, respiratory rate 16, and blood pressure is 130/80 mmHg. What is the next step in management?

Answer: B, Retrograde cystography

Explanation: Patient has suffered trauma to the pelvis, most likely from the steering wheel during rapid deceleration. There is severe pelvic laxity, which, in combination with suprapubic pain, indicates bladder rupture. Diagnosis can be made through retrograde cystography with pre- and postvoid imaging.

A. Immediate surgery → Incorrect. Surgery is not immediately indicated in this situation as long as the patient remains stable.

C. X-ray of the abdomen/pelvis → Incorrect. An x-ray will not accurately display bladder rupture.

D. MRI of the abdomen/pelvis → Incorrect. MRI will not accurately display bladder rupture.

E. CT of the abdomen/pelvis → Incorrect. CT is often used to evaluate trauma patients, but when bladder rupture is suspected, retrograde cystography is the first step.

Disorders of Pregnancy, Childbirth, and the Puerperium

Hao-Hua Wu, Kaitlyn Barkley, Leo Wang, Rebecca Gao, and DeCarla Albright

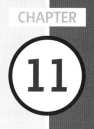

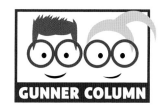

GUNNER COLUMN

Introduction

A little-known fact about the Surgery shelf is that 3%–7% of the questions will focus on disorders related to pregnancy, childbirth, and the puerperium, defined as the period of about 6 weeks after childbirth. The topics that most frequently appear on the Surgery shelf are covered here, including ectopic pregnancy, cervical insufficiency, Turner syndrome, Erb and Klumpke palsy, 22q11.2 deletion syndrome (aka DiGeorge syndrome), and congenital infections. The other disorders listed in the USMLE content outline are low-yield and rarely appear on the shelf. Anticipate spending no more than 2 hours on this chapter to peruse the material and complete the questions.

This chapter is divided into (1) Obstetric Complications, (2) Disorders of the Newborn, and (3) Gunner Practice. The diseases are presented in the following format: (1) Buzz Words, (2) Clinical Presentation, (3) Prophylaxis (PPx), (4) Mechanism of Disease (MoD), (5) Diagnostic Steps (Dx), and (6) Treatment and Management Steps (Tx/Mgmt).

Obstetric Complications

The most important obstetric complication to learn is ectopic pregnancy, which can also appear on the Ob/Gyn, Pediatrics, and Medicine shelf.

Ectopic Pregnancy

Buzz Words:
- Abdominal pain + amenorrhea + vaginal bleeding + palpable adnexal mass
- Beta hCG >2000 + thin endometrial stripe + "no adnexal masses" + no fetal pole in uterus
- **Ruptured ectopic:** Abdominal pain + amenorrhea + vaginal bleeding + orthostatic changes + hypovolemic shock

Clinical Presentation: Ectopic pregnancy is a condition in which the fertilized egg matures outside of the uterus (e.g., in the fallopian tube). This is particularly relevant on the Medicine shelf because it can present as lower right- or left-quadrant abdominal pain and be mistaken for a gastrointestinal (GI) disorder. Patients with hypotension or vital signs that suggest hypovolemic shock likely have ruptured ectopic pregnancies and require admission and surgery. The first test to be ordered is beta-hCG, which would show lower than expected levels. Diagnosis is confirmed with ultrasound. Patients with a history of previous pelvic/tubal surgery, pelvic inflammatory disorder, use of an intrauterine device (IUD), multiple sexual partners, infertility and in utero exposure to diethylstilbestrol (DES) are more at risk for ectopic pregnancy.

PPx: Avoid risk factors: previous ectopic/pelvic/tubal surgery, infertility treatment, IUD use, pelvic inflammatory disease (PID), multiple sexual partners.

MoD: Ectopic pregnancy is caused by failure of a fertilized egg to implant in the endometrium. Most often it occurs in the ampulla of the fallopian tube.

Dx:
1. Pelvic exam
2. Beta-hCG
3. Pelvic ultrasound

Tx/Mgmt:
1. If stable, methotrexate
2. Surgery for hemodynamically unstable patients

Cervical Insufficiency

Buzz Words: Preterm pregnancy + funneled lower uterine segment + open internal cervical os + fever + pelvic pressure + vaginal spotting (bleeding) for 7 days + hx of loop electrocautery excision procedure (LEEP)

Clinical Presentation: Cervical insufficiency is defined as the inability of the uterus to retain pregnancy in the absence of labor. Patients may typically present as pregnant mothers with a history of spontaneous abortion or multiple preterm births. Often, funneling at the internal uterine orifice or bulging of the amniotic sac can be seen on physical exam. There are certain measureable risk factors for cervical insufficiency (e.g., <25 mm cervical length before 24 weeks' gestation, aka short cervix) that are unlikely to be tested on the Surgery shelf. Transvaginal ultrasound is the gold standard for the evaluation of cervical incompetence, and cerclage wiring is the treatment and prophylactic management for this disorder (e.g., prevents uterus from expelling fetus before term!).

PPx: Cerclage wiring in early pregnancy

MoD: Can be caused by many different factors, including past gynecologic procedure (e.g., LEEP, cone biopsy), prior obstetric trauma, multiple gestation

Dx:

1. Pelvic exam
2. Transvaginal ultrasound

Tx/Mgmt: Cerclage wiring

Disorders of the Newborn

Turner Syndrome

Buzz Words: Amenorrhea + infertility + streak ovaries + short stature + coarctation of aorta (differences in BP among extremities) + webbed neck + cubitus valgus (when forearm is angled away from body to greater degree than normal when fully extended) + bicuspid aortic valve + horseshoe kidney + low hairline (where hair starts growing too close to eyebrows) + **osteoporosis** (due to ovarian dysgenesis) + lymphedema

Clinical Presentation: Turner syndrome, a genetic disorder, is high yield on the shelf. It affects only females (XO on chromosomal analysis and can present in many different ways): newborns may be found to have lower-than-normal blood pressure in the lower extremities (coarctation of aorta), toddlers may be found to have a webbed neck and to be below average in height, teenagers are found with amenorrhea (from streak ovaries), and adults may have cardiovascular problems due to a bicuspid aortic valve. Patients with Turner syndrome have normal cognitive abilities. Make sure to learn the Buzz Words, MoD, Dx, and Tx/Mgmt of this disease well as it can also appear on your Pediatrics, Ob/Gyn, and Medicine shelf.

MoD: XO genotype:

- Rib notching due to collateral vessels that develop to bypass coarctation of aorta
- Lymphedema due to dysgenesis of the lymphatic network

Dx:

1. Levels of follicle stimulating hormone (FSH) (likely will have high FSH and luteinizing hormone [LH] because of ovarian dysgenesis and no negative feedback)
2. Inhibin levels (will likely be low because inhibin → measure of ovarian function)
3. Estrogen/testosterone → lower estrogen and normal testosterone

QUICK TIPS

In males, the equivalent syndrome is Noonan except that the Buzz Word is cubitus valgus. Stem clues for Noonan syndrome: widely spaced nipples + dyslexia + amenorrhea + short + sexual immaturity + **face tapers from forehead to chin** + thickened neck + normal genotype (hard to differentiate except for build)

QUICK TIPS

Continuous murmur throughout chest + rib notching on chest x-ray = coarctation of aorta

4. Karyotpe analysis for definitive diagnosis
5. Electrocardiogram (ECG) and echocardiogram (echo) to screen for cardiac abnormalities
6. Baseline metabolic panel (BMP) to look at renal function

Tx/Mgmt:
1. Treatment for coarctation of aorta (e.g., indomethacin) and bicuspid aortic valve (e.g., valve replacement)
2. Recombinant human growth hormone

99 AR

Cochrane review on recombinant human growth hormone

Erb-Duchenne Palsy (Upper Trunk Lesion)

Buzz Words: Recently delivered infant + arm adducted, pronated, wrist flexed (Fig. 11.1)

Clinical Presentation: Erb palsy is a lesion of the upper trunk that can be caused by obstetric-related brachial nerve trauma or traumatic injury in an adult. For the Surgery shelf, it is more likely you'll see this in the setting of newborns because surgical management can be more successful for refractory cases. Patients with Erb palsy present with the "waiter's tip" or "bellman's" posture. If severe enough, Erb palsy can be associated with T1 avulsion and Horner syndrome.

PPx: Avoid shoulder dystocia

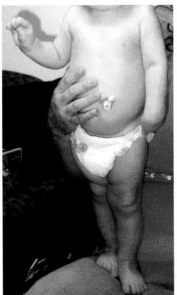
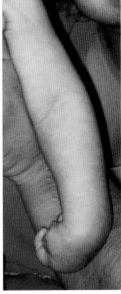

FIG. 11.1 Erb palsy. (From Graham JM, Sanchez-Lara PA: Brachial plexus palsy: Erb palsy, Klumpke palsy, obstetric palsy. In Graham JM, ed.: *Smith's recognizable patterns of human deformation*, 4th ed, Philadelphia, 2016, Elsevier.)

MoD: Traction on upper trunk (C5–C6) of brachial plexus due to shoulder dystocia → weakness of deltoid, biceps, infrapinatus, wrist extensors

Dx: Clinical diagnosis

Tx/Mgmt:
1. Conservative (gentle massage, physical therapy)
2. If T1 avulsion, Horner syndrome or no resolution of symptoms → neuroma excision and interpositional nerve grafting

99 AR

Review of nerve transfer indications in obstetrical brachial plexus palsy

Klumpke Palsy (Brachial Plexus Lower Trunk injury)

Buzz Words:
- Adult + grabbed branch during fall + atrophy of hypothenar muscles + sensory loss of pinky and lateral ring finger
- Recently delivered infant subject to upward force on arm during delivery + absent grasp reflex + claw hand (Fig. 11.2)

Clinical Presentation: Klumpke palsy is a lesion of the lower trunk that can be caused by obstetric-related brachial nerve trauma or traumatic injury in an adult. For the Surgery shelf, it is more likely you'll see this in the setting of newborns because surgical management in them can

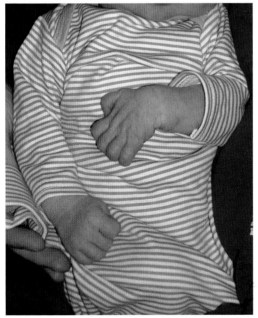

FIG. 11.2 Klumpke palsy. (From Buchanan EP, Richardson R, Tse R: Isolated lower brachial plexus [Klumpke] palsy with compound arm presentation: case report. *J Hand Surg Am* 38[8]:1567–1570, 2013.)

be more successful for refractory cases. Characterized by claw hand. If severe enough, can be associated with T1 avulsion and Horner syndrome.

PPx: Avoid stretch-like motion or shoulder dystocias

MoD: Traction on lower trunk (C8–T1) of brachial plexus due to shoulder dystocia → weakness of intrinsic hand muscles: lumbricals, interossei, thenar, hypothenar, sensory loss of ulnar distribution → extended wrist + hyperextended MCP joints + fixed interphalangeal joints + absent grasp reflex

Dx: Clinical diagnosis

Tx/Mgmt:

1. Conservative (gentle massage, physical therapy)
2. If T1 avulsion, Horner syndrome or no resolution of symptoms → neuroma excision and interpositional nerve grafting

22q11.2 Deletion Syndrome (aka DiGeorge Syndrome, aka Velocardiofacial Syndrome, aka Conotruncal Anomaly Face Syndrome)

Buzz Words: CATCH: Conotruncal cardiac defects (cyanotic disorders such as truncus arteriosus and tetralogy of Fallot) + Abnormal facies (low-set ears and micrognathia) + Thymic aplasia/hypoplasia + Cleft palate + Hypocalcemia (seizures, QT prolongation)

Clinical Presentation: 22q11.2 deletion syndrome is a genetic disorder that describes the phenotypical traits of a patient with a deletion at 22q11.2, which is the most common microdeletion in humans. This was formerly known as DiGeorge syndrome, velo-cardio-facial syndrome, or conotruncal anomaly face syndrome, but it was changed into a unifying name once it was clear the genetic abnormality was the same. Since many of the shelf questions were written a while ago, you may still see the terms *DiGeorge syndrome* or *velo-cardio-facial syndrome* pop up. Just be sure to know the distinguishing features of this syndrome: low-set ears, micrognathia, conotruncal abnormalities (e.g., tetralogy of Fallot, truncus arteriosus), immunodeficiency aplasia/hypoplasia, cleft palate, and hypocalcemia. One thing to be aware of is that the shelf presentation of 22q11.2 deletion syndrome could be very different from what you see clinically. Many patients with 22q11.2 deletion syndrome are now living into adulthood and have been found to suffer from concomitant psychiatric disease (e.g., schizophrenia), intellectual disability, autoimmune disorders, hypothyroidism, Parkinson disease, and neurodegenerative

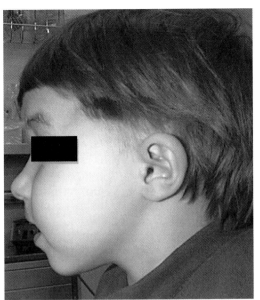

FIG. 11.3 Characteristic facies of 22q11.2 deletion syndrome, including micrognathia and low-set ears. (From Butts SC: The facial phenotype of the velo-cardio-facial syndrome. *Int J Pediatr Otorhinolaryngol* 73[3]:343–350, 2009.)

disease. These manifestations have not been classically seen on the shelf as Buzz Words for 22q11.2 deletion syndrome (aka DiGeorge aka velo-cardio-facial syndrome). However, as questions get updated, these adult manifestations may begin to appear as well (Fig. 11.3).

PPx: Avoid live vaccines such as rotavirus, yellow fever, and polio because of thymic aplasia → immunodeficiency; inactivated or killed vaccines are OK.

MoD: Chromosome 22q11.2 deletion causes defective development of pharyngeal pouches + hypocalcemia due to hypoplasia of parathyroid glands + cleft palate + congenital heart disease (truncus arteriosus) + immunodeficiency due to thymic aplasia/hypoplasia and resultant T-cell deficiency.

Dx:
1. BMP to assess for life-threatening hypocalcemia
2. CXR will show absent thymus
3. ECG and echo to assess cardiac defects
4. Chromosomal analysis

Tx/Mgmt:
1. Replete calcium if hypocalcemic
2. Surgical correction of conotruncal cardiac defects
3. Surgical correction of cleft palate
4. Genetic counseling

ON THE WARDS

Management of 22q11.2 deletion syndrome

Congenital Infections

You may be asked to identify a congenital infection on the Surgery shelf. Here are the seven most common ones tested. Be sure to know the difference between early and late congenital syphilis (<2 years old vs. ≥2 years old) as well what periventricular versus intracranial calcifications mean (former = congenital CMV; latter = congenital toxoplasmosis). PPx, MoD, Dx and Tx/Mgmt are unlikely to be tested on the Surgery shelf and are covered in Pediatrics and Ob/Gyn.

Disorders of Pregnancy, Childbirth, and the Puerperium Buzz Words

Buzz Words	Infection
Newborn + failure to thrive + lymphadenopathy + thrush + maternal IV drug use	Congenital HIV
Newborn + sensorineural hearing loss + patent ductus arteriosus murmur + cataracts (leukocoria) or glaucoma + hepatosplenomegaly + thrombocytopenic purpura (blueberry muffin rash)	Congenital rubella
Newborn + sensorineural hearing loss + no heart abnormality + periventricular calcifications + hepatosplenomegaly + chorioretinitis + microcephaly	Congenital CMV
≥2 years old + sensorineural hearing loss + no heart abnormality + saber shins + frontal bossing + interstitial keratitis + Hutchinson incisors + bulldog facies due to maldevelopment of maxilla + gummatous ulcers of nose and hard palate	Late congenital syphilis (≥2 years old)
<2 year old + runny nose + copper-colored macular rash on palms and soles + vesiculobullous eruptions + hepatosplenomegaly	Early congenital syphilis (<2 years old)
Newborn + microcephaly + limb hypoplasia + intrauterine growth restriction + cataracts + mother with pruritic vesicular rash	Congenital varicella syndrome
Newborn + **intracranial** calcifications + chorioretinitis + hydrocephalus + hepatosplenomegaly	Congenital toxoplasmosis

GUNNER PRACTICE

1. A 15-year-old girl is brought to the physician for a well visit. Her parents report that she has yet to have her period, like her friends, and that she is feeling "left out." She is also self-conscious about her height. Both her parents had reached at least 5′7″ by the age of 13, but she is still 5′0″ and has not grown since she was 9. Exam shows pubic hair development at Tanner stage 3 and breast development at Tanner stage 2. Pelvic exam shows no abnormalities. Her radial and brachial pulses feel stronger than her femoral, dorsalis pedis, and posterior tibialis pulse. Blood pressure taken at the ankle is 20 mm Hg lower than that in the ipsilateral arm. What is the likely diagnosis?
A. Constitutional pubertal delay
B. Normal development
C. Down syndrome
D. Turner syndrome
E. 22q11.2 deletion syndrome

2. A 3000-g baby delivered by a 28-year-old primagravida woman presents with an enlarged head. MRI shows that baby has intracranial calcifications. Examination shows an enlarged liver and spleen. What is the likely diagnosis?
A. Cytomegalovirus infection
B. Early-onset syphilis
C. Varicella infection
D. Toxoplasmosis infection
E. Congenital rubella

3. A newborn is brought in by his mother for concern about his arm. Since the delivery 24 hours earlier, the patient has not been able to move his left arm out of a fixed position by his side. His Apgar score was 8 and 9 at 1 and 5 minutes, respectively. He was able to demonstrate the grasp and Moro reflexes. On exam, the patient's left arm is found to be adducted and pronated, with the wrist in a flexed position. He is otherwise normal and feeding well. What is the most appropriate treatment for this patient?
A. Nerve transfer procedure
B. Forearm splint
C. Open reduction internal fixation
D. Closed reduction internal fixation
E. Reassurance and gentle massage

ANSWERS: What Would Gunner Jess/Jim Do?

1. WWGJD? A 15-year-old girl is brought into the physician for a well-visit. Her parents report that she has yet to have her period like her friends and that she is feeling "left out." She also is self-conscious about her height. Both her parents had reached at least 5'7" tall by the age of 13 but she is still 5'0" and has not grown since she was 9. Exam shows pubic hair development at Tanner stage 3 and breast development at Tanner stage 2. Pelvic exam shows no abnormalities. Her radial and brachial pulse feel stronger than her femoral, dorsalis pedis and posterior tibialis pulse. Systolic blood pressure taken at the ankle is 20 mmHg lower than the ipsilateral arm. What is the likely diagnosis?

Answer: D, Turner syndrome

Explanation: Patient is likely to have Turner syndrome given the Buzz Words of weak lower extremity pulses and decreased lower extremity BP compared with upper extremity BP. Patients with Turner syndrome also have pubertal delay due to ovarian dysgenesis, which would explain her amenorrhea. Definitive diagnosis is made with karyotype analysis. Chest x-ray would likely show notching ribs, which is pathognomonic for coarctation of the aorta, another classic feature of Turner syndrome.

A. Constitutional pubertal delay → incorrect. This would be more likely without the abnormal vascular discrepancy between the upper and lower extremities.

B. Normal development → incorrect. Given that patient is Tanner stage 3 and 2 for pubic hair and breast development, respectively, at the age of 15, we cannot conclude that this is normal development.

C. Down syndrome → incorrect. Down syndrome patients have cardiovascular abnormalities such as VSD and endocardial cushion defects but do not present with coarctation of the aorta.

E. 22q11.2 Deletion syndrome → incorrect. Patients with 22q11.2 deletion syndrome may exhibit conotruncal defects (e.g., tetralogy of Fallot, truncus arteriosus) that would likely require early surgery. Adolescent patients may exhibit symptoms from hypocalcemia and may have the classic facies of micrognathia and low-set ears.

2. WWGJD? A 3000-g baby delivered by a 28-year-old primagravida woman presents with an enlarged head.

MRI shows patient has intracranial calcifications. Examination shows an enlarged liver and spleen. What is the likely diagnosis?

Answer: D, Toxoplasmosis infection

Explanation: The only thing on the shelf that presents with "intracranial calcifications" on neuroimaging is toxoplasmosis infection. Be careful not to confuse this with periventricular calcifications, a finding that folks with congenital CMV may have. Toxoplasmosis can be spread to mom through contact with cats. Newborns with congenital toxoplasmosis can present with macrocephaly due to hydrocephalus and may require a neurosurgical consult.

A. Cytomegalovirus infection → incorrect. Congenital CMV infection is characterized by **periventricular** and not intracranial calcifications, along with chorioretinitis and sensorineural hearing loss.

B. Early-onset syphilis → incorrect. The hallmark of patients with early-onset syphilis (<2 years old) is a runny nose and rash on the palms and soles.

C. Varicella infection → incorrect. The typical presentation for congenital varicella is limb hypoplasia, cataracts, and intrauterine growth restriction.

E. Congenital rubella → incorrect. Congenital rubella is characterized by a blueberry muffin rash due to thrombocytopenic purpura as well as sensorineural hearing loss and a PDA murmur. This can be prevented if mom takes the MMR vaccine **before** the baby is conceived. Once pregnant, it is not advisable to give mom a live MMR vaccine.

3. WWGJD? A newborn is brought in by his mother for concern of his arm. Since the delivery 24 hours ago, patient has not been able to move his left arm out of a fixed position by his side. His APGAR score was 8 and 9 at 1 and 5 minutes, respectively. He was able to demonstrate the grasp and Moro reflex. On exam, patients left arm is found to be adducted and pronated with the wrist in a flexed position. He is otherwise normal and feeding well. What is the most appropriate treatment for this patient?

Answer: E, Reassurance and gentle massage

Explanation: Patient is likely suffering from Erb palsy due to shoulder dystocia during delivery. There are cases of Erb palsy that require surgery, as when Horner syndrome is present or if symptoms do not resolve within a year. However, most palsies caused by damage to the brachial plexus during birth are self-limited and can be treated with gentle massage and PT to prevent contractures.

A. Nerve transfer procedure → incorrect. Patient does not have any sign of Horner syndrome, which would be an indication for surgery.

B. Forearm splint → incorrect. Splints are not used for the treatment of Erb palsy. Gentle massage and reassurance are all that is needed.

C. Open reduction internal fixation → incorrect. There is no sign of fracture, so ORIF is unnecessary.

D. Closed reduction internal fixation → incorrect. There is no sign of fracture, so CRIF is unnecessary.

Diseases of the Skin and Subcutaneous Tissue

Rachel Dillinger, Kaitlyn Barkley, Hao-Hua Wu, Leo Wang, Rebecca Gao, and Temitayo Ogunleye

Introduction

Of the vast number of diseases and processes that have dermatologic manifestations, only a small fraction are eligible for surgical management. This makes it a quick topic in studying for the Surgical shelf. It is a good idea to quickly review the layers of the skin before reading on, so as to provide a frame of reference for where each disease takes place.

The organizing principle for this chapter is mechanism: neoplastic versus traumatic and mechanical injury. In studying, pay closer attention to the high-yield topics that pop up time and time again: malignancies (melanoma, squamous cell carcinoma, and basal cell carcinoma) and burn management. Less time can be devoted to topics like benign neoplasms and bites.

The chapter is divided into (1) Benign Neoplasms, (2) Malignant Neoplasms, (3) Traumatic and Mechanical Injury, and (4) Gunner Practice (application of the material learned).

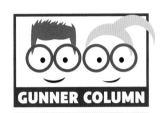

GUNNER COLUMN

Neoplasms

Benign Neoplasms

Epidermoid Cyst

Buzz Words: Flesh-colored, round, firm nodule + on the face/neck/extremities/scalp ± a central pore

Clinical Presentation: Epidermoid cysts are common, benign lesions can appear anywhere on the body but are most common on the face, neck, extremities, and scalp. There is a predilection for men in the third and fourth decades of life. Aesthetic concerns or suspicion for malignancy prompt patients to seek medical attention.

MoD: Epidermoid cysts arise from a proliferation of epidermal tissue in the dermis, likely from the infundibulum of a hair follicle. Human papillomavirus (HPV) and ultraviolet (UV) light exposure may also have a role. Additionally, these cysts can be part of Gardner syndrome (adenomatous colon polyps, various cysts, fibromas, and osteoma) or arise after local trauma such as surgery or slamming a finger in a car door.

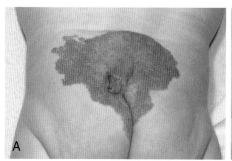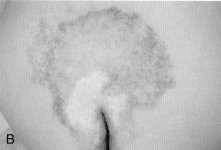

FIG. 12.1 Scoring of infantile hemangioma with the Hemangioma Activity Score (HAS) and Hemangioma Severity Scale (HSS) at *t* = 0 (age 4 months) (A) and 1 year after therapy (B). (From Janmohamed SR, de Waard-van der Spek FB, Madern GC, de Laat PC, Hop WC, Oranje AP: Scoring the proliferative activity of hemangioma of infancy: the Hemangioma Activity Score [HAS]. *Clin Exp Dermatol* 36:715–723, 2011.)

Dx: Appearance, history, and clinical suspicion

Tx/Mgmt: Surgical incision or excision of the cyst and entire cyst wall (to prevent recurrence)

Hemangiomas

Buzz Words:
- **Capillary hemangioma:** superficial pink/red lesion present on the head or neck of an infant + not present at birth + rapidly growing + blanches with pressure + epidermal involvement (Fig. 12.1)
- **Cavernous hemangioma:** Blue swollen lesion on the head or neck of an infant + not present at birth + rapidly growing + dermal and subcuticular involvement

Clinical Presentation: Hemangiomas are benign tumors that appear within the first month of life. They exhibit two phases: a rapid proliferative phase in the first year and a half followed by a gradual involution phase. They are classified based on the layer of skin affected.

MoD: Rapid proliferation of endothelial cells

Dx: Clinical, although magnetic resonance imaging (MRI)/computed tomography (CT)/ultrasound (US)/skin biopsy can confirm

Tx/Mgmt:
1. Observation, as most will spontaneously involute by 7 years of age.
2. If there is bleeding, interference with normal functioning, or malignancy, biopsy with possible excision.

Subcutaneous Lipoma

Buzz Words: Soft, lobulated mass + fluctuant + mobile (slippage sign) + 1–10 cm or more

Clinical Presentation: Lipomas are the most common soft tissue tumors and cause some patients mechanical

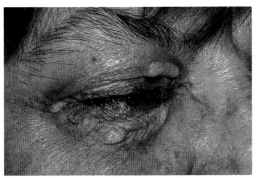

FIG. 12.2 Xanthelasma palpebrarum with typical yellowish hue. (From Bolognia JL, Schaffer JV, Duncan KO, Ko CJ: *Dermatology essentials*, Philadelphia, 2014, Elsevier.)

difficulty due to placement (e.g., a large medial upper-arm lipoma that interferes with arm movement past the trunk). Mostly they cause cosmetic concerns.

MoD: Subcutaneous lipomas are benign tumors of fat cells, for which the mechanism isn't entirely understood (though trauma has been proposed).

Dx: Clinical, although increasing size, symptoms, and firmness warrant biopsy.

Tx/Mgmt: Observation, unless the patient desires surgical excision due to cosmetic concerns or associated pain.

Cutaneous Xanthoma

Buzz Words: Yellowish, soft, flat, velvety papules + on the eyelids, extensor surfaces, or tendons (Fig. 12.2)

Clinical Presentation: In patients with hyperlipidemia, lipid-laden macrophages can accumulate in the skin, leading to the development of a xanthoma. They are further subdivided based on location and can include the eyelids, extensor surfaces, and subcutaneous tissues near tendons and ligaments.

PPx: Lipid control with agents such as statins, fibrates, bile acid–binding resins, etc. Familial testing if an inherited condition is suspected.

MoD: Elevated serum levels of lipoproteins lead to extravasation and accumulation around the dermal capillaries. Accompanying inflammation leads to the clinical presentation.

Dx:
1. Fasting lipid panel (markedly elevated lipoproteins)
2. Family hx of lipid metabolism disorders, myocardial infarction, aortic regurgitation, atherosclerosis
3. Shave, punch, or excisional biopsy showing foamy macrophages

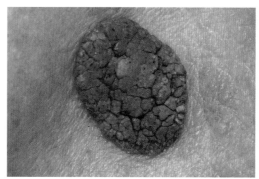

FIG. 12.3 Pigmented seborrheic keratoses. This is a gray-brown, thick, keratotic, stuck-on plaque. (From Brinster NK, Liu V, Diwan H, McKee PH: *Dermatopathology: high-yield pathology,* Philadelphia, 2011, Elsevier.)

Tx/Mgmt:

1. Lipid-lowering agents (statins, fibrates, bile acid binding resins, etc.) to decrease the size of the xanthoma(s) and lower risk of comorbidities.
2. Complete resolution often requires surgical excision, although uncontrolled hyperlipidemia can result in recurrence of the xanthoma.
3. Family testing if hyperlipidemia is suspected.

Seborrheic Keratosis

Buzz Words: Older patient + coin-like, waxy lesion on face or extremities + stuck on" appearance (Fig. 12.3)

Clinical Presentation: The incidence of seborrheic keratosis increases with age and fair complexion. The majority of older individuals will have at least one, so consistent dermatologic care to screen for complications is essential.

MoD: Benign clonal proliferation of a mutated keratinocyte

Dx: Clinical, although biopsy will show hyperplasia of benign, basaloid epidermal cells with horn pseudocysts

Tx/Mgmt:

1. Observe, excise, cryotherapy, curettage, or topical agents
2. Secondary tumors may arise within them, as in Bowen disease (squamous cell carcinoma [SCC] in situ) and malignant melanoma, although they themselves have no malignant potential.

Nevus

Buzz Words: Brown or black mole + sun-exposed sites + non-malignant

Clinical Presentation: The majority of patients will have numerous melanocytic nevi, especially Caucasian individuals. As ubiquitous as they are, epidemiologic factors do not aid in workup.

PPx: Avoid sunlight, use sunscreen

MoD: Benign proliferation of melanocytes that expand from the epidermis into the dermis, resulting in a raised lesion

Dx: Simple excisional biopsy

Tx/Mgmt:
1. Watchful waiting for any changes over time.
2. Excisional biopsy if malignancy is a concern.

Malignant Neoplasms

Basal Cell Carcinoma

Buzz Words: Sun-exposed areas + pink nodules + rolled edges + central crusting → BCC

Clinical Presentation: Incidence increases in individuals with a fair complexion, advanced age, male sex, and closer proximity to the equator.

PPx: Avoid direct sunlight and use sunscreen, avoid arsenic exposure

MoD: UV damage (UVA > UVB) induces mutations in the p53 tumor suppressor gene. Mutations in *PTCH*, a gene encoding a transmembrane protein in the hedgehog signaling pathway, lead to basal cell nevus syndrome and sporadic cutaneous BCCs.

Dx: Clinical suspicion with biopsy to confirm, which will show islands of proliferating epithelium resembling the basal layer of the epidermis.

Tx/Mgmt: Excision, curettage, cautery, deep cryotherapy, superficial radiation therapy, Mohs surgery

Squamous Cell Carcinoma

Buzz Words: Sun-exposed areas + red, ulcerative lesion ± scaling, ± draining sinus tract (Fig. 12.4)

Clinical Presentation: Incidence increases in individuals with a fair complexion, advanced age, male sex, and closer proximity to the equator.

PPx: Avoid direct sunlight and use sunscreen, minimize exposure to radiation from therapy and carcinogens

MoD: UV damage (UVA > UVB) induces mutations in the p53 tumor suppressor gene and the RAS mitogenic pathway.

Dx: Clinical suspicion and confirmed by biopsy, which shows atypical keratinocytes penetrating the basement membrane and proliferating into the dermis.

QUICK TIPS

BCC is the most common and least likely to metastasize, whereas melanoma is the least common and most likely to metastasize.

QUICK TIPS

Mohs surgery involves removing thin layers of skin until no cancer cells remain; it is effective for BCC and SCC.

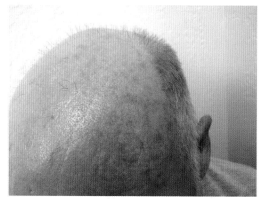

FIG. 12.4 Actinic keratosis. (From Wikimedia Commons. https://commons.wikimedia.org/wiki/File:Actinic_keratosis_on_balding_head.JPG. Used under Creative Commons Attribution-Share Alike 4.0 International license: https://creativecommons.org/licenses/by-sa/4.0/deed.en.)

Tx/Mgmt: Surgical excision, Mohs surgery. Lesions with high metastatic potential get additional radiation or chemo.

Melanoma

Buzz Words: The **ABCDEs**: **A**symmetry, irregular **B**orders, varying **C**olors, **D**iameter greater than 6 mm (approximately the size of an eraser), and **E**volution over time (including ulceration or bleeding)

Clinical Presentation: Incidence increases in individuals with a fair complexion, advanced age, and closer proximity to the equator. In younger patients, it is more common in women. In older patients, it is more common in men.

PPx: Avoid direct sunlight and use sunscreen

MoD: UV damage (UVA > UVB) induces mutations in the p53 tumor suppressor gene, activates the RAS mitogenic pathway, and/or inactivates the p16 tumor suppressor gene.

Dx:

1. Full-thickness biopsy ± sentinel lymph node biopsy
2. Recognition of subtype (Table 12.1, Fig. 12.5)

Tx/Mgmt: Based on depth of invasion (Table 12.2)

Kaposi Sarcoma

Buzz Words:

- **Non–AIDS-related**: elderly Jewish male from the Mediterranean/person from sub-Saharan Africa/transplant patient + flat, purple patches usually on the lower extremities → raised and rubbery (Fig. 12.6)
- **AIDS-related**: homosexual or bisexual males + AIDS + flat purple patches on perioral mucosa → raised + rubbery

Sentinel lymph node biopsy video

TABLE 12.1 Melanoma Subtypes

Subtype	Growth Pattern	Features
Superficial spreading	Superficially along the epidermis	Most common type, can arise from a benign mole
Lentigo maligna (an in situ lesion)	Superficially along the epidermis	Flat or mildly elevated mottled tan, brown, or dark brown discoloration
Acral lentigous melanoma	Superficially on the palms, soles, or underneath nails	Most common type in African Americans and Asians; can advance more quickly than the other superficial types
Nodular	Vertical	Typically invasive at the time of diagnosis

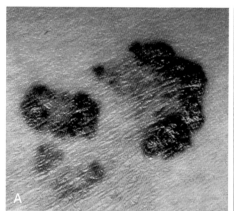
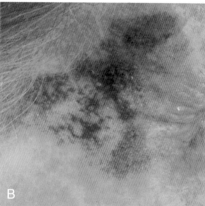
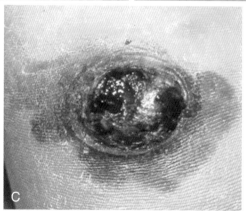

FIG. 12.5 Different melanoma subtypes: (A) superficial spreading; (B) lentigo maligna; and (C) nodular. (From Netscher DT: Skin tumors of the hand and upper extremity. In: Wolfe SW, ed.: *Green's operative hand surgery*, 7th ed, Philadelphia, 2017, Elsevier.)

TABLE 12.2 Surgical Margins

Breslow Thickness	Surgical Margin
≤1.0 mm	1 cm
1.01–2.0 mm	1–2 cm
≥2.0 mm	2 cm

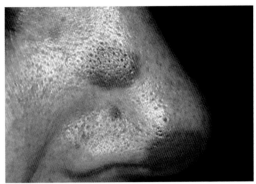

FIG. 12.6 Kaposi sarcoma. (From Sand M, Sand D, Thrandorf C, Paech V, Altmeyer P, Bechara FG: Cutaneous lesions of the nose. *Head Face Med* 6:7, 2010.)

Clinical Presentation: Kaposi sarcoma tends to arise in middle-aged adults regardless of the etiology. In the AIDS-related and Mediterranean subtypes, it is more common in men, while the African variant appears equally in men and women.

PPx: Immunosuppression (e.g., from antirejection medications for transplant patients or coinfection with HIV) increases the likelihood of sequelae.

MoD: HHV-8 infection

Dx: Clinical: Biopsy showing spindle cells and presence of LANA (viral protein) in the cells

Tx/Mgmt:

1. Local disease → surgical resection
2. Disseminated disease → liposomal doxorubicin and highly active antiretroviral treatment (HAART)

Cutaneous T-Cell Lymphoma/Mycosis Fungoides

Buzz Words: Psoriatic-appearing plaque → multicentric, confluent reddish-brown nodules + leonine facies

Clinical Presentation: There is a higher incidence in middle-aged and elderly populations as well as in men. It is exceedingly rare in younger patients.

MoD: Helper T cells congregate in the epidermis and gradually proliferate.

Dx: Clinical features and histology showing cerebriform lymphocytes

Tx/Mgmt:

1. Stage I (plaque stage) → topically with steroids, chemotherapy, psoralen plus ultraviolet A (PUVA)
2. Stage II (skin tumor stage) → systemically with steroids, chemotherapy, interferon, or monoclonal antibodies

QUICK TIPS
Sézary syndrome is another type of cutaneous T-cell lymphoma that, unlike mycosis fungoides, is malignant. It manifests with pruritic red rashes that cover most of the body and has a poor prognosis.

Trauma and Mechanical Injury

Burns

Buzz Words:
- **First-degree**—epidermis + red + pain + dry
- **Second-degree**—epidermis and dermis + red or white + pain ± blisters ± wet appearance ± blanching with pressure
- **Third-degree**—all layers of skin and extension into the subQ + black or white + leathery appearance + absence of pain + absence of blanching with pressure (Fig. 12.7)

Clinical Presentation: Burns have a characteristic look and presentation that is obvious to medical and nonmedical personnel alike. There are no real patterns affecting one group more than any other. As always, burns in a child should always raise clinical suspicion of child abuse, especially in the shape of cigarette butts and in locations that do not align with the provided history. Keep in mind that although third-degree burns are painless, they are often surrounded by first- and second-degree burns that are painful.

MoD:
- **Chemical**—irritation by chemicals caustic to the skin.
- **Circumferential**—increasing edema underneath an eschar that wraps around an extremity → blood supply is cut off.
- **Electrical**—lightning strike or contact with power lines creates entrance and exit wounds and, in passing between the two, injures deeper structures such as bone.
- **Respiratory**—inhalation of smoke in a house fire, for example, causes chemical injury to the lungs.
- **Thermal**—direct contact with open flame, scalding from steam, hot liquids, or contact with an object that has been heated, such as a frying pan.

Dx:
1. Clinical
2. Burns around the mouth or black soot in the throat → fiberoptic bronchoscopy can confirm respiratory burns in suspected patients.

Tx/Mgmt: See Fig. 12.8:
- **Chemical**—extensive irrigation with tap water in the shower, emergency eye wash, etc. (do NOT attempt to neutralize the burn); debridement and fluid resuscitation as necessary.

QUICK TIPS

Bone has the physical property of high resistance; when exposed to electricity, this leads to the generation of enough heat to melt the calcium phosphate matrix and/or cause periosteal necrosis. Keep this in mind in evaluating patients with electrical burns.

QUICK TIPS

Calculate the body area affected by using the rule of nines: If > 20% is affected, significant fluid may be lost and the prognosis begins to decline.

99 AR

Burn management

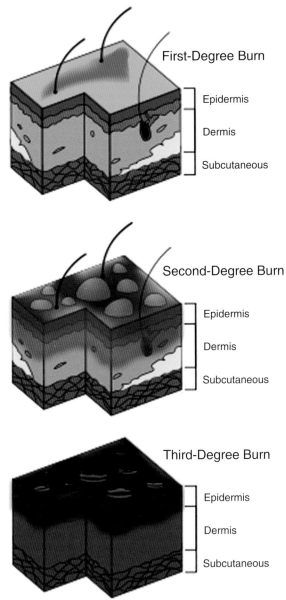

FIG. 12.7 Burns. (From K. Aainsqatsi at English Wikipedia (Original text: K. Aainsqatsi) - Transferred from en.wikipedia to Commons. (Original text: self-made), CC BY-SA 3.0, https://commons.wikimedia. org/w/index.php?curid=2584650.)

- **Circumferential**—if loss of blood flow is suspected → escharotomy
- **Electrical**—aggressive fluid resuscitation, potential debridement and amputation, and treatment of possible orthopedic injuries like posterior shoulder dislocation and compression of the vertebrae

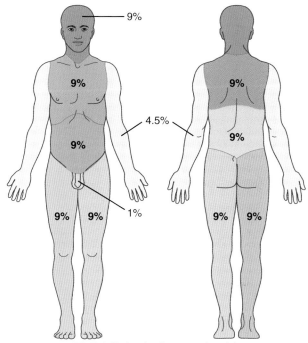

FIG. 12.8 Estimating burn area in adults.

- **Respiratory**—assess patency of airway (ABCs) → intubate if inadequate → assess ABGs and carboxyhemoglobin levels
- **Thermal**—aggressive fluid resuscitation, debridement, and skin grafting at sites where the skin has not regenerated after 2–3 weeks of wound care.

Bites and Stings

Dog/Animal Bite

Buzz Words: Bite marks on hands, extremities, or face

Clinical Presentation: Children are especially likely to suffer bites, as they are less likely to respect feeding or recognize that an animal's behavior is abnormal.

Dx: History and clinical presentation

Tx/Mgmt:
- Provoked bites: observe the dog for signs of rabies
- Unprovoked bites: immunoglobulin + vaccine + tetanus ppx + wound care

Human Bite

Buzz Words: "I punched a wall" + cuts over the knuckles + likely physical altercation (Fig. 12.9)

QUICK TIPS

Fluid resuscitation in patients with extensive burns is generally 1 L of lactated Ringer (without sugar) per hour, adjusted by urine output

QUICK TIPS

Rabid animals will act strangely, sometimes more aggressive or tentative than usual, and often will exhibit excess salivation. The only way to know for sure is to euthanize the animal and examine its brain.

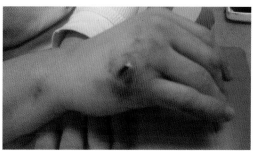

FIG. 12.9 Human bite. (From http://www.jailmedicine.com/case-study-i-fell-and-hurt-my-hand/.)

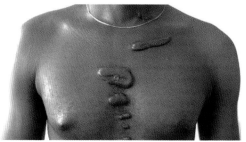

FIG. 12.10 Keloid. (From http://reichenbergerlab.uchc.edu/keloids/index.html.)

Clinical Presentation: Human bites are a surprisingly common occurrence, although the name is a bit misleading. Although the media occasionally report an individual who bites another person after ingesting bath salts, a "human bite" is most often secondary to a bar fight in which a punch to the face results in a laceration from contact with an opponent's teeth. Patients will typically obscure the true cause of the injury with a cover story ("I punched a wall"), so clinical suspicion is key for diagnosis, as untreated bites in which bacteria disseminate to the bone can cause osteomyelitis with serious sequelae.

PPx: Avoid contact between the fist and mouth

MoD: Bite from another person or knuckles being cut by teeth during a punch

Dx: History, clinical presentation, and physician judgment

Tx/Mgmt:
- Irrigation and surgical debridement
- Tetanus ppx

Snake Bite

Buzz Words: Outdoor activity + local pain, swelling, and discoloration within 30 minutes

Clinical Presentation: Although the vast majority of snake bites are innocuous, venomous species do exist, and the event itself can cause a great deal of distress. The prototypical patient is a young outdoorsman in a rural location.

Tx/Mgmt: Antivenom

Bee Sting

Buzz Words: Wheezing + rash + possible anaphylaxis and vasomotor shock

Clinical Presentation: Any individual who comes into contact with a hive is at risk, although fatal anaphylaxis is more common in older patients than in the young. It is important to discern between a regular sting, an allergic reaction, and anaphylaxis.

Dx: History and clinical presentation

Tx/Mgmt: Epinephrine + removal of stinger

Mechanical Injury

Decubitus Ulcers

Buzz Words: Bed sores + extended hospital stay ± wound breakdown

Clinical Presentation: Patients who are most at risk include thinner patients who don't have as much cushioning and therefore have more sensitive pressure points between their bones and skin.

PPx: Routinely moving bedridden patients, special beds that redistribute pressure, especially in thinner individuals

MoD: Continuous pressure on an area results in occlusion of the microvasculature, leading to ischemic necrosis of the surrounding tissues.

Dx: History and clinical appearance:
- Grade I: persistent redness
- Grade II: marked by ulceration
- Grade III: destruction of subQ structures like muscle or fat

Tx/Mgmt:
- Lower-grade lesions → wound care
- Higher-grade lesions → surgical debridement with adjuvant antibiotics ± amputation

QUICK TIPS

Keloids arise from excess collagen deposition beyond the margin of the original scar caused by trauma or surgery. Rates of recurrence after surgical resection range from ~50% to 100%.

QUICK TIPS

In frostbite management, the goal is to salvage as much tissue as possible. Rewarm affected areas in circulating water at 40°C and wait 3–4 weeks for clear demarcation of nonviable tissue, which can then be surgically debrided and/or amputated.

GUNNER PRACTICE

1. A 54-year-old, right-handed man comes into your office after his primary care provider discovered a suspicious lesion on his left arm. He owns a farm and has recently had to cut back on work due to weakness and clumsiness of his right hand, along with a left-sided headache

that bothers him in the mornings when he usually does his work. The lesion is 8-mm wide, in varying shades of brown, and slightly asymmetric. What is the best initial step?

A. PET scan of the head
B. Shave biopsy of the lesion
C. Sentinel lymph node biopsy of the axilla
D. Punch biopsy of the lesion
E. Observe and follow up in 3 months

2. A 30-year-old woman presents to your office for a general dermatologic exam. You notice a large scar covering her left leg and the patient reveals that she tripped and fell into a bonfire a few years earlier while on vacation. The rest of the exam is unremarkable. Before leaving, the patient asks if there's anything she should be concerned about, given the history of burn. You tell her to keep an eye out for:

A. A pearly-colored papule, possibly associated with telangiectasias
B. A small red nodule with scaling and/or a draining sinus tract
C. A pigmented lesion that lacks symmetry, regular borders, and uniform color
D. A reddish-purple cluster of plaques

3. During an apartment fire, a 21-year-old male and his three roommates are rescued by firemen; all have suffered varying levels of injury. In the ER, the patient is evaluated, and on primary survey is noted to have an intact airway, breathing, and circulation. His blood pressure is 130/92, respirations are 14/min, pulse is 86/min, and temperature is 99.1°F. Past medical history is unremarkable. Secondary survey reveals burns around the mouth and nose with dark residue inside the oral cavity. What is the next best step?

A. Supplemental oxygen via nasal cannula
B. Corticosteroids and antibiotics
C. Fiberoptic bronchoscopy
D. Endotracheal intubation
E. Tracheostomy

Notes

ANSWERS: What Would Gunner Jess/Jim Do?

1. WWGSD? A 54-year-old, right-handed man comes into your office after his primary care provider discovered a suspicious lesion on his left arm. He owns a farm and has recently had to cut back on work due to weakness and clumsiness of his right hand, along with a left-sided headache that bothers him in the mornings when he usually does his work. The lesion is 8-mm wide, in varying shades of brown, and slightly asymmetric. What is the best initial step?

Answer: D, Punch biopsy of the lesion

    Explanation: The patient has a lesion with features concerning for melanoma (>6 mm wide, color irregularities, and asymmetry) and a history of employment with frequent exposure to the sun (farming). The initial step in evaluation is to determine the depth of invasion by punch biopsy, which is key for prognosis.

    A. PET scan of the head → incorrect. Although the history revealed information concerning for a brain lesion (left-sided headache that is worse in the morning, along with weakness in the right hand) that could plausibly be from metastatic melanoma, a diagnosis of melanoma has yet to be made, and there are several steps before this answer choice would make sense.

    B. Shave biopsy of the lesion → incorrect. Shave biopsy will not allow for assessment of the full thickness, which is essential for staging melanoma.

    C. Sentinel lymph node biopsy of the axilla → incorrect. This is reasonable after a biopsy is taken, but not before.

    E. Observe and follow up in 3 months → incorrect. This patient has a suspicious lesion that needs further workup.

2. WWGJD? A 30-year-old woman presents to your office for a general dermatologic exam. You notice a large scar covering her left leg and the patient reveals she tripped and fell into a bonfire a few years ago while on vacation. The rest of the exam is unremarkable. Before leaving, the patient asks if there's anything she should be concerned about given the history of burn. You tell her to keep an eye out for a:

Answer: B, Small red nodule with scaling and/or draining sinus tract

    Explanation: This is a description of squamous cell carcinoma, for which old burns are a risk factor.

A. Pearly-colored papule, possibly associated with telangiectasias → incorrect. This is a description of basal cell carcinoma.

C. Pigmented lesion that lacks symmetry, regular borders, and uniform color → incorrect. This is a description of melanoma.

D. Reddish-purple cluster of plaques → incorrect. This is a description of Kaposi sarcoma.

3. WWGJD? After an apartment catches fire, a 21-year-old male and his three roommates are rescued by firemen and have suffered varying levels of injury. In the ER, he is in no apparent distress and on primary survey is noted to have intact airway, breathing, and circulation. His blood pressure is 130/92, respirations are 14/min, pulse is 86/min and temperature is 99.1°F. Past medical history is unremarkable. Secondary survey reveals burns around the mouth and nose with dark residue inside his oral cavity. What is the next best step?

Answer: C, Fiberoptic bronchoscopy.

Explanation: The patient likely suffered an inhalation injury from the fire given that he has burns around his mouth and soot within it. He is in no apparent distress and his vitals are stable, so fiberoptic bronchoscopy to visualize damage to the respiratory structures is the next step to confirm the diagnosis.

A. Supplemental oxygen via nasal cannula → incorrect. There is no indication that he needs oxygen at this point.

B. Corticosteroids and antibiotics → incorrect. In the setting of inhalation injury, this approach has been discredited.

D. Endotracheal intubation → incorrect. The patient is in no apparent distress, vitals are stable, and the primary survey raised no concern for securing an immediate airway. Subsequent ABG may reveal the need for intubation.

E. Tracheostomy → incorrect. See above. Also, there is no indication in the question stem that if intubation were necessary, endotracheal intubation would be difficult.

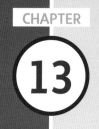
Diseases of the Musculoskeletal System and Connective Tissue

Hao-Hua Wu, Leo Wang, Rafael Madero-Marroquin, Kaitlyn Barkley, Rebecca Gao, and Neil Sheth

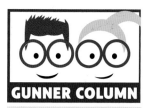

GUNNER COLUMN

99 AR
High-Yield Pediatric Orthopedics video

MNEMONIC

Seronegative spondyloar-
thropathies PAIR (Psoriatic
Arthritis, Ankylosing spondylitis,
Inflammatory bowel disease,
Reactive arthritis)

99 AR
Seronegative arthritis video

Introduction

Musculoskeletal (MSK) disease encompasses 3%–7% of the NBME Surgery shelf exam content. The most high-yield topics are the MSK disorders affecting the pediatric population, such as Perthes and Osgood-Schlatter (often seen in Pediatrics and Family Medicine as well).

Even though this is the Surgery shelf, you do NOT need to know the specifics of orthopedic procedures for the treatment of these diseases. As mentioned in the introduction, the Surgery shelf is much closer to the Medicine shelf in terms of tested concepts; thus, understanding the Buzz Words and the diagnostic/treatment steps are all you will need to ace this topic on exam day.

This chapter is divided into (1) Immunologic Disorders; (2) Infectious and Inflammatory Disorders, (3) Neoplasms; (4) Degenerative and Metabolic Disorders; (5) Traumatic and Mechanical Disorders; (6) Congenital Disorders; (7) Adverse Effects of Drugs on the Musculoskeletal System; and (8) Gunner Practice.

Immunologic Disorders

Seronegative Spondyloarthropathies

Ankylosing Spondylitis

Buzz Words: Young male + human leukocyte antigen (HLA)-B27 + back pain worse in the morning, better with activity + family history of spondyloarthritis

Clinical Presentation: Arthritis that affects the lower extremities and axial skeleton. Limitation of motion at the lumbar spine and limitation of chest expansion occur. Pain has good response to non-steroidal anti-inflammatory drugs (NSAIDs). Contrary to adult-onset ankylosing spondylitis, enthesitis (inflammation of the tendinous insertions on the bone) and peripheral arthritis are more common in children at disease onset. Patients with late-onset pauciarticular juvenile rheumatoid arthritis (JRA) are at high risk of developing this syndrome as adults. Elevated erythrocyte sedimentation rate (ESR) or C-reactive protein on lab exams.

MoD: Strong association with HLA-B27, infectious etiology has been suggested but not proven.

Dx: Clinical diagnosis is based on evidence of bilateral sacroilitis on imaging, back pain, and features of spondyloarthritis (enthesitis, uveitis, dactylitis, etc.)

Tx/Mgmt:

1. NSAIDs to control pain
2. Physical therapy
3. Glucocorticoids if NSAIDs fail
4. DMARDs to prevent joint damage

Arthritis of Inflammatory Bowel Disease

Buzz Words: Chronic arthritis + abdominal pain + erythema nodosum or pyoderma gangrenosum

Clinical Presentation: Inflammatory bowel disease (IBD) consists of ulcerative colitis and Crohn disease and can be associated with chronic arthritis. Patients may present with a pattern indistinguishable from ankylosing spondylitis. The presence of erythema nodosum or pyoderma gangrenosum in a patient with chronic arthritis should raise the suspicion of IBD.

MoD: Underlying Crohn disease or ulcerative colitis

Dx: Underlying disease confirmed with small bowel imaging and endoscopy with biopsies

Tx/Mgmt: Treat underlying IBD

> **QUICK TIPS**
> Primary sclerosing cholangitis is a Buzz Word for ulcerative colitis.

Reactive Arthritis (aka Reiter Disease/Reiter Arthritis)

Buzz Words: Conjunctivitis + urethral discharge + artharlgia + pericarditis/aortic regurg + history of sexually transmitted infection (STIs) or gastrointestinal (GI) infection + HLA B27

Clinical Presentation: Reactive arthritis is one of the seronegative spondyloarthropathies, which means an arthritis that does not have an anti-IgG antibody (non-rheumatoid). It is associated with HLA-B27, and has a classic triad of conjunctivitis, urethritis, and arthritis (can't see, can't pee, can't climb up a tree). Know how to identify reactive arthritis on the shelf, and keep a keen eye out for antecedent infections, such chlamydia (STI) and bacterial GI infections (*Campylobacter, Shigella, Salmonella*).

PPx: Avoid chlamydia and GI infections

Mechanism of Disease (MoD): Unknown, but can be triggered by an STI (*Chylamydia trachomatis*) or a GI infection (*Campylobacter jejuni, Salmonella* or *Shigella*).

> **MNEMONIC**
> Can't see, can't pee, can't climb up a tree → reactive arthritis (conjunctivitis, urethritis, arthralgia)

QUICK TIPS

Other HLA-B27 diseases aside from reactive arthritis: Psoriatic arthritis, ankylosing spondylitis and inflammatory bowel disease associated with arthritis

Dx:
1. Complete blood count/basic metabolic panel (CBC/BMP)
2. XR of affected arthritic joints
3. Fundoscopic exam for conjunctivitis
4. UA/UCx for urethritis
5. Genetic testing for HLA-B27

Tx/Mgmt:
1. Antibiotics
2. Steroids

Psoriatic Arthropathy

Buzz Words: DIP arthritis + nail-pitting + onycholoysis (lifting of nail plate) + dactylitis (sausage fingers) + itchy rash with silvery plaques + chronic uveitis

Clinical Presentation: Psoriatic arthropathy is a seronegative arthropathy that presents as arthritis in the setting of chronic psoriasis. Knees, ankles, fingers, and toes may be involved. Arthritis is asymmetric and affects four or fewer joints at presentation. DIP arthritis is uncommon but highly suggestive of this diagnosis. Higher risk of axial involvement if the patient if HLA-B27+.

MoD: Unknown but related to HLA-B27

Dx:
1. XR (erosions seen in the joint since this is an inflammatory arthritis)
2. HLA-B27
3. RA and ANA to r/o other forms of inflammatory arthropathy

Tx/Mgmt:
1. NSAIDs
2. Methotrexate
3. Tumor necrosis factor (TNF)-alpha inhibitors

Juvenile Idiopathic Arthritis

Buzz Words: Articular pain for >3 months + morning stiffness that improves throughout the day + salmon-colored rash

Clinical Presentation: This is an umbrella term that includes different causes of chronic arthritis. Clinical presentation varies by subtype (Table 13.1).

MoD: Unclear: Alterations in both humoral and cell-mediated immunity occur. Th1 lymphocytes play a central role (TNF-alpha), although B-cell activation, immune complex formation, and complement activation also promote inflammation.

TABLE 13.1 Juvenile Idiopathic Arthritis Subtypes

Subtype	Clinical Presentation
Oligoarthritis	• ≤4 joints within the first 6 months • Predominantly large joints and lower extremities • Persistent oligoarticular if >4 joints are never involved • Extended oligoarticular if >4 joints are eventually affected, worse prognosis • 30% have uveitis or iridocyclitis • Most cases resolve in less than 6 months
Polyarthritis	• ≥5 joints in both upper and lower extremities • RF positive polyarthritis resembles adult rheumatoid arthritis with rheumatoid nodules on extensor surfaces • Micrognathia reflects chronic temporomandibular joint disease • 60% enter remission within 15 years • Worse prognosis with older onset
Systemic (Still's disease)	• Arthritis • Fever: spiking, twice-daily, ≥39°C (102.2°F) • Rash: salmon-colored trunk and proximal extremities, evanescent • Hepatosplenomegaly, lymphadenopathy, serositis • Variable course, 50% will eventually achieve remission

Dx:
- XR of joint (osteopenia and subchondral sclerosis around involved joints).
- Might be ANA+, RF+ or have an >ESR but these tests are not diagnostic.

Tx/Mgmt: Goal is to prevent joint damage and induce disease remission. Treatment plan is tailored to the specific subtype of juvenile idiopathic arthritis (JIA). NSAIDs and steroids are prescribed.

Dermatomyositis and Polymyositis

Buzz Words:
- **Polymyositis:** proximal muscle weakness + no rash
- **Dermatomyositis:** proximal muscle weakness + heliotrope rash + Gottron's papules

Clinical Presentation: Dermatomyositis and polymyositis both predominantly affect proximal muscles, leading to issues with stair climbing or lifting things above the level of the shoulder. Dermatomyositis also presents skin alterations, like periorbital violaceous heliotrope rash

Dermatomyositis of the hand

and erythematous and hypertrophic skin over metacarpal and PIP joints (Gottron's papules). May present with constitutional symptoms like weight loss, fever, fatigue, or headache.

PPx: Vitamin D and calcium, sunscreen

MoD: Diabetes mellitus (DM) is primarily a capillary vasculopathy, whereas PM involves direct T cell invasion of muscle fibers, similar to that seen in adult polymyositis. HLA B8/DR3 and HLA DQalpha*0501 are associated with higher risk of DM and are sometimes associated with a viral illness.

Dx:
1. Muscle strength testing
2. Increased muscle enzymes (CPK, lactic acid dehydrogenase [LDH], alanine transaminase [ALT], aspartate aminotransferase [AST], aldolase)
3. Electromyography
4. Muscle biopsy:
   - EMG and muscle biopsy should only be used when the diagnosis remains uncertain.

Tx/Mgmt:
1. Corticosteroids
2. Immunosuppressive agents (methotrexate, intravenous immunoglobulin [IVIG], cyclosporine, cyclopohosphamide)
3. Physical therapy

Polymyalgia Rheumatica

Buzz Words: Proximal muscle stiffness/pain + female + ≥50 years old + temporal arteritis + elevated ESR + normal creatine kinase (CK)

Clinical Presentation: Polymyalgia rheumatica is a musculoskeletal disorder of unknown origin that presents in elderly females who complain of muscle pain with normal CK labs. Its claim to fame on the shelf is its association with temporal arteritis. This disorder will be rarely tested by itself, so feel free to skip as long as you know the diagnostic and treatment steps for temporal arteritis.

Dx:
1. CBC/BMP
2. ESR/CRP (elevated)
3. CK (normal)
4. Temporal artery biopsy (if temporal arteritis has still not been r/o)

Tx/Mgmt: Steroids

Infectious and Inflammatory Disorders

Gangrene

Buzz Words: Pain out of proportion to signs of disease

Gangrenous foot

- **Dry gangrene:** clinical features of vascular obstruction, such as pale/blue/gray/purple coloration, numbness, decreased perfusion, common on ends of fingers and toes
- **Wet gangrene:** bullae, ecchymosis, crepitation of gas, cutaneous anesthesia
- **Gas gangrene (clostridial myonecrosis):** crepitation with palpation, bronze skin discoloration, tense bullae, serosanguineous or dark fluid and necrotic areas

Clinical Presentation: Gangrene is the localized death of body tissue. Most high-yield concept to know for the shelf is gas gangrene.

PPx: Prevention of risk factors, especially, diabetes, peripheral vascular disease, and trauma

MoD:
- **Dry gangrene:** insufficient blood supply
- **Wet gangrene:** necrotizing bacterial infection
- **Gas gangrene:** *Clostridium perfringens* infection of tissue releases alpha toxin, a lecithinase (phospholipase) that degrades tissue and cell membranes → gas bubble formation → gas gangrene (myonecrosis)

Dx: Clinical diagnosis:
- **Dry gangrene:** peripheral vascular disease work up: reduced ABI (<0.4), absence of vascular flow on ultrasound
- **Gas gangrene:** Gram-positive or Gram variable stain, few polys, bacteremia in 15%, gas dissecting into muscle on radiographs

Tx/Mgmt:
- **Dry:** Revascularization if feasible
- **Gas:** Antibiotics and wound debridement (surgical removal of dead tissue):
  1. Hyperbaric oxygen or maggot debridement therapy
  2. Amputation

Necrotizing Fasciitis

Buzz Words: Cellulitic skin + intense disproportionate pain + SIRS (acutely ill); initially hyperesthetic, later anesthetic, bullae, and darkening of skin to bluish-gray + dirty dishwater fluid

Clinical Presentation: Necrotizing fasciitis is emergent and has a roughly 30% mortality rate.

QUICK TIPS
Fournier's gangrene: necrotizing fasciitis of the male or female genitalia

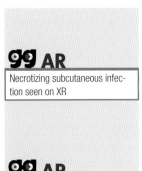

gg AR

Necrotizing subcutaneous infection seen on XR

gg AR

Necrotizing fasciitis on CT scan

MoD: Tissue ischemia 2/2 occlusion of small subcutaneous vessels → skin infarction and necrosis → infection of deep soft tissues that rapidly tracks along fascial planes

Dx:

1. CBC (high white blood cell [WBC] count)
2. XR of affected area can show gas

Tx/Mgmt: Broad-spectrum intravenous (IV) antimicrobials AND urgent surgical exploration and excision of devitalized tissue

Osteochondritis Dissecans

Buzz Words: Young male athlete + deep knee pain that is worsened by exercise + magnetic resonance imaging (MRI) shows lesion in bone beneath cartilage

Clinical Presentation: Osteochondritis dissecans is condition in which the bone underneath the cartilage of a given joint becomes necrotic, leading to knee pain and debility from sport. Patients can present with vague or deep knee pain that may localize along the medial or lateral joint line. If the fragment of dead bone with overlying cartilage becomes unstable, there may be locking of the joint. Boys are more commonly affected than girls. The knee is the most commonly affected joint, followed by the elbow and ankle.

PPx: N/A

Dx:

- Plain radiograph shows a subchondral bony fragment surrounded by a crescent-shaped radiolucency; however, radiographs can be normal.
- MRI if plain radiography is normal and there is persistence of clinical symptoms.

Tx/Mgmt:

1. Non-weight bearing and immobilization
2. Physical therapy
3. Surgery:
   - Skeletal immaturity, smaller lesion size, and absence of mechanical symptoms or pain have been associated with a higher likelihood of healing with non-operative treatment
   - Unstable lesions will not usually heal with conservative treatment

Transient Synovitis (Toxic Synovitis)

Buzz Words: Six year old boy + hip pain + history of upper respiratory infection 1–2 weeks prior to presentation

Clinical Presentation: Transient synovitis is the inflammation of the synovium of the hip joint capsule 2/2 viral infection. Patients experience acute onset of pain in the groin, anterior thigh, or knee, and can present with a painful, limping gait. It is often afebrile, contrary to septic arthritis.

Dx:
1. CBC (slightly elevated)
2. ESR/CRP (slightly elevated)
3. Rule out septic arthritis with blood cultures and aspiration of the joint, as the consequences of misdiagnosed septic arthritis can be serious.

Tx/Mgmt: NSAIDs, bed rest, and observation: Most children recover completely within 3–6 weeks.

Septic Arthritis

Buzz Words: Acute onset of fever + exquisite joint tenderness with micromotion + unilateral erythema + aspiration

Clinical Presentation: Septic arthritis is the infection of a joint and requires emergent treatment. Classic presentation is a painful, swollen joint that exhibits pain even with slightest amount of motion (e.g., tenderness with micromotion). The hip is most commonly affected in younger children, whereas the knee is commonly affected in older children. Complications include avascular necrosis and cartilaginous damage.

MoD: Hematogenous seeding of the synovial space occurs. Less often, it can be the result of direct inoculation or extension from a contiguous focus. *Staphylococcus aureus* and *Streptococcus pyogenes* are the most common organisms. *Neisseria gonorrhoeae* may cause septic arthritis in adolescents.

Dx:
1. CBC
2. ESR/CRP
3. Blood culture
4. Synovial fluid aspiration and culture (organisms and elevated WBC count)

Tx/Mgmt: Empiric IV antibiotics that cover Gram-positive organisms for 4–6 weeks

Osteomyelitis

Buzz Words: Infant or 10-year-old boy + fever + recent injury in which skin was penetrated (e.g., stepped on a nail) + XR/MRI show lesions of the bone:
- Osteomyelitis + sickle cell anemia → *Salmonella*
- Osteomyelitis + stepped on a nail → *Pseudomonas*

Osteomyelitis video

Clinical Presentation: Osteomyelitis is the bacterial infection of bone. It can present as fever, bone pain, erythema, swelling and induration. Refusal to move the involved limb in younger children; painful limp in older children.

MoD: It is most commonly an acquired infection through hematogenous seeding. *S. aureus* and *S. pyogenes* are the most common organisms. *Salmonella* in the case of sickle cell anemia. *Pseudomonas aeruginosa* in children who step on a nail. Fractures that require surgical reduction are a risk factor.

Dx:
1. CBC
2. ESR/CRP
3. XR
4. MRI
5. Blood and wound cultures

Tx/Mgmt:
1. IV or high-dose oral antibiotics given for 4–6 weeks (broad-spectrum antistaphylococcal agents and vancomycin for methicillin-resistant Staphylococcus aureus (MRSA)
2. Surgical debridement

Myofascial Pain Syndrome

Buzz Words: Muscle pain and spasms that worsen when carrying heavy backpacks

Clinical Presentation: Myofascial pain syndrome is pain in the muscles that occurs when a non-related pressure/trigger point is pressed. It is characterized by tender points in the affected muscles, as well as muscle spasms. Pain is often caused by poor body posture, repetitive use of a part of the body, or carrying heavy backpacks. The diagnosis of juvenile fibromyalgia may be made when there are multiple tender points.

Dx: Clinical diagnosis

Tx/Mgmt:
- Pregabalin and duloxetine
- Physical therapy

Neoplasms

Imaging of pediatric bone tumors video

Benign Neoplasms

Osteoid Osteoma

Buzz Words: Older teen + bone pain that is worse at night + **relieved by aspirin** + small round lucency with sclerotic margin on XR

Clinical Presentation: Osteoid osteoma is a benign bone tumor of osteoblasts that presents as bone pain worse at night and **relieved by aspirin.** It is more common in boys than girls. Most commonly affects the proximal femur and tibia, vertebral lesions can cause scoliosis. Palpation of the area does not alter the discomfort.

MoD: Benign, bone-forming tumor that produces high levels of prostaglandins

Dx: XR of affected bone (small, round lucency with a sclerotic margin)

Tx/Mgmt:
1. NSAIDs
2. Percutaneous radiofrequency ablation
3. Surgical resection/curettage

Osteoblastoma

Buzz Words: Older teen with chronic bone pain + does not respond to aspirin + lytic lesion with radiolucent nidus

Clinical Presentation: It is a more aggressive version of osteoid osteoma. Presents with insidious onset of dull aching pain. Predilection for the vertebrae. Unlike an osteoid osteoma this lesion is not self-limited, and may produce symptoms of cord compression if in the vertebrae.

MoD: Benign, bone-producing tumor

Dx:
1. XR and computed tomography (CT)
2. Bone scan

Tx/Mgmt: Surgical removal of the tumor (curettage/marginal excision with bone grafting): Untreated osteoblastoma will continue to enlarge and may damage bone and adjacent tissues.

Osteochondroma

Buzz Words: Older teen + hard painless mass that has not changed in years + sessile or pedunculated lesion on surface of bone

Clinical Presentation: Osteochondromas are neoplasms of cartilage and the most common benign bone tumor. Presents as painless mass near a joint, or painful mass related to local trauma. Some patients can have multiple hereditary exostoses, which can impair limb-growth, so they must be monitored during growth. One of the most common benign bone tumors in children.

MoD: Occur spontaneously, but have been reported following radiotherapy. Bony spur with a cartilaginous cap that overlies it and is the source of growth.

Dx:
1. XR
2. CT/MRI

99 AR
Osteoblastoma review

99 AR
Osteochondroma review

FOR THE WARDS
Multiple osteochondromas = multiple hereditary exostosis

Tx/Mgmt: Observation, surgical resection only if symptomatic

Enchondroma

Buzz Words: Older teen + discovery of bone mass after fracture + lucent, central medullary lesions on XR

Clinical Presentation: Enchondromas are tumors composed of hyaline cartilage. Most enchondromas are asymptomatic unless a fracture is present. They are often incidental findings. When symptomatic there may be widening of the bone, deformity, and limb-length discrepancy. Ollier syndrome presents with multiple enchondromas, malignant transformation occurs in 10%–25% of cases. Maffucci syndrome presents with multiple enchondromas, soft tissue hemangiomas, and malignant transformation to chondrosarcoma occurs in nearly 100% of cases.

MoD: Benign lesion of hyaline cartilage that occurs centrally in the bone.

Dx:

1. XR (oval, well-circumbscribed, central lucent lesion, with or without matrix calcifications)
2. Bone scan
3. MRI
4. Core needle-biopsy to r/o chondrosarcoma

Tx/Mgmt: Observation w/XR at 6 and 12 months, surgical removal if large and/or symptomatic

Giant Cell Tumor

Buzz Words: Soap-bubble appearance on XR, pain, swelling, and limited ROM at epiphyseal end of distal femur or proximal tibia

Clinical Presentation: A benign tumor of the bone that has a histological presentation of many giant cells. Very rarely tested in the shelf exam, and if it is tested, will likely only be the diagnosis of the disease (e.g., "soap-bubble" appearance).

Dx:

1. XR soap-bubble appearance
2. CT scan
3. Giant cells seen in histological specimen

Tx/Mgmt:

1. Bisphosphonates
2. Denosumab
3. Wide resection

Malignant Neoplasms of Bone and Muscle

Osteosarcoma

Buzz Words: Male adolescent + palpable, painful mass + history of retinoblastoma + sunburst appearance on imaging

Clinical Presentation: Osteosarcoma is malignant tumor of osteoblastic proliferation. Pain and localized swelling occur without systemic manifestations. It is most frequent in adolescents. Most common in the distal femur, proximal tibia, and proximal humerus, mainly involving the metaphysis of these long bones. There may be limited motion, joint effusion, tenderness and warmth.

MoD: Malignant tumor of the bone-producing mesenchymal stem cells: Associated with previous **retinoblastoma**, Paget's disease of bone, Li-Fraumeni syndrome, radiation therapy, and fibrous dysplasia

Dx:

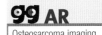
Osteosarcoma imaging

1. XR (sunburst appearance)
2. MRI
3. Biopsy

Tx/Mgmt: Chemotherapy + surgical removal, with amputation or limb-sparing surgery

Ewing's Sarcoma

Buzz Words: Male adolescent + pain and localized swelling + systemic manifestations + onion-skin appearance on imaging

Clinical Presentation: Ewing's sarcoma is a round cell tumor that has a very characteristic onion-skin appearance on XR. Patients present with bone pain, swelling, soft tissue mass, fever, malaise, weight loss, leukocytosis, and elevated ESR. Unlike osteosarcoma, in which long bones are predominantly involved, Ewing's sarcoma can affect both flat and long bones.

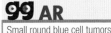
Small round blue cell tumors

MoD: Unknown, but 95% have a chromosomal translocation between chromosomes 11 and 22.

Dx:
1. XR (onion-skin appearance)
2. MRI
3. Biopsy

Tx/Mgmt: Chemotherapy is prescribed due to high risk of metastasis, followed by surgical excision. Radiation therapy is used when complete excision is impossible.

Rhabdomyosarcoma

Buzz Words: Child <10 year old + painless enlarging mass on the back of the neck

Clinical Presentation: Rhabdomyosarcoma is a malignant tumor of the striated muscle. Two-thirds occur in children younger than 10 years of age. Most commonly present as a painless soft tissue mass. Symptoms are caused by compression of adjacent structures, which depends on the region it is affecting and include cranial nerve palsies, proptosis, and obstruction of the oropharynx. They most commonly arise from the head and neck; the second most common site is the genitourinary tract; and the third most common site of involvement is the extremities.

MoD: Unknown, arises from the same embryonic mesenchyme as striated skeletal muscle. It is associated with neurofibromatosis and Li-Fraumeni syndrome.

Dx: XR

Tx/Mgmt: Complete surgical resection, if possible, plus radiotherapy and chemotherapy to eradicate metastasis and prevent recurrence

99 AR

3D model of the Knee

Degenerative and Metabolic Disorders

Degenerative

Patellofemoral Syndrome (Formerly Patellar Chondromalacia)

Buzz Words: Knee pain + worse when descending stairs + patella in a lateral position

Clinical Presentation: Pain comes from contact of the patella with the femur. Presents as knee pain that is difficult to localize; pain is often worse when climbing stairs, squatting, running, or sitting for prolonged periods. Physical examination may show the patella in a lateral position.

MoD: Joint malalignment and excessive use

Dx: Physical exam (medial patellar tenderness or pain with compression of the joint confirms the diagnosis in the absence of a significant effusion and other positive findings).

Tx/Mgmt: Rest, stretching, and strengthening of the medial quadriceps

Intervertebral Disc Herniation

Buzz Words:

- **Lumbar:** Positive straight leg test + pain shooting down leg from back + paresthesias and weakness of lower extremity + unilateral
- **Cervical:** Positive Spurling test + pain shooting down arm + paresthesias and weakness of upper extremity + unilateral
- L3–L4 disc: weakness of knee extension, decreased patellar reflex
- L4–L5 disc: weakness of dorsiflexion, difficulty in heel-walking
- L5–S1 disc: weakness of plantarflexion, difficulty in toe-walking, decreased Achilles reflex (Table 13.2)

TABLE 13.2 Disc Herniation: Cervical and Lumbar Radiculopathy

Disc	Root	Pain/Paresthesias	Sensory Loss	Motor Loss	Reflex Loss
C4–C5	C5	Neck, shoulder upper arm	Shoulder	Deltoid, biceps, infraspinatus	Biceps
C5–C6	C6	Neck, shoulder, lat. arm, radial forearm, thumb, and index finger	Lat. arm, radial forearm, thumb, and index finger	Biceps, brachioradialis	Biceps, brachioradialis, supinator
C6–C7	C7	Neck, lat. arm, ring and index finger	Radial forearm, index and middle fingers	Triceps, extensor carpi ulnaris	Triceps, supinator
C7–T1	C8	Ulnar forearm and hand	Ulnar half of ring finger, little finger	Intrinsic hand muscles, wrist extensors, flexor digitorum profundus	Finger flexion
L3–L4	L4	Anterior thigh, inner shin	Anteriomedial thigh and shin, inner foot	Quadriceps	Patella
L4–L5	L5	Lat. thigh and calf, dorsum of foot, great toe	Lat. calf and great toe	Extensor hallucis longus, foot dorsiflexion, inversion and eversion	None
L5–S1	S1	Back of thigh, lateral posterior calf, lat. foot	Posterolat. calf, lat. and sole of foot, smaller toes	Gastrocnemius, foot eversion	Achilles

Clinical Presentation: Due to desiccation of the annulus fibrosus, nucleus pulposus of intervertebral disc can herniate outward and compress the nerve of the superior vertebrae (e.g., intervertebral herniation of L4–L5 will compress L4 root). Patients present with back pain and pain radiating into the legs (oftentimes the leg pain is worse than the back pain). Pain is often made worse by coughing, or sitting, and it may be relieved by standing up. Lumbar region is most commonly affected. Patient may lean toward the unaffected side to relieve pressure on the spinal cord.

MoD: Tear in the annulus fibrosus occurs, which allows protrusion of the nucleus pulposus. Unlike adults, in children it is mostly caused by repetitive activity, and rarely by trauma.

Dx: MRI (best study) shows loss of lumbar lordosis due to muscle spasm, sometimes a mild lumbar scoliosis, as well as loss of intervertebral disc height.

Tx/Mgmt:
1. Rest and PT
2. NSAIDs
3. Steroid injections
4. Surgery

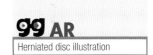
99 AR
Herniated disc illustration

Osgood-Schlatter's disease review

Osgood-Schlatter Disease

Buzz Words: Twelve-year-old boy + basketball player + pain over the tibial tuberosity

Clinical Presentation: Osgood-Schlatter disease is inflammation of the patellar tendon at the insertion of the tibial tubercle (e.g., apophysitis). Patient presents with swelling of the tibial tuberosity with pain and tenderness over the tibial tubercle that is exacerbated with activity and relieved with rest. Most common in 10- to15-year-old boys who participate in sports involving repetitive jumping. Usually asymmetric, but can be bilateral.

MoD: Overuse of the extensor mechanism of the patella, causing traction apophysitis at the insertion of the patellar tendon to the proximal tibia

Dx: Clinical diagnosis: Imaging is not necessary unless the patient has unusual complaints.

Tx/Mgmt:

1. Activity modification, rest, ice after exercise
2. Arotective pad can be used over the tibial tubercle to protect from direct trauma
3. If severe, immobilization of the joint

Osteoarthritis

Heberden and Bouchard nodes - osteoarthritis review

Buzz Words: Joint crepitus with motion + pain worse with motion + joint stiffness after inactivity + osteophyte enlargement of DIP joints (Heberden nodes), PIP joints (Bouchard nodes) + joint space narrowing on radiographs

Clinical Presentation: Osteoarthritis is the most common chronic degenerative condition of the joints, and occurs due to non-inflammatory breakdown of articular cartilage. This results in pain, stiffness, and loss of joint mobility, most commonly in hip, knee, back, PIP, and DIP. The pain is worse with the use of the joint and improves with rest.

PPx: Maintain healthy weight, engage in physical activity

MoD: Non-inflammatory progressive articular cartilage degeneration at weight-bearing joints: femoral head, knee, cervical, and lumbar vertebrae

Dx: Clinical diagnosis: XR may show joint space narrowing, subchondral sclerosis, osteophyte formation, and subchondral cysts.

Tx/Mgmt:

1. Heat, decreased weight bearing, PT
2. Use of a cane and brace
3. Analgesics (NSAIDs)
4. Steroid injection
5. Surgery (arthroplasty, aka joint replacement)

Metabolic

Legg-Calvé-Perthes Disease

Buzz Words: Four- to ten-year-old boy + insidious hip/knee pain with painful limp

Clinical Presentation: Legg-Calve-Perthes disease is an idiopathic avascular necrosis of the proximal femoral epiphysis and affects children from 4 to 10 years of age. It can begin as painless but will progress to a mildly painful limp, usually related to activity. Decreased internal rotation and abduction of the hip occur. Pain may be referred to the knee or the groin. Has been found to be associated with attention deficit hyperactivity disorder (ADHD) and delayed bone age. High yield for the Pediatrics shelf.

MoD: Temporary interruption of blood flow to the femoral epiphysis, causing avascular necrosis. Etiology is unknown.

Dx:

1. XR: AP and frogleg lateral views
2. Bone scan
3. MRI
4. Arthrogram

Affected femoral head appears small, shows sclerotic bone and widened joint space. Presence of a crescentic subchondral fracture in the femoral head is termed the "crescent sign."

Tx/Mgmt: Principle of treatment is to contain the femoral head within the acetabulum, which prevents deformation of the femoral head:

1. Non-weight bearing, PT
2. NSAIDs
3. Surgery

99 AR

XR of Perthes disease

Osteodystrophy

Buzz Words: CKD + osteitis fibrosa cystica (cystic bone spaces filled with "brown tumor" consisting of osteoclasts and deposited hemosiderin from hemorrhages) + osteopenia and "Looser zones" (pseudofractures) in osteomalacia

Clinical Presentation: Osteodystrophy is a general term for dystrophic growth of the bone, most commonly due to renal disease or disturbances in calcium and phosphorus metabolism. It is manifested by (1) osteomalacia (decreased mineralization of bone due to decreased calcium and 1,25-[OH]$_2$D); and (2) osteitis fibrosa cystica (due to increased PTH).

MoD:

- Renal failure → decreased vitamin D → decreased mineralization of bone → osteomalacia
- Renal failure → increased PTH → osteitis fibrosa cystica

Dx:
1. CMP (hypocalcemia, hyperphosphatemia, decreased vitamin D, increased parathyroid hormone, increased alkaline phosphatase)
2. Bone biopsy

Tx/Mgmt:
1. Vitamin D and/or calcium supplementation
2. Treat chronic kidney disease (CKD)

Osteomalacia/Rickets

Buzz Words: Waddling gait + difficulty walking, soft, bending bones, vitamin D deficiency, bone pain, and muscle weakness

Clinical Presentation: Osteomalacia refers to a softening of the bones, most commonly caused by vitamin D deficiency. Rickets = soft bone in **children** 2/2 vitamin D deficiency; osteomalacia = vitamin D induced bone softening in **adults.** Most common chief complaint is bone pain and muscle weakness. Osteomalacia and rickets are associated with vitamin D deficiency, CKD, hypocalcemia.

PPx: Vitamin D and calcium

MoD: Defective mineralization of osteoid growth plates

Dx:

Osteomalacia XR

1. CMP (decreased serum calcium and phosphate, increased alkaline phosphatase [ALP] and PTH)
2. XRs show osteopenia and "Looser zones" (pseudofractures)

Tx/Mgmt: Vitamin D supplementation

Avascular Necrosis of Femoral Head

Buzz Words: Trauma + corticosteroids + excessive alcohol intake + recent total hip replacement + crescent sign (subchondral radiolucency)

Clinical Presentation: Avascular necrosis is due to death of bone tissue caused by a lack of blood supply, resulting in arthritis. On the shelf, remember the risk factors for avascular necrosis, and be able to identify its appearance on radiograph. Risk factors: trauma, corticosteroids, excessive alcohol intake, recent total hip replacement, lupus, sickle cell patient.

MoD: Compromise of bone vasculature 2/2 multiple predisposing etiologies

Dx:

Avascular necrosis of femoral head xrays

1. MRI for early detection due to high sensitivity
2. Anterior-posterior and frogleg lateral XR showing mild density changes, or pathognomonic crescent sign (subchondral radiolucency) in later phases

Tx/Mgmt:
1. Supportive
2. Surgery (core decompression) if severe
3. If refractory, then total hip replacement

Osteopenia/Osteoporosis

Buzz Words: Elderly lady + hip fractures

Osteoporosis gudelines

Clinical Presentation: Osteopenia and osteoporosis are diseases that fall on a spectrum of decreased bone mineral density, where osteopenia can sometimes be considered to be a precursor to osteoporosis. To be diagnosed with osteopenia, the bone mineral density T-score falls between −1.0 and −2.5, while to be diagnosed with osteoporosis, the bone mineral density T-score is less than −2.5. Osteopenia is a sign of normal aging, in contrast to osteoporosis, which is present in pathologic aging. It is important to also realize that osteoporosis in question stems may refer to secondary osteoporosis, caused by excess steroids, Cushing syndrome, hyperthyroidism, long-term heparin, hypogonadism, or vitamin D deficiency.

PPx: Calcium, vitamin D, weight-bearing exercise, smoking cessation

MoD: Rate of bone resorption exceeds rate of bone formation after peak bone mass is attained. Associated with low estrogen (menopause), calcium/vitamin D deficiency, decreased physical bone mass, hypogonadism, hyperthyroidism, smoking, alcohol abuse, corticosteroids, prolonged heparin use, Cushing syndrome.

Dx: Dual energy x-ray absorptiometry (DEXA) scan:
- Osteopenia: DEXA Bone Mineral Density T-score between −1.0 and −2.5
- Osteoporosis: DEXA Bone Mineral Density T-score < −2.5

Tx/Mgmt:
1. Non-pharmacologic—adequate calorie, calcium, and vitamin D, weight-bearing exercise, smoking cessation, reduce EtOH intake
2. For established osteoporosis or high-risk osteopenia, bisphosphonates
3. PTH therapy for 24 months

Osteitis Deformans (Paget Disease of Bone)

Buzz Words: Increased hat size + hearing loss + pathologic fractures + osteogenic sarcoma + heart failure due to arteriovenous malformations (AVMs) in vascular bone

Clinical Presentation: Paget disease of bone is common in aging bone, and the majority of patients are asymptomatic. In patients that are symptomatic, it is important to remember pathognomonic clues, such as increased hat size, in combination with hearing loss or pathologic fractures. Sometimes, the only abnormality in work-up will be increased ALP.

MoD: Increased osteoclastic activity is followed by increased osteoblastic activity, forming poor-quality bone in pelvis, skull, and femur.

Dx:
1. CMP (normal serum calcium, phosphorus, and PTH, but **increased ALP**)
2. XRs show thickened bone with shaggy areas of radiolucency
3. Bone scans show "hot spots"

Tx/Mgmt: Bisphosphonates and calcitonin

Spondylolisthesis

Buzz Words: Radiographic Scotty dog sign seen on oblique films + low back pain during lumbar extension + minimal tenderness

Clinical Presentation: Spondylolisthesis is a common cause of low back pain in athletes, and refers to anterior slippage of one vertebrae over another. It is caused by repetitive hyperextension creating shear of posterior elements (diving, weightlifting, wrestling, gymnastics). Its precursor is spondylosis (a vertebral crack or stress fracture); if the spondylosis weakens the bone sufficiently, then vertebral slippage (spondylolisthesis) will occur.

PPx: Avoid repetitive hyperextension

MoD: Bilateral pars defects (spondylolysis) leads to slippage forward of an upper vertebral segment on the lower segment, most commonly L5–S1, then L4–L5, then L3–L4.

Dx:
1. Clinical diagnosis
2. XR ("Scotty the dog" sign)

Tx/Mgmt:
1. Restriction of aggravating activities
2. NSAIDs, and cast or thoracic-lumbar-sacral orthosis, physical therapy

Gout

Buzz Words: Negatively birefringent crystals + recent large meal or alcohol consumption, swollen, red, and painful MTP joint of big toe (podagra) + tophus formation on external ear, olecranon bursa, or Achilles tendon

Clinical Presentation: Gout, also known as monosodium urate crystal deposition disease, is caused by hyperuricemia, and is manifested by recurrent attacks of acute inflammatory arthritis, chronic arthropathy, accumulation of urate crystals, uric acid nephrolithiasis, most commonly in the MTP of the big toe. On the shelf, be able to distinguish this from other arthritides, as well as pseudogout. It is associated with underexcretion of uric acid (lead poisoning, alcoholism, excess red meat, seafood, beer, thiazides), overproduction of uric acid (Lesch-Nyhan syndrome, PRPP excess, increased cell turnover from leukemia or psoriasis treatment).

PPX: Avoid excess red meats, seafood, alcohol, thiazides

MoD: Prolonged hyperuricemia → tissue deposition of monosodium urate

Dx:
1. Uric acid levels (elevated)
2. CBC (absolute neutrophilic leukocytosis)
3. Confirm with joint aspiration showing negatively birefringent MSU crystals

Tx/Mgmt:
1. Acute flare—NSAIDs (indomethacin, ibuprofen), glucocorticoids, colchicine
2. Chronic: xanthine oxidase inhibitors such as allopurinol, febuxostat

Pseudogout (Calcium Pyrophosphate Dihydrate Deposition Disease)

Buzz Words: Positively birefringent crystals + acute pain, redness, swelling, limited ROM in joint + chondrocalcinosis

Gout and pseudogout mnemonic

Clinical Presentation: In calcium pyrophosphate dihydrate deposition disease (CPPD), calcium pyrophosphate crystals deposit in joints, leading to inflammation. Deposition is common in elderly patients with degenerative joint disease, and increases with age and osteoarthritis of the joints. In most cases, the cause of deposition is unknown, but joint trauma, hemochromatosis, hemosiderosis, hyperparathyroidism, and Bartter syndrome are risk factors. On the shelf, it is important to be able to distinguish the crystals of CPPD from gout.

MoD: Deposition of calcium pyrophosphate in tissues and cartilage (chondrocalcinosis)

Dx:
1. XR (chondrocalcinoisis)
2. Joint aspiration showing rhomboid crystals, weakly birefringent under polarized light

Tx/Mgmt:
1. NSAIDs, colchicine, glucocorticoids
2. Arthroscopic surgery

Dupuytren's Contracture

Dupuytren's contracture images

Buzz Words: Painless stiffness of fingers + nodules on palmar fascia + contractures (baseline flexion at MCP or PIP joint) + palpable cord running longitudinally in subcutaneous tissue, which puckers the skin and limits extension

Clinical Presentation: Dupuytren's contracture is a contracture of the proliferated longitudinal bands of the palmar aponeurosis lying between the skin and flexor tendons in the distal palm and fingers, most commonly in the ring and small fingers. It begins as a nodule and progresses to fibrous bands, with contracture of the fingers. Associated with diabetes, cigarettes, alcohol use, repetitive hand use, familial history of contracture.

MoD: Slowly progressive fibroblastic proliferation and disorderly collagen deposition with fascial thickening

Dx: Clinical diagnosis

Tx/Mgmt:
1. Glove with padding, or modifying tools with cushions
2. Glucocorticoid injection (triamcinolone acetonide and lidocaine)
3. Collagenase injection
4. Surgery (fasciotomy)

Myositis Ossificans

Buzz Words: Upper or lower extremity mass at site of known blunt trauma + radiographs showing formation with peripheral calcification and a lucent center

Clinical Presentation: Myositis ossificans is a reactive process of heterotopic bone formation that occurs after an episode of blunt trauma. This will most likely appear as an answer choice on the shelf, so be able to rule this out based on history.

MoD: Heterotopic ossification of skeletal muscle following muscular trauma

Myositis ossicicans radiographs

Dx: XR

Tx/Mgmt: Symptomatic treatment

Rhabdomyolysis

Buzz Words: Myalgias + weakness + myoglobinuria + AKI + elevated CPK + hyperkalemia, hypocalcemia, hyperuricemia

Clinical Presentation: Rhabdomyolysis is the breakdown of muscle tissue, which leads to release of muscle contents into blood, most notably myoglobin, which is toxic to the kidneys. On the shelf, recognize that rhabdomyolysis will be a result of some pathologic process, and be able to recognize and manage this problem. Patients may present with myalgias, weakness, red to brown urine following trauma, crush injuries, prolonged immobility, seizures, snake bites, or daptomycin.

MoD: Skeletal muscle breakdown, release of myoglobin into bloodstream → AKI, elevated CPK, hyperkalemia, hypocalcemia, hyperuricemia

Dx:
1. Serum CK > 5X ULN (usually >5000 IU/L)
2. UA dipstick

Tx/Mgmt: IV fluids, mannitol (osmotic diuretic), bicarbonate (drives K back into cells)

QUICK TIPS
Key diagnostic laboratory studies: CK, UA dipstick, and microscopy.

Traumatic and Mechanical Disorders
Subluxation of the Radial Head (Nursemaid's Elbow)

Buzz Words: Child <6 years old + arm pulled by caretaker + pain with flexed elbow

Clinical Presentation: Pain and persistence of elbow flexion even though the patient's hand function is normal. Usually presents after a strong, pulling force is exerted on the arm in patients younger than 6 years of age. High-yield for the Pediatrics shelf.

MoD: Sudden, strong, upward pulling of the arm causing rapid extension of the elbow. This causes a dislocation of the annular ligament into the joint and between the radial head and the humerus.

Dx: Clinical diagnosis: Radiographs are usually normal because the subluxation is usually inadvertently reduced by the technician while positioning the arm for imaging.

Tx/Mgmt: **Rotation of the forearm into supination while pressuring the radial head.** A successful reduction can usually be felt as a click, after which the child recovers movement of the joint and the pain is relieved.

99 AR
Nursemaid elbow reduction techniques

Anterior Dislocation of the Shoulder

Buzz Words: Athlete with severe pain + shoulder "popped" out of place + abduction and external rotation mechanism

Clinical Presentation: Severe pain, patients usually notice that the humeral head is out of place. Some athletes that are prone to this injury are gymnasts, football players, and wrestlers.

MoD: Forceful abduction, extension and external rotation of the shoulder

Dx: Post-reduction radiographs may show a posterior lateral humeral head impaction fracture (Hill-Sachs lesion). Sensation of the lateral deltoid region and the extensor surface of the proximal forearm should be verified, as they are altered with injury to the axillary nerve or the musculocutaneous nerve, respectively.

Tx/Mgmt: Immobilization after closed reduction. There is a high rate of recurrence, and rehabilitation focuses on strengthening the rotator cuff, deltoid, and pericapsular muscles.

Anterior shoulder dislocation video

Adam's forward bend test video

Scoliosis

Buzz Words: Asymmetry of the shoulders or iliac crests + bump in the back while bending down

Clinical Presentation: Scoliosis presents as asymmetry of shoulder height, scapular position, and iliac crests. Adam's forward bend test is performed by having the child bend forward from the waist, while the examiner looks for a lower back prominence representing posterior displacement of the spine. Scoliosis is typically painless, and the presence of pain may indicate an underlying disorder that should be investigated.

MoD: Most cases are idiopathic; however, it can be caused by leg length discrepancy, neuromuscular disorders, vertebral anomalies, connective tissue disorders, or genetic syndromes.

Dx: PA and lateral XR of the spine are used to calculate the Cobb angle, which measures the angle between the superior and inferior vertebrae tilted into the curve.

Tx/Mgmt:
1. Bracing
2. Surgery

Flexible Kyphosis and Scheuermann Kyphosis

Buzz Words: Patient brought by family members concerned about "hunched back" + voluntary correction (flexible kyphosis) or stiffness (Scheuermann kyphosis)

Clinical Presentation: It is usually detected by family or friends. Flexible kyphosis is benign and can be corrected voluntarily, while Scheuermann kyphosis is structural and stiff.

Dx: Clinical for flexible scoliosis. Scheuermann disease is defined by wedging >5 degrees of three or more consecutive vertebral bodies, so standing lateral spine radiographs are necessary for the diagnosis.

Tx/Mgmt: Flexible kyphosis does not require treatment. Scheuermann kyphosis can be treated with strengthening and stretching exercises, analgesics, and avoidance of precipitance. Bracing or surgical correction is done if the pain persists or if the kyphosis is >90 degrees.

Slipped Capital Femoral Epiphysis

Buzz Words: Overweight 12-year-old + dull pain in the hip that worsens with physical activity

Clinical Presentation: Non-radiating, dull, aching pain in the hip, groin, thigh, or knee that causes an altered gait. Internal rotation, flexion, and abduction are usually decreased in the affected hip. Pain is usually increased with physical activity. Risk factors include obesity, hypothyroidism, hypopituitarism, and renal osteodystrophy. Very high-yield for the Pediatrics shelf.

Dx: AP and frogleg lateral radiographs reveal posterior displacement of the femoral epiphysis. Earliest changes include widening and irregularity of the physis, with thinning of the proximal epiphysis.

99 AR
Slipped capital femoral epiphysis radiograpbs

Tx/Mgmt: The goal is to prevent further progression of the slip and to stabilize the physis. This is done by pinning the epiphysis with a single, large screw. Osteonecrosis and chondrolysis are the two most serious complications.

Erb-Duchenne Palsy (Upper Trunk Lesion)

Buzz Words: Recently delivered infant + arm adducted, pronated, wrist flexed

Clinical Presentation: Erb palsy is a lesion of the upper trunk that can be caused by obstetrical-related brachial nerve trauma or traumatic injury as an adult. For the Surgery shelf, it is more likely you'll see this in the setting of newborns because surgical management can be more successful for refractory cases. Patient's with Erb palsy present with the "Waiter's Tip" or "Bellman's" posture. If severe enough, can be associated with T1 avulsion and Horner syndrome.

MoD: Traction on upper trunk (C5–C6) of brachial plexus 2/2 shoulder dystocia → weakness of deltoid, biceps, infrapinatus, wrist extensors.

Dx: Clinical diagnosis

Tx/Mgmt:
1. Conservative (gentle massage, physical therapy)
2. If T1 avulsion, Horner syndrome or no resolution of symptoms, neuroma excision, and interpositional nerve grafting

99 AR
Review of Nerve Transfer Indications in Obstetrical Brachial Plexus Palsy

Klumpke's Palsy (Brachial Plexus Lower Trunk Injury)

Buzz Words:
- Adult + grabbed branch during fall + atrophy of hypothenar muscles + sensory loss of pinky and lateral ring finger
- Recent delivered infant subject to upward force on arm during delivery + absent grasp reflex + claw hand

Clinical Presentation: Klumpke's palsy is a lesion of the lower trunk that can be caused by obstetrical-related brachial nerve trauma or traumatic injury as an adult. For the surgery shelf, it is more likely you'll see this in the setting of newborns because surgical management can be more successful for refractory cases. It is characterized by claw hand. If severe enough, can be associated with T1 avulsion and Horner syndrome.

MoD: Traction on lower trunk (C8–T1) of brachial plexus 2/2 shoulder dystocia→ weakness of intrinsic hand muscles: lumbricals, interossei, thenar, hypothenar, sensory loss of ulnar distribution → extended wrist + hyperextended MCP joints + fixed interphalangeal joints + absent grasp reflex

Dx: Clinical diagnosis

Tx/Mgmt:
1. Conservative (gentle massage, physical therapy)
2. If T1 avulsion, Horner syndrome or no resolution of symptoms, neuroma excision and interpositional nerve grafting

Congenital Disorders

Achondroplasia/Dwarfism

99 AR
Achondroplasia video

Buzz Words: Large head + short arms and legs

Clinical Presentation: Patient has disproportionate short stature with rhizomelic shortening of the arms and legs. Kyphoscoliosis and lumbar lordosis may be pronounced. Homozygotes have increased susceptibility to pulmonary complications and brainstem and spinal cord compression.

MoD: **Autosomal dominant** mutation in the FGFR3 gene

Dx: Clinical diagnosis

Tx/Mgmt: Goal is to maximize functional capacity and to monitor and prevent potential complications.

Developmental Dysplasia of the Hip

99 AR
Developmental Dysplasia of the Hip video

Buzz Words: Joint laxity/clicking + breech delivery + positive Barlow and Ortolani maneuvers

Clinical Presentation: It is asymptomatic in infants, careful examination will reveal hip dislocation using Ortolani and Barlow maneuvers. In infants greater than 3 months of age, the dislocation can become relatively fixed, and the Galeazzi test should be used. There is increased risk in the newborn with breech presentation, positive family history, females, and first-born children.

PPx: The typical physical examination of the newborn includes the use of Ortolani and Barlow maneuvers, this is because an earlier detection of this condition leads to a better clinical outcome.

MoD: Abnormality in stability or shape of the femoral head and acetabulum

Dx:
1. Physical examination demonstrates hip instability, asymmetry, or limited abduction.
2. Imaging may be helpful to confirm the diagnosis, ultrasound is used for infants younger than 6 months of age because the hip and pelvis are not yet ossified at that age.
3. AP radiographs may be used in infants greater than 6 months of age.

Tx/Mgmt:
1. Pavlik harness for infants younger than 6 months
2. Reduction if the diagnosis is not made until after 6 months of age
3. Monitoring with regular hip radiographs until the child is skeletally mature

Genu Valgum (Knock-Knee)/Genu Varum (Bow-Leg)

Buzz Words:
- **Physiologic varus/valgus:** Symmetric, normal stature + no thrusts with ambulation + tibiofemoral angle within two standard deviations of the mean for age
- **Pathologic varus:** Unilateral, short stature, asymmetry, lateral knee-joint protrusion (thrust) with walking + progressive bowing + <6 cm between femoral condyles with patella facing forward and medial malleoli together
- **Pathologic valgus:** Unilateral, short stature, asymmetry, medial knee-joint protrusion (thrust) with walking + >8 cm between medial malleoli with patellas facing forward and femoral condyles together + progressive deformity after age 4–5
- **Pathologic valgus:** Mucopolysaccharidosis

Clinical Presentation: Varus and valgus refer to angulation or bowing within the shaft of a bone or at a joint. Varus is the term for inward angulation of the distal segment of a bone or joint, and valgus is the term for outward angulation of the distal segment of a bone or joint. Pathologic varus: Blount disease. Pathologic valgus: Mucopolysaccharidosis.

Dx: Clinical diagnosis

Tx/Mgmt:

- **Physiologic varus/valgus:** observation and parental reassurance
- **Pathologic varus/valgus:** imaging, bracing, medical therapy for primary disease if available, then surgical therapy if refractory

Tibia Vara (Blount Disease)

Buzz Words: Overweight 3-year-old African-American girl + bowlegs + lateral thrust with gait

Clinical Presentation: Risk factors include: African-American females, being overweight, starting to walk early in life, and having an affected family member. Presents as progressive, unilateral bowing, or persistent bowing after 2 years of age.

MoD: Abnormal endochondral ossification of the medial aspect of the proximal tibial physis

Dx: Weight-bearing AP and lateral views of the lower extremities

Tx/Mgmt: Brace treatment for 1 year should be started by 3 years of age. If the deformity does not resolve with bracing, surgical therapy is required. Surgical intervention should be performed before 4 years of age to reduce the risk of recurrence. In the case of adolescent Blount disease, surgical management is the preferred treatment.

Metatarsus Adductus

Buzz Words: First-born child + C-shaped foot that can be straightened by manipulation

Clinical Presentation: Presents as medial curvature of the mid-foot that can be straightened to a certain degree. Incidence is higher in first-borns and twins. Commonly bilateral, but affects the left leg more commonly than the right in unilateral cases.

MoD: Usually caused by intrauterine constraint

Dx: Clinical diagnosis

Tx/Mgmt: Self-limited: Corrective casting is required in severe cases that cannot be passively corrected to the midline.

Talipes Equinovarus (Club Foot)

Buzz Words: Chromosomal syndrome + rigid ankle fixed in plantarflexion

Clinical Presentation: Patient has plantarflexion and inversion of the ankle with a medially curved forefoot. Usually rigid, with little range of motion and calf atrophy.

MoD: Multifactorial, but it can present as part of another syndrome such as chromosomal syndromes, myelodysplasia, and arthrogryposis.

Dx: Clinical diagnosis

Tx/Mgmt: Serial casting, surgery if necessary

Osteogenesis Imperfecta

Buzz Words: Blue sclerae + fractures with minimal trauma

Clinical Presentation: Patient presents with bone fragility, short stature, blue sclerae, scoliosis, hearing loss, teeth that wear quickly, and easy bruisability. It may be confused with child abuse.

MoD: Most commonly caused by autosomal dominant mutations in genes encoding type I collagen (COL1A1 and COL1A2). Classified into different subtypes based on the genetic, radiographic, and clinical characteristics.

Dx: Clinical diagnosis

Tx/Mgmt:
1. Activity restriction and surgical correction of misalignments
2. Biphosphonates may be given to reduce the risk of fractures

Muscular Dystrophy (Duchenne and Becker)

Muscular dystrophy video

Buzz Words: Four-year-old boy + enlarged calves + trouble catching up with his friends + family history of a muscular disease

Clinical Presentation: Patient presents with slow, progressive weakness of the proximal muscles, which may present with Gower sign. **Duchenne muscular dystrophy has an earlier onset and is more severe than Becker muscular dystrophy** (BMD). Patients with DMD lose the ability to walk by 10 years of age, while patients with BMD are usually able to walk until they are 20 years old. Patients also present with pseudohypertrophy of the calves, caused by replacement of muscular tissue with lipids.

MoD: X-linked disorder caused by mutation of the dystrophin gene.

Dx:
1. Elevated CK levels
2. EMG with small muscle potential with normal nerve conduction
3. DNA testing reveals gene deletion
4. Western blot (decreased dystrophin)

5. Muscle biopsy to confirm the diagnosis if the genetic studies are negative

Tx/Mgmt:

1. Oral steroids can improve muscle strength in the early stages
2. Physical therapy and respiratory support when needed

McArdle Disease (Glycogen Storage Disease V or GSD V)

Buzz Words: Myoglobinuria with exercise + muscle biopsy with biochemical testing showing myophosphorylase deficiency + periodic acid-Schiff stain showing increased glycogen

Clinical Presentation: McArdle disease is an autosomal recessive disease caused by mutations in the muscle phosphorylase on chromosome 11, and presents with exercise intolerance, fatigue, myalgia, cramps, myoglobinuria, poor endurance, muscle swelling, and fixed weakness. On the shelf, be able to distinguish this from rhabdomyolysis, weakness, and other causes of fatigue. Can also present with arrhythmia from electrolyte abnormalities.

MoD: Autosomal recessive deficiency of skeletal muscle glycogen phosphorylase (myophosphorylase) → increased glycogen in muscle, unable to be broken down

Dx:

1. Non-ischemic forearm exercise test
2. Muscle biopsy, periodic acid-Schiff (PAS) stain
3. Genetic testing

Tx/Mgmt:

1. Carbohydrate-rich diet
2. Ingestion of sucrose 5 minutes before aerobic exercise, warm-up, and moderation in physical activity

Mitochondrial Myopathies

Buzz Words:

- **Isolated myopathy**: exercise intolerance, fatigue, weakness
- Chronic progressive external ophthalmoplegia (CPEO): gradual EOM paresis, bilateral ptosis

Most common syndromes are:

- **Leigh syndrome (subacute necrotizing encephalomyelopathy):** developmental delay, ataxia, dystonia, external ophthalmoplegia, seizures, lactic acidosis, vomiting, weakness
- **MELAS (mitochondrial encephalomyopathy with lactic acidosis and stroke-like episodes):** Hallmark of this syndrome is stroke-like episodes that cause hemiparesis, hemianopia, cortical blindness

- Other features include seizures, headaches, vomiting, short stature, hearing loss, muscle weakness

Clinical Presentation: Mitochondrial myopathies are rare and variable diseases that typically present with a constellation of symptoms from various organ systems. The shelf likely will not test these directly, but rather a specific mitochondrial myopathy may appear as an answer choice for a clinical scenario relating to fatigue, or weakness. Common mitochondrial myopathies can be ruled out in the absence of multisystem disease.

MoD: Mitochondrial DNA mutations

Dx:
1. Muscle biopsy
2. Genetic testing

Tx/Mgmt:
1. Supportive
2. Supplementation with coenzyme Q10, creatine, and L-carnitine

Adverse Effects of Drugs on the Musculoskeletal System

Drug-induced Myopathy

Buzz Words: Steroids, statins, cocaine, AZT, antimalarials (chloroquine), colchicine, ipecac, chemo, interferon, antipsychotics associated with NMS

Clinical Presentation: Above are the drugs that can cause myopathy. Just be familiar with these to rule out answer choices. No need to memorize as you need to for step 1.

PPx: Avoid drugs that induce myopathy

MoD: Varied, including direct myotoxicity, immunologically induced, indirect muscle damage

Dx: CK elevation, severe myopathy will show rhabdomyolysis

Tx/Mgmt: Stop offending agent

Malignant Hyperthermia

Buzz Words: Within 1 hour of anesthesia induction → onset of hypercapnia, tachycardia, **muscle rigidity**, rhabdomyolysis, arrhythmia, high temperature

Clinical Presentation: Malignant hyperthermia is an adverse reaction to succinylcholine, which is given during anesthesia.

MoD: Susceptibility is inherited as autosomal dominant with variable penetrance. Mutations in voltage-sensitive ryanodine receptor cause increase calcium release from sarcoplasmic reticulum.

Dx: Clinical presentation

99 AR

Malignant hyperthermia guidelines

Tx/Mgmt:

1. Discontinue inhaled anesthetic, switch to propofol if surgery cannot be halted
2. Dantrolene (ryanodine receptor antagonist)
3. Add charcoal filters to anesthesia breathing circuit
4. 100% FiO_2
5. Assess for cardiac dysrhythmias
6. Supportive care in the intensive care unit for more than 24 hours

GUNNER PRACTICE

1. A 75-year-old nursing home resident presents to the emergency department with altered mental status. She has baseline dementia but has been increasingly confused according to staff. She is unable to provide any history in the emergency department. While obtaining a urine sample via straight cath, a nurse notices an erythematous, fluctuant area just inferior to the left labia majora. The area is surgically explored. Upon incision, "dirty dishwater" fluid is released and the tissue is debrided. Which of the following is the most likely diagnosis?
   A. Bartholin cyst
   B. *N. gonorrhea*
   C. *C. trachomatis*
   D. Fournier's gangrene
   E. Lichen planus
   F. Lichen sclerosis

2. A 31-year-old male with history of sickle cell anemia presents with left knee pain and swelling for 2 days. The pain is worse with movement and is associated with some redness as well. The patient has tried acetaminophen with only some relief. On exam, temperature is 38.5°C, pulse 103/min, respiratory rate 16/min, and blood pressure 145/87. The joint space is palpated and sterilely aspirated. What microbe is most likely to be isolated?
   A. *C. jejuni*
   B. *Escherichia coli*
   C. *Klebseilla pneumoniae*
   D. *Listeria monocytogenes*
   E. *Legionella pneumophilia*
   F. *P. aeruginosa*
   G. *Proteus vulgaris*
   H. *Salmonella enterica*
   I. *Shigella dysenteriae*

3. A 15-year-old male presents with right arm pain for 3 months that is preventing him from completing his schoolwork and playing football. His pediatrician orders an XR, which reveals an "onion-skin" lesion on the diaphysis. Which of the following is most likely?
   A. Chondrosarcoma
   B. Giant cell tumor
   C. Osteosarcoma
   D. Ewing sarcoma
   E. Metastatic lesion

ANSWERS: What Would Gunner Jess/Jim Do?

1. WWGJD? A 75-year-old nursing home resident presents to the emergency department with altered mental status. She has baseline dementia but has been increasingly confused according to staff. She is unable to provide any history in the emergency department. While obtaining a urine sample via straight cath, a nurse notices an erythematous, fluctuant area just inferior to the left labia majora. The area is surgically explored. Upon incision, "dirty dishwater" fluid is released and the tissue is debrided. Which of the following is the most likely diagnosis?

Answer: D, Fournier's gangrene

The term "dirty dishwater" is a Buzz Word for necrotizing fasciitis or gangrene. The fluid is a combination of intravascular fluid that enters the interstitium and products of metabolism by the anaerobic bacteria infecting the area. Fournier's gangrene is necrotizing fasciitis in the perineum and is associated with poor hygiene and may be due to elderly neglect.

A. Bartholin cyst → Incorrect. This is more common in young, sexually active women and would be intravaginal, not inferior to the labia.

B. *N. gonorrhea* → Incorrect. This is more common in young, sexually active women and would be intravaginal, not inferior to the labia.

C. *C. trachomatis* → Incorrect. This is more common in young, sexually active women and would be intravaginal, not inferior to the labia.

E. Lichen planus → Incorrect. This is an inflammatory skin disorder that would not cause "dirty dishwater" fluid.

F. Lichen sclerosis → Incorrect. This is an inflammatory skin disorder that would not cause "dirty dishwater" fluid.

2. WWGJD? A 31-year-old male with history of sickle cell anemia presents with left knee pain and swelling for 2 days. The pain is worse with movement and is associated with some redness as well. The patient has tried acetaminophen with only some relief. On exam, temperature is 38.5°C, pulse 103/min, respiratory rate 16/min, and blood pressure 145/87. The joint space is palpated and sterilely aspirated. What microbe is most likely to be isolated?

Answer: H, *Salmonella enterica*

There is a strange association between sickle cell anemia and *Salmonella* joint infections. The most likely joint infections in this population are still Gram-positive cocci including MSSA and MRSA. However, neither of those were choices. Of the Gram-negative rods listed, *Salmonella enterica* is the one associated with sickle cell anemia.

A. *C. jejuni* → Incorrect.

B. *Escherichia coli* → Incorrect.

C. *Klebseilla pneumoniae* → Incorrect.

D. *Listeria monocytogenes* → Incorrect.

E. *Legionella pneumophilia* → Incorrect.

F. *Pseudomonas aeruginosa* → Incorrect.

G. *Proteus vulgaris* → Incorrect.

H. *Shigella dysenteriae* → Incorrect.

3. WWGJD?: A 15-year-old male presents with right arm pain for 3 months that is preventing him from completing his schoolwork and playing football. His pediatrician orders an XR, which reveals an **"onion-skin"** lesion. Which of the following is most likely?

Answer D, Ewing sarcoma

Knowing Buzz Words for the shelf exam is very helpful. Sometimes the question only gives you one Buzz Word; for example, "onion-skin," and you have to pick the associated disease. The tumor associated with "onion-skin" appearance on XR is Ewing sarcoma.

A. Chondrosarcoma → Incorrect. Chondrosarcomas are rarely found at the diaphysis because cartilage is usually only present near the epiphysis and metaphysis.

B. Giant cell tumor → Incorrect. Giant cell tumors have a "soap-bubble" appearance.

C. Osteosarcoma → Incorrect. Osteosarcoma has a "sunburst" appearance.

E. Metastatic lesion → Incorrect. Metastatic tumors can be osteolytic or osteoblastic but are not associated with an "onion-skin" appearance and would be very uncommon in a 15-year-old male.

Endocrine and Metabolic Disorders

Jonathan Hunt, Hao-Hua Wu, Leo Wang, Rebecca Gao, and Sean Harbison

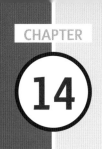

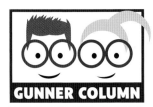

GUNNER COLUMN

Introduction

Endocrine organs assess environmental inputs and secrete hormonal outputs into the circulatory system to regulate growth, metabolism, and sexual development and function. Endocrine disorders represent a disruption of these normal processes. They are not the most heavily tested material on the shelf exam, but will surely factor into 5–10 questions with an emphasis on recognition and work-up. As a result, the highest yield material from this section includes being able to identify unique Buzz Words (e.g., necrolytic migratory erythema in glucagonoma, or a tender goiter in Dequervain's thyroiditis) in the context of multiple normal and abnormal hormone concentrations, which you will need to be able to confidently interpret. Since a sturdy understanding of pathophysiology of each disease is essential to properly interpret these combinations of hormonal variations, this section spends a lot of time addressing the mechanism of each disease, and how it ties into the clinical presentation. For the most part, work-up comes secondary to understanding the disease process, but it is extremely high-yield to commit to memory the work-up algorithms for common nebulous findings (e.g., thyroid nodules, adrenal incidentaloma, pituitary adenoma). Although understanding the mechanisms of every endocrine disease process may sound daunting, mechanism is less heavily emphasized on the Surgery shelf than on USMLE Step 1.

To provide a framework for study, the disorders are grouped by organ system as endocrine gland hyposecretion disorders, endocrine gland hypersecretion disorders, and endocrine gland neoplasms. Once you understand how each endocrine disorder ties into its category, the Buzz Words should then help you distinguish it from other disorders within the same category. As you read through the disorders of the endocrine pancreas, the thyroid and parathyroids, the hypothalamic-pituitary-adrenal axis, and the congenital syndromes, make sure to revisit basic physiology. This will provide context to the clinical picture, work-up, and management of the disorder in isolation, and in the setting of surgery both as the target of therapy and as a complicating factor.

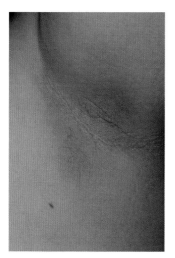

FIG. 14.1 Acanthosis nigricans are velvety, hyperpigmented plaques found on the neck and axilla, associated with a 2× risk of type 2 diabetes as compared to unaffected individuals. (From Wikimedia Commons: https://commons.wikimedia.org/wiki/File:Acanthosis-nigricans4.jpg. Used under Creative Commons Attribution-Share Alike 3.0 Unported license: https://creativecommons.org/licenses/by-sa/3.0/deed.en.)

Diabetes Mellitus and Other Disorders of the Endocrine Pancreas

Diabetes Mellitus

Type 2 Diabetes Mellitus

Buzz Words: Obese pt >40 years old + family hx + recent weight loss + polyuria + polydipsia + fatigue + acanthosis nigricans (see Fig. 14.1) + signs of underlying disease (Table 14.1)

PPx: Lifestyle modification (diet, exercise, stop smoking)

MoD: Peripheral insulin resistance → Increased pancreatic insulin synthesis → Progressive pancreatic β-cell failure 2/2 IAPP (amylin) deposition

Dx:
- Sx of hyperglycemia + random plasma glucose greater than 200 mg/dL
- Two separate fasting plasma glucose greater than 126 mg/dL
- Two separate 2-hour post-oral glucose challenges greater than 200 mg/dL

Two separate HbA1C greater than 6.5%

Tx/Mgmt:
- Pre-op, d/c oral hypoglycemic agents and take ½ morning dose of insulin on day of surgery
- Peri/post-op strict glycemic control (see Table 14.1)

99 AR

Type 1 vs. type 2 diabetes mellitus

TABLE 14.1 Acute and Chronic Complication of Diabetes Mellitus

Complication	Acute or Chronic	Buzz Words	MoD	PPx	Dx	Tx/Mgmt
Diabetic coma (HHNS)	Acute	Elderly DM2 with limited ability to drink	Hyperglycemia → osmotic diuresis → dehydration	(1) Glycemic control, (2) hydration	(1) Hyperglycemia, (2) hyperosmolarity, (3) pH WNL	(1) Absolute CI to surgery, (2) rehydrate w/ IV fluids + insulin
Diabetic ketoacidosis	Acute	DM1 with insulin noncompliance or stress (infection) + Fruity breath + DKA: Delirium/Dehydration + Kussmaul breathing + Abdominal pain (N/V)	Unmet insulin demand → hyperglycemia (osmotic diuresis) + ketogenesis (metabolic acidosis) → elevated serum K+ in setting of lower total K+	Glycemic control	(1) Hyperglycemia, (2) Anion gap metabolic acidosis, (3) Ketonuria	(1) Absolute CI to surgery, (2) IV fluids (with dextrose) + insulin gtt + supplement potassium, (3) follow anion gap
Hypoglycemic shock	Acute	Sympathetic (diaphoresis, tachycardia) + CNS (diplopia, cognitive impairment, seizure, coma) + vasomotor (syncope)	Refer to Table 14.2	Address underlying cause	Measure plasma glucose, insulin, C-peptide, proinsulin, β-hydroxybutyrate, and oral hypoglycemic agents	(1) PO glucose; (2) if unconscious, IV dextrose; (3) If unconscious and no IV access, SubQ/IM glucagon; (4) address underlying cause
Cerebral edema	Acute	DKA + CNS changes during treatment (altered mental status, headache)	DKA → ischemia (cytotoxic edema), increased BBB permeability (vasogenic edema), fluid therapy (osmotic edema) → cerebral edema	Avoid DKA	Altered mental status in setting of DKA treatment	(1) Reduce rate of IV fluid administration, (2) mannitol

CNS, Central nervous system; *IM*, intramuscular; *IV*, intravenous.

Complication	Acute or Chronic	Notes
Accelerated atherosclerosis	Chronic	False ABIs (due to calcification of arterial wall); Increased p(CAD, PVD, stroke) → Tx w/ risk factor reduction
Autonomic dysfunction	Chronic	Gastroparesis (early satiety + N/V → evaluated with upper endoscopy to r/o obstruction → confirm diagnosis with gastric emptying study → Tx w/ metoclopramide); impotence; masks abdominal pain and MI; neurogenic bladder
Diabetic foot	Chronic	Neuropathy → ulcers at pressure points (heel, metatarsal head, and tips of toes) that fail to heal → Tx w/ wound cleaning, elevation, and amputation if worsens; prevent with regular foot exams by podiatrist
Infections	Chronic	Fournier's gangrene—def. perineal infection of diabetic perinea → Tx w/ triple antibiotics + wide debridement; increased p(infection: mucormycosis, pseudomonas malignant otitis externa, sepsis, UTIs)
Nephropathy	Chronic	Arteriosclerosis in efferent tubules → increased GFR in glomeruli → nodular glomerular sclerosis (Kimmelstiel-Wilson nodules) → progressive proteinuria → CRF (slow progression with ACE-inhibitor); MCC kidney transplant; Renal papillary necrosis with NSAIDs or sickle cell disease
Ocular complications	Chronic	Retinopathy (non-proliferative – microaneurysms → flame hemorrhage, hard exudate, and macular edema; proliferative—def. retinal neovascularization → Tx w/ retinal photocoagulation, surgery, and anti-VEGF Bevacizumab); cataracts; glaucoma; blindness; prevent with regular ophthalmology exams (newly diagnosed DM2 need immediate ophthalmologic evaluation)
Oculomotor neuropathy	Chronic	Deep fibers of CN3 affected while superficial fibers spared → CN3 palsy sparing the pupil
Peripheral neuropathy	Chronic	Paresthesias; decreased DTRs; decreased DCML sensation; Tx w/ duloxetine (SNRI), NSAIDs, and gabapentin
Wound healing impairment	Chronic	—

TABLE 14.2 Causes of Hypoglycemia in Adults

Ill or Medicated Individual

1. Drugs
Insulin or insulin secretagogue
Alcohol
Others (refer to UpToDate table on drugs that cause
   hypoglycemia)

2. Critical illnesses
Hepatic, renal, or cardiac failure
Sepsis (including malaria)
Inanition

3. Hormone deficiency
Cortisol
Glucagon and epinephrine (in insulin-deficient diabetes
   mellitus)

4. Nonislet cell tumor

Seemingly Well Individual

5. Endogenous hyperinsulinism
Insulinoma
Functional beta cell disorders (nesidioblastosis)
   Noninsulinoma pancreatogenous hypoglycemia
   Post gastric bypass hypoglycemia
Insulin autoimmune hypoglycemia
   Antibody to insulin
   Antibody to insulin receptor
Insulin secretagogue
Other

6. Accidental, surreptitious, or malicious hypoglycemia

Reproduced with permission from: Cryer PE, Axelrod L, Grossman AB, et al.
Evaluation and management of adult hypoglycemic disorders: an Endocrine
Society Clinical Practice Guideline. *J Clin Endocrinol Metab.* 2009;94:709.
Copyright © 2009 The Endocrine Society.

Islet Cell Disorders—Hypoglycemia

Insulinoma

Buzz Words: Whipple's triad = hypoglycemia + central nervous
system (CNS) and sympathetic/vasomotor symptoms
(syncope, diaphoresis, cognitive impairment, seizure,
coma) + relief of symptoms after glucose administration

Clinical Presentation: Patient is 50 years old with MEN1 family
hx (6%).

MoD: Pancreatic β-islet cell (Fig. 14.2) neoplasm → Secretes
insulin

Dx:

1. Elevated serum insulin and C-peptide levels (Fig. 14.3)
   despite fast (as opposed to surreptitious insulin use)
2. Fasting insulin-to-glucose ratio >0.4
3. Triphasic computed tomography (CT) scan to localize

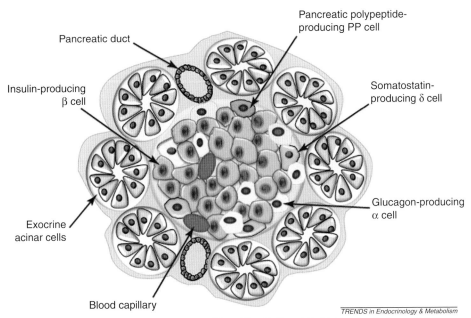

FIG. 14.2 Anatomy of the islets of Langerhans. (From Efrat S, Russ HA: Making β cells from adult tissues. *Trends Endocrinol Metab* 23[6]:278–285, 2012.)

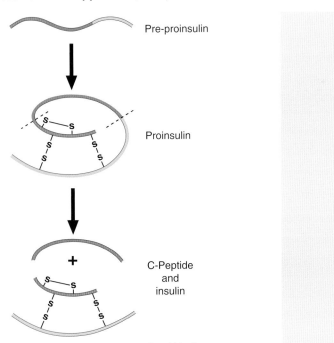

FIG. 14.3 C-peptide is cleaved from proinsulin within the secretory vesicle, which allows physicians to determine whether or not an elevated insulin level is due to endogenous hypersecretion or exogenous administration. (From Gaw A, Murphy MJ, Cowan RA, O'Reilly DStJ, Stewart MJ, Shepherd J, eds: *Clinical biochemistry: an illustrated colour text*, ed 5. London, 2013, Elsevier.)

Tx/Mgmt:
1. Surgical resection
2. If unresectable, diazoxide (suppresses insulin secretion)
3. If refractory to diazoxide, octreotide

Nesidioblastosis

Buzz Words: Infant with macrosomia + hypoketotic hypoglycemia within first few hours of life

Clinical Presentation: Isolated population presents with consanguinity or founder effect (e.g., Saudi Arabia, central Finland).

MoD: AR inactivating mutation of ATP-sensitive potassium channels in pancreatic β-islet cells → Persistent depolarization of β-islet cells → Constant hypersecretion of insulin

Dx: Elevated serum insulin and C-peptide levels despite fast

Tx/Mgmt: Near-total (95%) pancreatectomy

Other Causes of Hypoglycemia

Dx: Adrenal insufficiency (elevated plasma ACTH), liver failure (elevated LFTs), sepsis (fever), surreptitious insulin use (elevated serum insulin level, low C-peptide level), surreptitious sulfonylurea use (elevated serum insulin and C-peptide levels).

Islet Cell Disorders—Hyperglycemia

Glucagonoma

Buzz Words: Mild diabetes with weight loss + necrolytic migratory erythema (Fig. 14.4) + chronic diarrhea + neuropsychiatric symptoms (e.g., depression)

Clinical Presentation: Patient is 50 years old with MEN1 family hx (20%).

MoD: Pancreatic α-islet cell neoplasm → Secretes glucagon → Hyperglycemia + increased catabolic consumptive processes (→ normochromic normocytic anemia, hypoaminoacidemia, and decreased levels of antithrombin III[1] causing venous thrombosis)

Dx:
1. Elevated serum glucagon levels
2. Triphasic CT scan to localize

Tx/Mgmt:
1. If tumor is localizable, surgical resection
2. If unresectable, octreotide (somatostatin analogue) + intravenous (IV) amino and fatty acid infusions

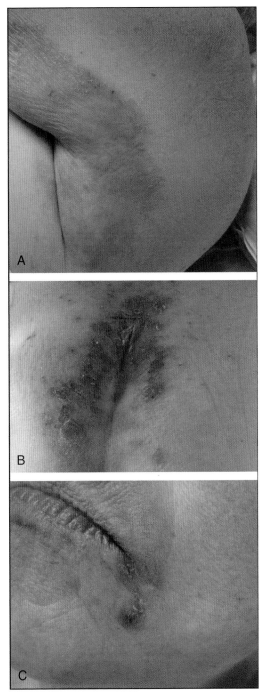

FIG. 14.4 Necrolytic migratory erythema is an inflammatory dermatosis, classically characterized as a blistering red rash involving the face, perineum, and extremities. Associated signs include glossitis, angular cheilitis, and stomatitis. A physical examination of this patient revealed widespread, circumscribed, bilateral, and symmetric erythematous eroded plaques with scale. (A) Lesions were located primarily in the axilla. (B) Her trunk, groin, and gluteal cleft were affected, as were her upper legs. (C) Erythematous scaly plaques were also noted in continuity with the oral labial commissures, consistent with angular cheilitis. (From Compton NL, Chien AJ: A rare but revealing sign: necrolytic migratory erythema. *Am J Med* 126[5]:387–389, 2013.)

Somatostatinoma

Buzz Words: Diabetes + gallstones + steatorrhea

Clinical Presentation: Patient is 50 years old with MEN1 family hx (45%) or NF-1.

MoD: Pancreatic δ-islet cell neoplasm → Secretes somatostatin → Inhibits gastrointestinal (GI) hormones (cholecystokinin → cholelithiasis, gastrin → hypochlorhydria, insulin → diabetes, secretin → steatorrhea)

Dx:
1. Elevated serum somatostatin level
2. Triphasic CT scan to localize

Tx/Mgmt:
1. If tumor is localizable, surgical resection
2. If unresectable, chemotherapy (for cure) and octreotide (for symptomatic relief)

Islet Cell Disorders—Non-Glycemic

Gastrinoma (Zollinger-Ellison Syndrome)

Buzz Words: Refractory/recurrent peptic ulcer disease extending beyond first portion of duodenum + watery diarrhea + MEN-1 symptoms in 25% (hypercalcemia, hypophosphatemia)

Clinical Presentation: Males 20 to 50 years old with MEN1 family hx (25%)

MoD: Pancreatic or duodenal G-cell neoplasm → Secretes gastrin → High gastric acid output → Excess acid causes: recurrent ulcers in duodenum and jejunum, low pH inactivates pancreatic enzymes → Steatorrhea and malabsorption → Weight loss, low pH causes bile salts to precipitate out → Osmotic diarrhea → Abdominal pain

Dx:
1. Upper endoscopy to evaluate ulcers
2. Elevated fasting serum gastrin level
3. If equivocal, secretin stimulation test (secretin inhibits gastrin secretion from normal G-cells, but stimulates gastrin secretion from gastrinoma cells)
4. Triphasic CT scan to localize

Tx/Mgmt:
1. If tumor is localizable, surgical resection
2. If non-localizable, exploratory surgery and proximal gastric vagotomy if not found
3. If metastatic (liver) or not surgical candidate, omeprazole (PPI) + octreotide (Fig. 14.5)

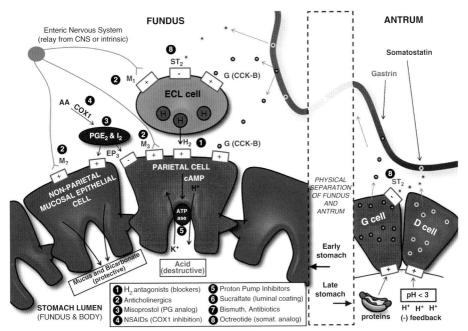

FIG. 14.5 Regulation of parietal cell acid secretion. *cAMP*, Cyclic adenosine monophosphate; *CNS*, central nervous system; *NSAID*, nonsteroidal anti-inflammatory drug. (From Wikimedia Commons: https://commons.wikimedia.org/wiki/File:Determinants_of_Gastric_Acid_Secretion.svg. Created by Adam L. VanWert, PharmD, PhD. Used under Creative Commons Attribution 3.0 Unported license. https://creativecommons.org/licenses/by/3.0/deed.en.)

Vasoactive Intestinal Polypeptide Tumor (VIPoma, Watery Diarrhea, Hypokalemia, and Achlorhydria Syndrome, Pancreatic Cholera)

Buzz Words: Watery diarrhea despite fasting + hypokalemia + achlorhydria

Clinical Presentation: Patient is 2 to 4 years old or 30–50 years old with MEN1 family hx (5%) and have metastasized by time of diagnosis (70%).

MoD: Pancreatic islet cell neoplasm → VIP activates adenylate cyclase to increase cAMP → Net fluid/electrolyte secretion into GI lumen (secretory diarrhea, hypokalemia) + vasodilation (facial flushing) + inhibition of gastric acid secretion (achlorhydria)

Dx:
1. Elevated serum VIP level
2. Triphasic CT scan to localize

Tx/Mgmt:
1. Fluid resuscitation and electrolyte repletion
2. If tumor is localizable, surgical resection
3. If unresectable, octreotide
4. If refractory to somatostatin analogs, glucocorticoids

99 AR

Mechanism for increase of gastrin release by secretin in Zollinger-Ellison syndrome

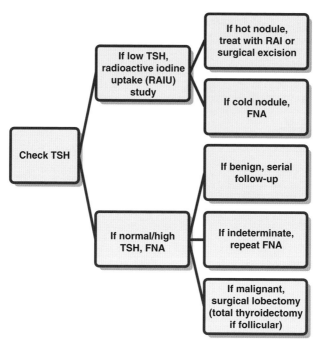

FIG. 14.6 Algorithm for workup of a thyroid nodule. *FNA*, Fine-needle aspiration; *TSH*, thyroid-stimulating hormone.

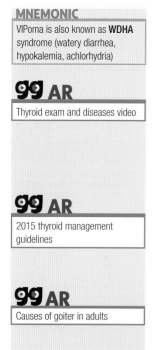

MNEMONIC

VIPoma is also known as **WDHA** syndrome (watery diarrhea, hypokalemia, achlorhydria)

99 AR
Thyroid exam and diseases video

99 AR
2015 thyroid management guidelines

99 AR
Causes of goiter in adults

Thyroid and Parathyroid Disorders

Thyroid—Structural

Thyroid Nodule Workup

Goiter

Buzz Words: Enlarged thyroid ± thyroid dysfunction ± obstructive sx (exertional dyspnea, obstructive sleep apnea, hoarseness, dysphagia, Horner syndrome (Fig. 14.6)

PPx: Adequate iodine intake (for goiters 2/2 iodine deficiency)

MoD: High thyroid-stimulating hormone (TSH) or TSH-like stimulation of thyroid (2/2 to iodine deficiency, thyroiditis, or autoimmune etiologies) → Diffuse goiter

Dx: See Fig. 14.7 for workup algorithm

Tx/Mgmt:

- If nodular goiter, fine-needle aspiration (FNA) and surgically excise if indicated
- If diffuse goiter with cosmetic deformity or compressive symptoms, surgically excise

Thyroid—Endocrine (Hypo)

Hypothyroidism

Buzz Words: Slowing down (hyporeflexia, bradycardia, dyspnea on exertion, constipation, weight gain, fatigue)

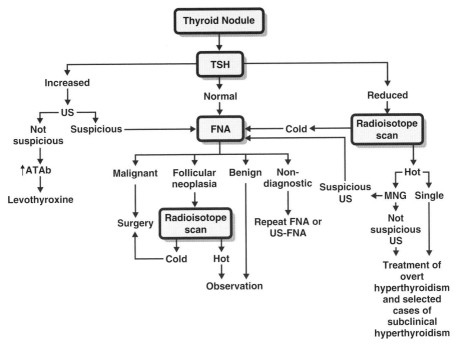

FIG. 14.7 Algorithm for workup of goiter. *FNA*, Fine-needle aspiration; *TSH*, thyroid-stimulating hormone. (From Dominguez LJ, Bevilacqua M, Dibella G, Barbagallo M: Diagnosing and managing thyroid disease in the nursing home. *J Am Med Dir Assoc* 9[1]:9–17, 2008.)

+ percussion myoedema (increased CK) + periorbital myxedema + brittle hair + cold intolerance

Clinical Presentation: Women who have small body size at birth and during childhood.

MoD: Insufficient T3/T4 → Decreased β1 receptors (bradycardia, DOE), decreased Na$^+$/K$^+$-ATPase activity (cold intolerance, weight gain, fatigue, hyporeflexia, constipation), decreased LDL receptors (hypercholesterolemia)

Dx:
1. Elevated TSH
2. Subclinical hypothyroidism if TSH elevated but serum free T3/T4 not low

Tx/Mgmt:
1. Lifelong levothyroxine (T4)
2. If compressive sx from goiter, thyroidectomy

Hashimoto's Thyroiditis

Buzz Words: Female 30–50 years old with hx of autoimmune disorders + hypothyroidism sx + non-tender goiter + association with non-Hodgkin lymphoma

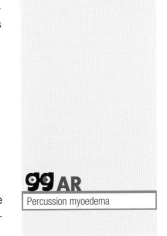

Percussion myoedema

Clinical Presentation: Women (7:1) who have history of autoimmune disorders and children.

MoD: Autoimmune lymphocytic infiltration of thyroid gland with germinal centers

Dx:

1. Elevated TSH
2. Confirm diagnosis with antithyroglobulin (anti-TG) and antimicrosomal (anti-TPO) antibodies

Tx/Mgmt: Same as hypothyroidism Tx/Mgmt

Euthyroid Sick Syndrome

Buzz Words: Critically ill patient (cancer, MI, CHF, CRF, sepsis) + low TSH + low T3/T4

Clinical Presentation: Intensive care unit (ICU) patient who has no PMH of thyroid illness.

MoD: Critically ill state → Elevated endogenous serum cortisol → Inhibits 5'-monodeiodinase, stimulates 5-monodeiodinase → Decreased conversion of T4 to T3, increased conversion of T4 to reverse T3 (Fig. 14.8)

Dx: Low TSH and serum free T3/T4 levels with elevated reverse T3 level

Tx/Mgmt:

1. Retest full thyroid panel after resolution of illness
2. If clinical evidence of hypothyroidism in critically ill pts (myxedema coma) → Levothyroxine

Thyroid—Endocrine (Hyper)

Hyperthyroidism

Buzz Words: Speeding up (hyperreflexia, tachycardia and atrial fibrillation/flutter, diarrhea, weight loss despite increased appetite, hyperactivity, tremor) + fine hair + heat intolerance

99 AR

More testable causes of hypothyroidism

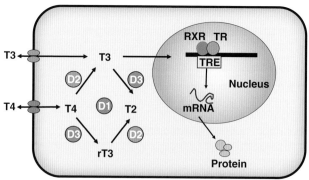

FIG. 14.8 Thyroid hormone conversion pathways. (From Gurnell M, Visser TJ, Beck-Peccoz P, Chatterjee VK: Resistance to thyroid hormone. In Jameson JL, ed: *Endocrinology: adult and pediatric* ed 7, Philadelphia, 2016, Elsevier.)

Clinical Presentation: Older women (5:1) who have smoking history.

MoD: Excessive T3/T4 → Increased β1 receptors (tachycardia, arrhythmias), increased Na^+/K^+-ATPase activity (heat intolerance, weight loss, hyperactivity, tremor, hyperreflexia, diarrhea), increased LDL receptors (hypocholesterolemia)

Dx:

1. Low TSH
2. Subclinical hyperthyroidism if TSH low but serum free T3/T4 not elevated

Tx/Mgmt:

1. β-blocker and Saturated Solution of Potassium Iodide (SSKI; Wolff-Chaikoff effect) as bridge to long-term therapy.
2. Radioiodine therapy or surgical resection, followed by lifelong levothyroxine (preferred if unable to tolerate thionamides).
3. Medical management (Fig. 14.9) prefers methimazole (inhibits TPO, more rapid action with less side effects) over PTU (inhibits TPO and 5′-deiodinase), except in the first trimester of pregnancy where methimazole can cause aplasia cutis.

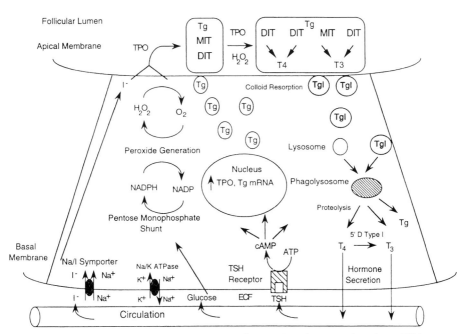

FIG. 14.9 Thyroid hormone synthesis pathway. *cAMP*, Cyclic adenosine monophosphate; *TSH*, thyroid-stimulating hormone. (From Brent G: Thyroid hormones [T4, T3]. In: Conn PM, Melmed S, eds: *Endocrinology: basic and clinical principles*, Totowa, NJ, 1997, Humana Press.)

Graves Disease

Buzz Words: MCC hyperthyroidism + stressed out (e.g., pregnant) female with autoimmune hx + diffuse goiter + exophthalmos + pretibial myxedema

Clinical Presentation: Younger women who have history of autoimmune disorders.

MoD: Anti-TSH receptor IgG antibodies (type II hypersensitivity) → Stimulate TSH receptors on follicular cells of thyroid (goiter, hyperthyroidism) and on dermal fibroblasts → Increased fibroblast secretion of GAGs in shins (pretibial myxedema) and in retro-orbital space (exophthalmos)

Dx:

1. Low TSH and elevated serum free T3/T4
2. Anti-TSH receptor antibodies
3. Diffuse radioactive iodine uptake (Fig. 14.10)

Tx/Mgmt: Same as hyperthyroidism Tx/Mgmt. Surgical resection via bilateral subtotal thyroidectomy.

Thyroid Storm

Buzz Words: Hyperthyroid pt + acute stress (infection, trauma, surgery, pregnancy) + tachyarrhythmia + hyperpyrexia + altered mental status (delirium, coma)

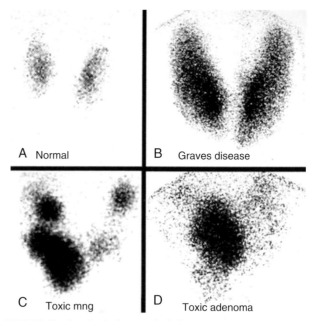

A Normal   B Graves disease

C Toxic mng   D Toxic adenoma

FIG. 14.10 Radioactive iodine uptake in hyperthyroidism. (From Medscape, http://img.medscapestatic.com/pi/meds/ckb/67/30867tn.jpg.)

PPx: Proper recognition and treatment of hyperthyroid condition

MoD: Hyperthyroid state sets context of increased responsiveness to catecholamines → Acute stress introduces catecholamine overload → Overstimulation of β1 receptors (tachyarrhythmia), Na⁺/K⁺-ATPase channels (hyperpyrexia/altered mental status, N/V, diarrhea)

Dx: Clinical diagnosis of life-threatening sx in setting of low TSH and elevated serum free T3/T4

Tx/Mgmt:

1. β-Blocker (propanolol) to control heart rate
2. PTU + SSKI to inhibit thyroid synthesis and release
3. Steroids to inhibit peripheral conversion of T4 to T3
4. Cooling blanket to address hyperpyrexia
5. Radioactive iodine therapy as preferred long-term therapy to prevent recurrence

Thyroid—Neoplasm

Papillary Carcinoma (MC)

Buzz Words: Female who is 30 to 40 years old + hx of childhood head/neck radiation + palpable lymph nodes

PPx: Avoid childhood head/neck radiation

MoD: Increased risk with activation mutations of RET and BRAF, lymphatic spread (slow) to lymph nodes and lungs

Dx: Refer to Fig. 14.6 for workup of thyroid nodule. Histology includes psammoma bodies (concentric lamellated calcifications), "Orphan Annie" eye nuclei (nuclei with central clearing), and papillary finger-like organization (Fig. 14.11).

Thyroid storm 5-minute lecture

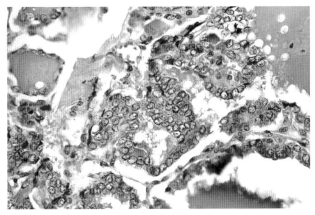

FIG. 14.11 Histology of papillary thyroid carcinoma. (From Maitra A: The endocrine system. In Kumar V, ed: *Robbins and Cotran pathologic basis of disease*, ed 9, Philadelphia, 2015, Elsevier.)

Tx/Mgmt:
1. Pre-op ultrasound (US) evaluation of central and lateral lymph nodes
2. If less than 1.5 cm and no neck radiation hx, unilateral lobectomy with isthmusectomy; else, total thyroidectomy
3. If central or lateral lymph nodes palpable or suspicious under US, central or ipsilateral neck dissection respectively indicated
4. Postoperative levothyroxine (replace normal hormone and suppress tumor regrowth) and radioactive iodine (for patients with intermediate or high risk of recurrence)

Follicular Carcinoma

Buzz Words: Female who is 40 to 60 years old + distal metastases (bone/lung)
MoD: Increased risk with RAS oncogene mutation, hematogenous spread to bones (lytic) and lungs
Dx: Refer to Fig. 14.6 for workup of thyroid nodule. **Since FNA cannot distinguish follicular carcinoma from follicular adenoma, diagnostic surgery is indicated.**
Tx/Mgmt:
1. Total thyroidectomy
2. Postoperative radioactive iodine for ablation of any remaining functional tissue
3. Postoperative levothyroxine (replace normal hormone and suppress tumor regrowth)

Medullary Carcinoma

Buzz Words: Hypocalcemia + family hx (of medullary carcinoma, MEN 2A, or MEN 2B; 10%) + MEN IIA or IIB sx (pheochromocytoma, hyperparathyroidism)
PPx: Avoid childhood head/neck radiation
MoD: Increased risk with autosomal dominant activation mutation of RET proto-oncogene → Neuroendocrine tumor of calcitonin-secreting parafollicular C cells → Elevated calcitonin levels may produce hypocalcemia and deposit as amyloid stroma (Fig. 14.12).
Dx: Refer to Fig. 14.6 for workup of thyroid nodule. Histology includes sheets of cells in amyloid stroma (apple-green birefringence on Congo red stain).
Tx/Mgmt:
1. In MEN II syndrome, operate on any existing pheochromocytoma first
2. Total thyroidectomy with bilateral dissection of central lymph node compartment
3. Postoperative levothyroxine (replace normal hormone and suppress tumor regrowth)

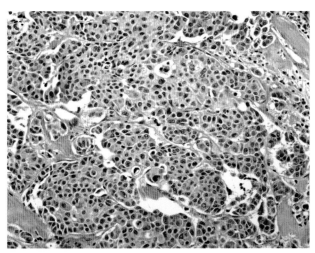

FIG. 14.12 Histology of medullary thyroid carcinoma. (From Albores-Saavedra J, Dorantes-Heredia R, Chablé-Montero F, Córdova-Ramón JC, Henson DE: Association of urothelial carcinoma of the renal pelvis with papillary and medullary thyroid carcinomas. A new sporadic neoplastic syndrome? *Ann Diagn Pathol* 18[5]:286–290, 2014.)

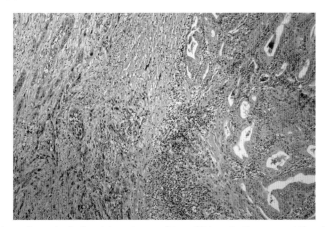

FIG. 14.13 Histology of anaplastic thyroid carcinoma. (From Wikimedia Commons: https://commons. wikimedia.org/wiki/File:Anaplastic_thyroid_carcinoma_low_mag.jpg. Used under Creative Commons Attribution-Share Alike 3.0 Unported license: https://creativecommons.org/licenses/by-sa/3.0/deed.en.)

Anaplastic Carcinoma

Buzz Words: Male who is older than 60 years + rapidly enlarging asymmetric non-tender neck mass + compression/ invasion of upper aerodigestive tract (dyspnea, dysphagia, hoarseness)

MoD: Dedifferentiation of antecedent differentiated thyroid cancer (p53 mutation). Invades local structures (extremely aggressive).

Dx: Refer to Fig. 14.6 for workup of thyroid nodule. Histology includes pleomorphic undifferentiated cells (Fig. 14.13)—distinguishes from the inflammatory fibrosis characteristic of Riedel thyroiditis (Fig.14.14).

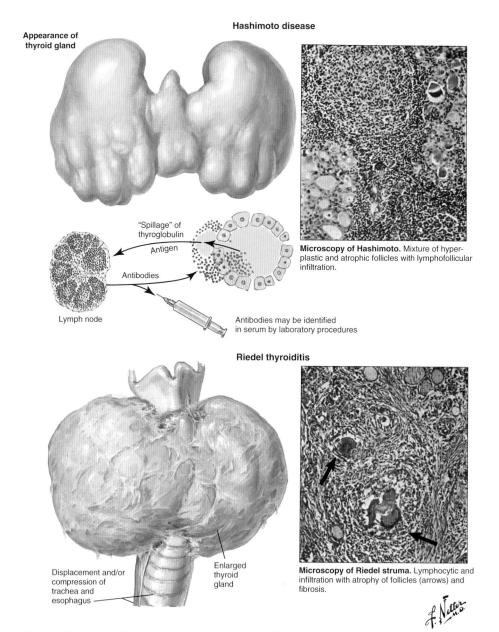

Hashimoto disease

Appearance of thyroid gland

"Spillage" of thyroglobulin

Antigen

Antibodies

Lymph node

Antibodies may be identified in serum by laboratory procedures

Microscopy of Hashimoto. Mixture of hyperplastic and atrophic follicles with lymphofollicular infiltration.

Riedel thyroiditis

Displacement and/or compression of trachea and esophagus

Enlarged thyroid gland

Microscopy of Riedel struma. Lymphocytic and infiltration with atrophy of follicles (arrows) and fibrosis.

FIG. 14.14 Histology of Riedel thyroiditis. (Copyright 2017 Elsevier Inc. All rights reserved. www.netterimages.com.)

Tx/Mgmt:

1. If operable, total thyroidectomy followed by chemoradiation
2. If inoperable because locally advanced, neoadjuvant therapy followed by total thyroidectomy if responsive
3. If metastatic, palliative care (locoregional resection and tracheostomy to relieve aerodigestive obstruction)

Parathyroid

Hypoparathyroidism

Buzz Words: Post-(para)thyroidectomy + perioral numbness/tingling + tetany (Trousseau sign, Chvostek sign) + prolonged QT interval on electrocardiogram

Clinical Presentation: Patient status is post thyroid, parathyroid, or radical neck surgery.

PPx: (1) Parathyroidectomy: radioguided parathyroidectomy with pre-op sestamibi scan (Fig. 14.15) and intraoperative PTH monitoring. (2) Thyroidectomy: parathyroid autotransplantation into sternocleidomastoid or forearm.

MoD: Accidental surgical excision of parathyroid glands, autoimmune destruction, or DiGeorge syndrome → Absence of parathyroid glands → Decreased PTH (Fig. 14.16) → Hypocalcemia (paresthesias, tetany)

Dx: Inappropriately low/normal PTH level in setting of hypocalcemia and hyperphosphatemia (in the absence of hypomagnesemia)

Tx/Mgmt:

1. Acutely, IV calcium gluconate
2. Chronically, PO calcium and calcitriol (vitamin D)

99 AR
Thyroid carcinoma summary image

99 AR
Chvostek's sign and Trousseau's sign

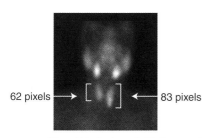
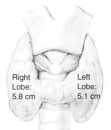
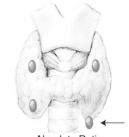

62 pixels → [ ] ← 83 pixels	Right Lobe: 5.8 cm Left Lobe: 5.1 cm	
Thyroid Lobe Length Ratio from Sestamibi: 62 pix/83 pix = 0.75	Thyroid Lobe Length Ratio from Ultrasound: 5.8 cm/5.1 cm 1.14	Absolute Ratio Difference between Sestamibi and Ultrasound: |0.75-1.14| = 0.39
A	B	C

FIG. 14.15 Sestamibi scan for localizing abnormal parathyroid gland. (From Nagar S, Walker DD, Embia O, Kaplan EL, Grogan RH, Angelos P: A novel technique to improve the diagnostic yield of negative sestamibi scans. *Surgery* 156[3]:584–590, 2014.)

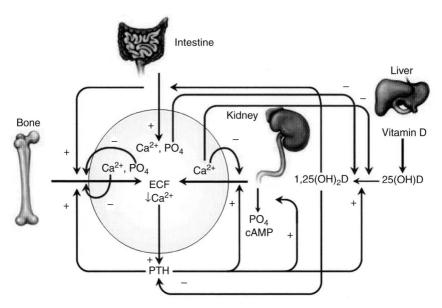

FIG. 14.16 The calcium homeostasis system. (Reproduced in modified form with permission from Brown EM: Mechanisms underlying the regulation of parathyroid hormone secretion in vivo and in vitro. *Curr Opin Nephrol Hypertens* 2:541–551, 1993. As modified in Brown EM: Role of the calcium-sensing receptor in extracellular calcium homeostasis. *Best Pract Res Clin Endocrinol Metab* 27[3]:333–343, 2013, Copyright © 2013 Elsevier Ltd.)

Primary Hyperparathyroidism

Buzz Words: Stones (kidney stones) + bones (osteitis fibrosa cystica) + groans (constipation) + psychiatric overtones (depression) + acute pancreatitis

Clinical Presentation: Patient may have familial or past medical history that is concerning for MEN syndromes.

MoD: Parathyroid adenoma/hyperplasia → Increased PTH → Activates adenylate cyclase to increase cAMP (measurable in urine) → Increased calcium bone resorption of calcium and phosphate, increased kidney resorption of calcium at distal convoluted tubule, decreased kidney resorption of phosphate at proximal convoluted tubule → Increased ALP (osteitis fibrosa cystica, see Fig. 14.17), hypophosphatemia, hypercalcemia (weakness, constipation, acute pancreatitis, depression), and hypercalciuria (kidney stones)

Dx:

1. Inappropriately elevated PTH level in setting of hypercalcemia and hypophosphatemia
2. Twenty-four-hour urinary calcium excretion to r/o familial hypocalciuric hypercalcemia
3. Sestamibi scan to distinguish adenoma (85%) from hyperplasia (10%) and localize adenoma

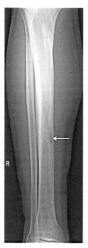

FIG. 14.17 Osteitis fibrosa cystica (also known as brown tumors) are cystic bone spaces created by the increased osteoclast activity of hyperparathyroidism, with hemorrhage into the cystic space depositing brown-pigmented hemosiderin. (From Wikimedia Commons: https://commons.wikimedia.org/wiki/File:Osteitis_fibrosa_cystica_tibiae_X-ray.jpg. In the public domain.)

Tx/Mgmt:
1. If symptomatic, IV fluids and furosemide (loop diuretics lose calcium) to bridge until definitive treatment
2. If adenoma, surgical resection with intraoperative PTH monitoring
3. If hyperplasia, parathyroid exploration and resection of 3½ parathyroid glands, with autograft of remaining parathyroid tissue to nondominant forearm for easier future access if necessary

Secondary Hyperparathyroidism
Buzz Words: Chronic renal failure + bone pain (renal osteodystrophy)

MoD: Chronic renal failure → Compromised kidney response to PTH → Hypovitaminosis D, hyperphosphatemia, and hypocalcemia → Reactive parathyroid gland hyperplasia → Hyperparathyroidism → Induced osteoblastic RANK-L secretion (Fig. 14.18) → Increased osteoclastic activity causes renal osteodystrophy (bone lesions)

Dx: Elevated PTH, hypocalcemia, hyperphosphatemia, and hypovitaminosis D in setting of chronic renal failiure

Tx/Mgmt:
1. Dietary phosphate restriction, with refractory hyperphosphatemia addressed with phosphate binders
2. Vitamin D supplementation
3. Cinacalcet to sensitize Ca^{2+}-sensing receptor in parathyroid gland

Secondary hyperparathyroidism - causes, symptoms, & treatment

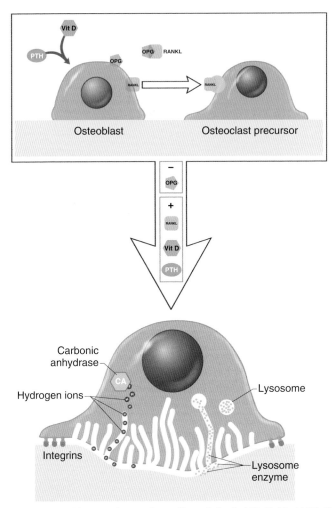

FIG. 14.18 PTH effect on osteoblasts and osteoclasts. (From Schmitz MR, DeHart MM, Qazi Z, Shuler FD: Basic sciences. In: Miller MD, Thompson SR, eds: *Miller's review or orthopaedics*, ed 7, Philadelphia, 2016, Elsevier.)

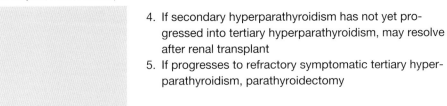

4. If secondary hyperparathyroidism has not yet progressed into tertiary hyperparathyroidism, may resolve after renal transplant
5. If progresses to refractory symptomatic tertiary hyperparathyroidism, parathyroidectomy

Adrenal Disorders

Non-Neoplastic

Adrenal Insufficiency

Buzz Words:
- **Adrenal insufficiency:** Fatigue + hypotension + sugar/salt cravings (Fig. 14.19)

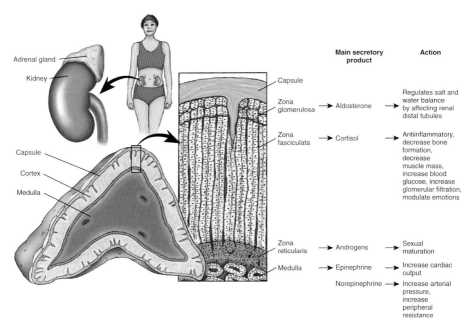

FIG. 14.19 Adrenal gland zone anatomy. (Modified from Thibodeau GA, Patton KT: *Anatomy and physiology*, ed 7, St Louis, 2010, Mosby. As adapted in Little JW, Falace DA, Miller CS, Rhodus NL: *Little and Falace's dental management of the medically compromised patient*, ed 8, St Louis, 2013, Mosby.)

- **Primary adrenal insufficiency:** Hypoaldosteronism (hyponatremia, hyperkalemia, metabolic acidosis) + skin/mucosal hyperpigmentation
- **Tertiary adrenal insufficiency:** Exogenous steroid use (e.g., athletes)

Clinical Presentation:
- Younger women with history of autoimmune disorders → Primary
- Immigrant with suspected tuberculosis with hematogenous spread → Primary
- College student with recent history of *Neisseria meningitidis* → Primary
- Postpartum women with extensive intrapartum bleeding → Secondary (Sheehan)
- Patient who suddenly stops using steroids → Tertiary

PPx: Taper steroid withdrawal to prevent tertiary adrenal insufficiency

MoD:
- Primary
- Acute (Waterhouse-Friedrichsen syndrome—def. acute adrenal hemorrhage 2/2 *N. meningitidis* endotoxic shock or DIC)

- Chronic (Addison disease – def. adrenal atrophy 2/2 auto-immune or TB) → Hypoaldosteronism + hypocortisolism → Increased ACTH (cleaved from POMC, creating MSH byproduct to hyperpigment skin/mucosa – see Fig. 14.20)
- **Secondary:** Hypopituitarism → Decreased ACTH → Hypocortisolism with aldosterone WNL
- Tertiary: Chronic exogenous steroid administration → Decreased CRH synthesis, secretion, and action at anterior pituitary → Decreased ACTH → Hypocortisolism with aldosterone WNL

Dx:
1. 8 AM serum cortisol and plasma ACTH → If low cortisol and high ACTH, primary adrenal insufficiency
2. If low cortisol and low ACTH, CRH stimulation test → If subnormal ACTH response, secondary adrenal insufficiency; if exaggerated ACTH response, tertiary adrenal insufficiency

Tx/Mgmt:
1. Addisonian crisis: IVF D5NS + IV dexamethasone (doesn't interfere with plasma cortisol measurement)
2. Before surgery, stress dose hydrocortisone
3. Typical management includes glucocorticoid (hydrocortisone) and mineralocorticoid (fludrocortisone) replacement

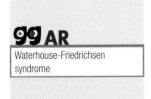

99 AR

Waterhouse-Friedrichsen syndrome

Hypercortisolism

Buzz Words: BAM CUSHINGOID – Buffalo hump + amenorrhea (hirsutism) + moon facies/myopathy (proximal) + crazy (psychosis, depression) + ulcers + skin changes (acne, purple striae, easy bruising) + hypertension (refractory) + infection + osteoporosis/obesity (truncal) + immunosuppression + diabetes (insulin resistance)

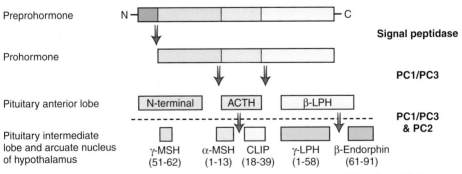

FIG. 14.20 POMC cleavage into ACTH and MSH. (Courtesy Dr. Malcolm Low, University of Michigan, Ann Arbor, MI. From Cone RD, Elmquist JK: Neuroendocrine control of energy stores. In Melmed S, Polonsky K, Larsen PR, Kronenberg H, eds: *Williams textbook of endocrinology*, ed 13, Philadelphia, 2016, Elsevier.)

Clinical Presentation:

- Patient on steroids → Iatrogenic
- Male smoker with hemoptysis, cough, and weight loss → Small cell lung cancer paraneoplastic syndrome
- Women 25–45 years old → Cushing disease
- Women 40–60 years old → Adrenal tumors

PPx: Avoid exogenous corticosteroids

MoD:

- Iatrogenic (exogenous corticosteroids) → Low ACTH → Bilateral adrenal atrophy
- Adrenal hyperplasia/adenoma/carcinoma → Low ACTH → Unilateral adrenal atrophy of uninvolved gland
- Cushing disease (ACTH-secreting pituitary adenoma) or ectopic ACTH (paraneoplastic syndrome 2/2 SCLC) → High ACTH → Bilateral adrenal hyperplasia

Dx:

1. Overnight low-dose dexamethasone suppression test (DST) to rule out normal
2. Plasma ACTH to distinguish exogenous glucocorticoids and adrenal tumor (low ACTH) from other causes
3. Overnight high-dose DST distinguishes Cushing disease (adequate suppression) from ectopic ACTH secretion (no suppression)—see Fig. 14.21
4. Localize pituitary adenoma with magnetic resonance imaging (MRI) or adrenal adenoma with CT

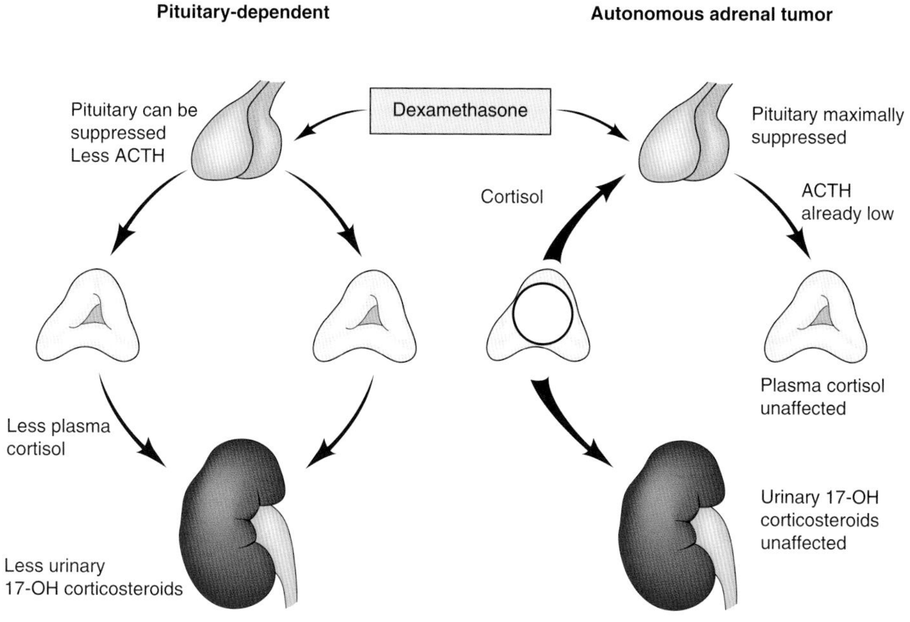

Pituitary-dependent   **Autonomous adrenal tumor**

Pituitary can be suppressed Less ACTH

Dexamethasone

Pituitary maximally suppressed

Cortisol

ACTH already low

Less plasma cortisol

Plasma cortisol unaffected

Less urinary 17-OH corticosteroids

Urinary 17-OH corticosteroids unaffected

FIG. 14.21 Cushing syndrome suppression test. (From Lennard TWJ: Endocrine surgery. In Garden OJ, ed: *Principles and practice of surgery*, ed 6, London, 2012, Elsevier.)

Tx/Mgmt:

- Exogenous corticosteroids → Taper
- Adrenal adenoma → Unilateral adrenalectomy
- If adrenal carcinoma → Surgical excision if operable
- Ectopic ACTH-secreting tumor, surgical excision if operable
- Cushing disease, transsphenoidal adenomectomy
- Medical management if surgery is delayed, contra-indicated, or unsuccessful (ketoconazole—inhibits cholesterol desmolase, metyrapone—inhibits 11β-hydroxylase, mitotane—adrenocorticolytic)

Neoplastic

Adrenal Neuroblastoma

Buzz Words: Pediatric + abdominal mass that crosses the midline + opsoclonus-myoclonus ("dancing eyes, dancing feet")

MoD: N-myc oncogene activation → Embryonic SRBC tumor of neural crest cells located along the sympathetic chain (50% in adrenal medulla) → Transverse myelitis (spinal cord compression), Horner syndrome (cervical location), opsoclonus-myoclonus syndrome (paraneoplastic), and hypertension (catecholamine secretion)

Dx:

1. Twenty-four-hour urine catecholamine metabolites (HVA, VMA) and metanephrines
2. CT scan to localize
3. 123I-MIBG body scan to evaluate for metastases

Tx/Mgmt: Surgical resection ± chemoradiation

Pheochromocytoma

Buzz Words: Hyperadrenergic episodes (headache, diaphoresis, tachycardia) + refractory hypertension + MENII

Clinical Presentation: A 40- to 60-year-old patient presents with history suspicious for MENII, VHL, or neurofibromatosis.

MoD: Tumor of chromaffin neural crest cells in adrenal medulla → Secretes catecholamines → Episodic hyperadrenergic states

Dx:

1. Twenty-four-hour urine catecholamines, VMA, and metanephrine
2. CT or MRI to localize lesions
3. I-123-MIBG body scan or positron emission tomography (PET) scan to evaluate for metastases if non-localizable or suspicious (e.g., paraganglioma, of large diameter)

Tx/Mgmt:

1. To avoid hypertensive crisis, preoperative irreversible α-blockade (phenoxybenzamine) followed by β-blockade (propanolol)
2. Laparoscopic adrenalectomy
3. Adequate fluid replacement to avoid postoperative hypotension from catecholamine-withdrawal vasodilation

Adrenal Incidentaloma

Buzz Words: Asymptomatic patient + adrenal mass incidentally found on abdominal CT scans

MoD: MCC non-functioning adenoma (>75%)

Dx:

1. Overnight DST to r/o subclinical Cushing syndrome
2. Twenty-four-hour urine catecholamines and metanephrine to r/o pheochromocytoma
3. If hypertension or hypokalemia, plasma aldosterone and renin to r/o primary hyperaldosteronism
4. CT without contrast, followed by MRI if inadequate

Tx/Mgmt:

- If less than 4 cm and non-suspicious, CT follow-up within 1 year
- If known primary malignancy elsewhere, FNA biopsy (after excluding pheochromocytoma) to r/o metastatic disease
- If bilateral, investigate for congenital adrenal hyperplasia
- If none of the above, unilateral adrenalectomy (>4 cm, suspicious, grows >1 cm in 1 year, or functioning)

Pituitary Disorders: (See Fig. 14.22)
Hypopituitarism

Diabetes Insipidus (Central)

Buzz Words: Polyuria + nocturia + polydipsia + hypernatremia

MoD: Brain trauma, neoplasm, infection, or surgical damage → Decreased ADH secretion from posterior pituitary → Decreased ability to concentrate urine in collecting tubule (low urine specific gravity) → Hyperosmotic volume contraction (hypernatremia)

Dx: Water deprivation test shows greater than 50% rise in urine osmolarity with ADH administration

Tx/Mgmt:

1. Desmopressin/DDAVP (synthetic ADH substitute with no vasopressor activity)
2. Fluid replacement with D5NS to prevent cerebral edema while hypernatremia corrects

Primary Hypogonadism

Buzz Words: Delayed puberty + decreased testosterone + increased luteinizing hormone (LH)

AR
Catecholamine breakdown pathways

AR
Adrenal mass differential diagnosis

MNEMONIC
The Awesome Frats Love Beer – TSH, ACTH, FSH, LH = Basophils

MNEMONIC
Good Hippies Pop Acid – GH, PRL = Acidophils

MNEMONIC
ADH, SON = ADH is synthesized in the supraoptic nucleus

AR
Mechanism of ADH at collecting duct principal cells

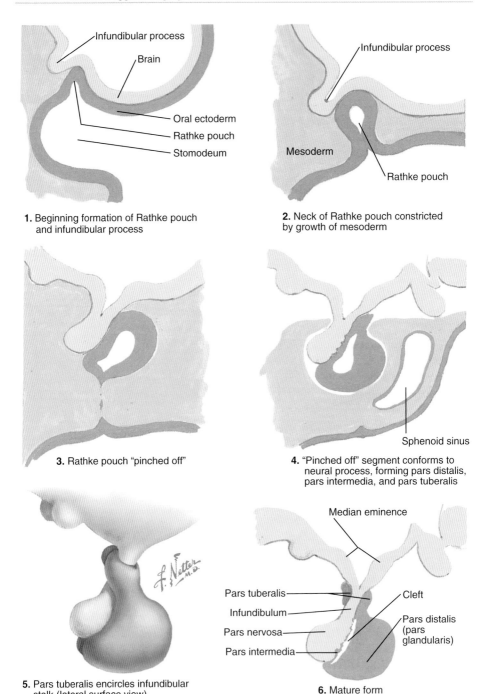

1. Beginning formation of Rathke pouch and infundibular process

2. Neck of Rathke pouch constricted by growth of mesoderm

3. Rathke pouch "pinched off"

4. "Pinched off" segment conforms to neural process, forming pars distalis, pars intermedia, and pars tuberalis

5. Pars tuberalis encircles infundibular stalk (lateral surface view)

6. Mature form

FIG. 14.22 Hypothalamus-pituitary axis. (Copyright 2017 Elsevier Inc. All rights reserved. www.netterimages.com.)

PPx: MMR vaccine, avoid testicular radiation exposure

MoD:

- Klinefelter syndrome → Testicular atrophy
- Cryptorchidism or varicocele → Increased scrotal temperature → Induction of apoptosis → Loss of germ cell mass
- Disorder of androgen synthesis
- Myotonic dystrophy
- Mumps → Orchitis
- Testicular torsion
- Radiation

Dx:

1. Low morning serum total testosterone (make sure to consider that SHBG increases with aging and decreases with obesity)
2. High LH and follicle-stimulating hormone (FSH) concentrations

Tx/Mgmt: Males with non-functioning testicular tissue should undergo orchiectomy

Hypogonadotropic Hypogonadism

Buzz Words:

1. Decreased testosterone + decreased LH → Secondary hypogonadism

MoD:

- Isolated gonadotrophic-releasing hormone (GnRH) deficiency (Kallmann syndrome)
- GnRH suppression (hyperprolactinemia, excess glucocorticoids, GnRH analogs)
- Hypothalamic damage (neoplasms, infections, apoplexy, trauma, surgery, or radiation in the sellar region)

Dx:

- Low morning serum total testosterone (make sure to consider that SHBG increases with aging and decreases with obesity)
- Low LH and FSH concentrations

Tx/Mgmt:

- Males with nonfunctioning testicular tissue should undergo orchiectomy
- Treat hyperprolactinemia with bromocriptine or cabergoline (dopamine agonist), and transsphenoidal pituitary adenoma surgical resection if refractory to medical management
- Treat non-operable hypothalamic damage with sex steroid replacement, with pulsatile GnRH for induction of ovulation/spermatogenesis

Laron Syndrome

Buzz Words: Dwarfism + small head

MoD: Defective GH receptor → Decreased linear growth

Dx:

1. Elevated GH level
2. Low IGF level

Tx/Mgmt: Recombinant insulin-like growth factor (IGF)

Panhypopituitarism

Buzz Words: Secondary hypocortisolism + hypothyroidism + hypogonadotropic hypogonadism + short stature (if pediatric) + impaired lactation

MoD: Craniopharyngioma, metastases, pituitary apoplexy, empty sella syndrome, trauma, radiation, infiltration → Decreased secretion of pituitary hormones (GH, PRL, TSH, ACTH, FSH, LH, ADH, oxytocin—Fig. 14.23)

Dx: MRI

Tx/Mgmt: Hormone replacement therapy (thyroxine, glucocorticoids, sex steroids, GH)

Pituitary Apoplexy (e.g., Sheehan Syndrome)

Buzz Words: Acute headache + ophthalmic findings (diplopia, bitemporal hemianopsia) + impaired lactation + refractory hypotension + postpartum woman

MoD:

- Hemorrhage of pituitary tumor → Destruction of pituitary gland + mass effect (CN III – diplopia) → Hypopituitarism
- Sheehan syndrome—def. peripartum pituitary enlargement because of increased lactotrophs → Postpartum hemorrhage yields hypovolemic shock → Pituitary infarction → Hypopituitarism

Dx: MRI

Tx/Mgmt:

1. If severe visual or neurological symptoms, surgical decompression
2. Hormone replacement therapy (thyroxine, glucocorticoids, sex steroids, GH)

99 AR

MRI series of Sheehan Syndrome

Hyperpituitarism

Gigantism/Acromegaly

Buzz Words: Large tongue + macrognathia (large jaw) + enlarged hands/feet (increasing hat, glove, shoe, or ring size) + deepening of the voice + frontal bossing + new-onset diabetes → Acromegaly (Fig. 14.24)

Severe anterior pituitary deficiency

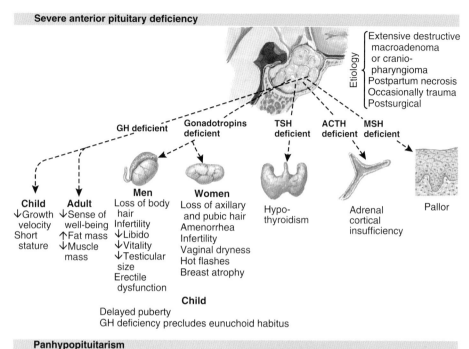

Etiology
{ Extensive destructive
macroadenoma
or cranio-
pharyngioma
Postpartum necrosis
Occasionally trauma
Postsurgical

GH deficient — Gonadotropins deficient — TSH deficient — ACTH deficient — MSH deficient

Child
↓Growth velocity
Short stature

Adult
↓Sense of well-being
↑Fat mass
↓Muscle mass

Men
Loss of body hair
Infertility
↓Libido
↓Vitality
↓Testicular size
Erectile dysfunction

Women
Loss of axillary and pubic hair
Amenorrhea
Infertility
Vaginal dryness
Hot flashes
Breast atrophy

Hypo-thyroidism

Adrenal cortical insufficiency

Pallor

Child
Delayed puberty
GH deficiency precludes eunuchoid habitus

Panhypopituitarism

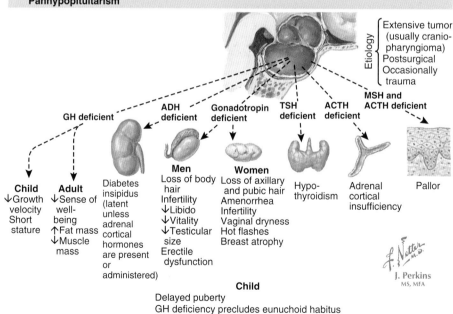

Etiology
{ Extensive tumor
(usually cranio-
pharyngioma)
Postsurgical
Occasionally
trauma

GH deficient — ADH deficient — Gonadotropin deficient — TSH deficient — ACTH deficient — MSH and ACTH deficient

Child
↓Growth velocity
Short stature

Adult
↓Sense of well-being
↑Fat mass
↓Muscle mass

Diabetes insipidus (latent unless adrenal cortical hormones are present or administered)

Men
Loss of body hair
Infertility
↓Libido
↓Vitality
↓Testicular size
Erectile dysfunction

Women
Loss of axillary and pubic hair
Amenorrhea
Infertility
Vaginal dryness
Hot flashes
Breast atrophy

Hypo-thyroidism

Adrenal cortical insufficiency

Pallor

f. Netter
MD
J. Perkins
MS, MFA

Child
Delayed puberty
GH deficiency precludes eunuchoid habitus

FIG. 14.23 Panhypopituitarism. *TSH,* Thyroid-stimulating hormone. (Copyright 2017 Elsevier Inc. All rights reserved. www.netterimages.com.)

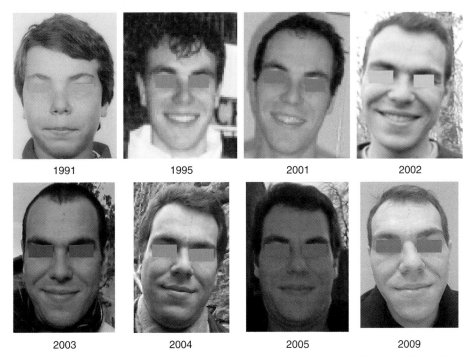

1991   1995   2001   2002

2003   2004   2005   2009

FIG. 14.24 Acromegaly picture series. (From Chanson P, Salenave S, Kamenicky P, Cazabat L, Young J: Acromegaly. *Best Pract Res Clin Endocrinol Metab* 23[5]:555–574, 2009. Copyright © 2009 Elsevier Ltd.)

MoD:

- GH-secreting pituitary adenoma before epiphyseal fusion → Increased linear bone growth → Gigantism
- GH-secreting pituitary adenoma after epiphyseal fusion → Generalized enlargement of bone (facial and extremity characteristics) and soft tissue (deep voice, hypertrophy of left ventricle) + mass effect of pituitary adenoma at optic chiasm (bitemporal hemianopsia) + increased IGF-1 (insulin resistance, diastolic hypertension)

Dx:

1. Elevated serum IGF-1
2. Inadequate suppression of serum GH following oral glucose tolerance test
3. Pituitary MRI to localize

Tx/Mgmt:

1. Transsphenoidal surgical resection of pituitary adenoma
2. If non-resectable or not cured post-operatively, octreotide (somatostatin analog)
3. If refractory to octreotide, add pegvisomant (GH receptor antagonist)

Prolactinoma

Buzz Words: Galactorrhea + hypogonadism + bitemporal hemianopsia

MoD: PRL-secreting pituitary adenoma → PRL stimulates milk production (galactorrhea) + suppresses GnRH synthesis and release (hypogonadism) + mass effect of pituitary adenoma near optic chiasm (bitemporal hemianopsia, oculomotor nerve palsy, hypopituitarism)

Dx:
1. Pregnancy test
2. Elevated serum prolactin
3. Pituitary MRI to localize

Tx/Mgmt:
1. Bromocriptine or cabergoline (dopamine agonist) to suppress PRL levels
2. If refractory to medical management, transsphenoidal resection
3. If non-resectable, radiation

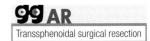
Transsphenoidal surgical resection

Nelson Syndrome

Buzz Words: Post-bilateral adrenalectomy + bitemporal hemianopsia + hyperpigmentation (see Fig. 14.25)

PPx: Properly identify Cushing disease before therapeutic bilateral adrenalectomy with MRI, pituitary radiation

MoD: Bilateral adrenalectomy for refractory Cushing syndrome when pt actually has Cushing disease → Loss of negative feedback by cortisol → Enlargement of ACTH-secreting pituitary adenoma → Increased ACTH (cleaved from POMC, creating MSH byproduct to hyperpigment skin/mucosa) + mass effect of pituitary adenoma at optic chiasm (bitemporal hemianopsia)

Dx:
1. Elevated ACTH level
2. Enlarging pituitary adenoma on MRI

Tx/Mgmt:
1. Transsphenoidal resection
2. If resection fails, pituitary irradiation

Regulators of prolactin secretion

Syndrome of Inappropriate ADH (SIADH)

Buzz Words: Euvolemic hyponatremia (confusion, convulsion, coma)

Clinical Presentation: Patient presents with history of CNS disturbance (e.g., stroke, head trauma), small cell lung cancer, or drugs (e.g., carbamazepine, cyclophosphamide, selective serotonin reuptake inhibitors [SSRIs]).

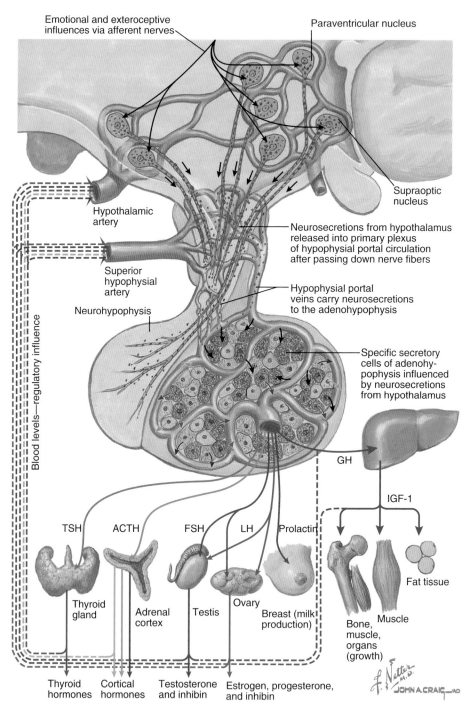

FIG. 14.25 Nelson syndrome. *FSH,* Follicle-stimulating hormone; *IGF,* insulin-like growth factor; *LH,* luteinizing hormone; *TSH,* thyroid-stimulating hormone. (Copyright 2017 Elsevier Inc. All rights reserved. www.netterimages.com.)

MoD:
- SCLC paraneoplastic syndrome → Ectopic ADH secretion
- CNS disturbance (trauma, stroke, etc.) → Enhance ADH release
- Drugs (carbamazepine, cyclophosphamide, SSRIs) → Enhance ADH release or effect

Dx:
- Hypotonic hyponatremia
- Elevated urine osmolarity

Tx/Mgmt:
- Treat the underlying disease
- Fluid restriction
- IV hypertonic saline if severe hyponatremia
- Demeclocycline (diminish collecting tubule responsiveness to ADH by inhibiting V2-receptor associated adenylyl cyclase activation)

Neoplastic

Craniopharyngioma
Buzz Words: Hypopituitarism + bitemporal hemianopsia (Fig. 14.26)

> **MNEMONIC**
> Drugs that cause SIADH –
> "Can't Concentrate Serum
> Sodium" – Carbamazepine,
> Cyclophosphamide, SSRIs

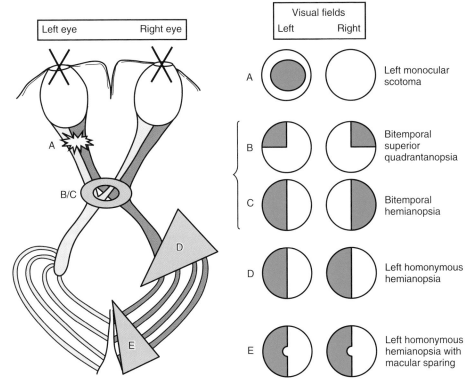

FIG. 14.26 Bilateral hemianopsia diagram. (From Kaufman MD, Milstein MJ. Kaufman's clinical neurology for psychiatrists, ed 7, Philadelphia, 2013, Elsevier.)

Clinical Presentation: (1) Hypopituitarism in children 5–14 years old. (2) Hypopituitarism in adults 50–75 years old.

MoD: Benign suprasellar tumor (adjacent to optic chiasm), derived from Rathke pouch (oral ectoderm) → Mass effect of pituitary adenoma on optic chiasm (bitemporal hemianopsia) and on pituitary (hypopituitarism, diabetes insipidus)

Dx:
1. Calcified parasellar cystic lesion on MRI or CT
2. Preoperative endocrine testing (adrenal and thyroid function) and visual field testing to establish baseline

Tx/Mgmt:
1. Neurosurgical resection
2. If incomplete resection or recurrence, postoperative radiation therapy

MRI series of craniopharyngiomas

Multiple Endocrine Neoplasias

MEN I

Buzz Words: Refractory peptic ulcer disease (ZES) + kidney stones (hyperparathyroidism)

PPx: (1) DNA screening for at-risk family members, (2) Screen pts with MEN I, known *MEN1* mutation carriers, and at-risk family members for hypercalcemia to detect asymptomatic hyperparathyroidism.

MoD: AD mutation of *MEN1* (tumor suppressor) → Pituitary tumors (prolactinoma, acromegaly) + pancreatic islet cell tumors (Zollinger-Ellison syndrome, glucagonoma, insulinoma, VIPoma) + parathyroid adenomas

Dx:
- 2+ primary MEN I tumors
- 1+ primary MEN I tumor + first-degree family history
- Germline *MEN1* (menin—tumor suppressor) mutation

Tx/Mgmt: Treat respective neoplasias as described previously in this section

MEN II

Buzz Words:
- **MEN IIA:** MTC or pheochromocytoma <35 years old + family history → MEN IIA
- **MEN IIB:** MTC or pheochromocytoma <35 years old + oral/intestinal ganglioneuromas + marfanoid habitus (lanky)

PPx:
- Screen pts with MEN II with plasma metanephrine to r/o pheochromocytoma
- Screen serum calcium to r/o hyperparathyroidism

- Screen pts serum calcitonin + thyroid US to r/o MTC
- Prophylactic thyroidectomy in children with *RET* mutation

MoD:
- MEN IIA: AD mutation of *RET* in neural crest cells →
  Parathyroid hyperplasia + MTC + pheochromocytoma
- MEN IIB: AD mutation of *RET* in neural crest cells →
  MTC + pheochromocytoma + oral/intestinal ganglio-
  neuromas + marfanoid habitus

Dx:
- 1+ primary MEN II classical features + germline *RET*
  mutation
- 2+ primary MEN II classical features in absence of *RET*
  mutation

Tx/Mgmt: Treat respective neoplasias as described previously in this section

Congenital Disorders

Congenital Hypothyroidism (Cretinism)

MEN syndrome Venn diagram

Buzz Words: Infant 6 to 12 weeks old + developmental delay
+ umbilical hernia + protuberant tongue + hypotonia +
prolonged jaundice (see Fig. 14.27)
PPx: (1) Adequate maternal iodine intake, (2) newborn TSH
screening required by law
MoD: Etiologies include primary (MCC thyroid dysgenesis,
dyshormonogenesis, resistance to thyroid hormone) or
transient (iodine deficiency/excess, maternal antibody-
mediated) hypothyroidism
Dx: Elevated blood TSH
Tx/Mgmt:
1. Levothyroxine to keep free T4 WNL
2. Reevaluate thyroid function at 3 years old to distinguish
   permanent versus transient hypothyroidism by discon-
   tinuing therapy for 30 days, then measuring TSH and fT4
3. Surgical repair of umbilical hernia if persists in patients
   older than 2 years old

Congenital Adrenal Hyperplasia

Buzz Words:
1. Diffuse skin pigmentation + bilateral adrenal
   enlargement
   - **17-Hydroxylase deficiency:** CAH + hypernatremic
     hypertension + puberty delay
   - **21-Hydroxylase deficiency :** CAH + hyponatremic
     hypotension + precocious puberty
   - **11-Hydroxylase deficiency :** CAH + hypernatremic
     hypertension + precocious puberty

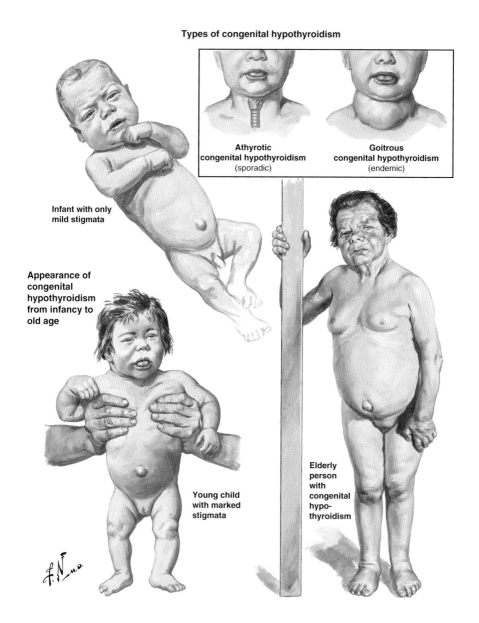

Types of congenital hypothyroidism

Athyrotic
congenital hypothyroidism
(sporadic)

Goitrous
congenital hypothyroidism
(endemic)

Infant with only
mild stigmata

Appearance of
congenital
hypothyroidism
from infancy to
old age

Young child
with marked
stigmata

Elderly
person
with
congenital
hypo-
thyroidism

FIG. 14.27 Cretinism. (Copyright 2017 Elsevier Inc. All rights reserved. www.netterimages.com.)

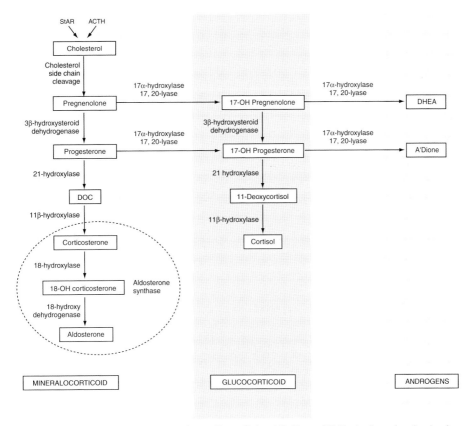

FIG. 14.28 Adrenal steroid synthesis pathway. (From Guber HA, Farag AF: Evaluation of endocrine function. In McPherson RA, ed: *Henry's clinical diagnosis and management by laboratory methods*, ed 23, St. Louis, 2017, Elsevier.)

Clinical Presentation: Eskimos or Caucasians present with precocious or delayed puberty.

MoD: Congenital adrenal enzyme deficiency → Increased products proximally in synthesis pathway, decreased products distally in synthesis pathway (Fig. 14.28) → Increased mineralocorticoids (aldosterone or 11-deoxycortisone) cause hypernatremic hypertension, decreased mineralocorticoids cause hyponatremic hypotension, increased sex hormones causes virilization and precocious puberty, decreased sex hormones cause ambiguous genitalia and delayed puberty

Dx:

- **17-Hydroxylase deficiency:** Elevated corticosterone levels + low aldosterone and renin levels
- **21-Hydroxylase deficiency:** Elevated 17-hydroxyprogesterone concentration
- **11-Hydroxylase deficiency:** Elevated 11-deoxycortisosterone and DHEAS levels

Tx/Mgmt:
- **17-Hydroxylase deficiency**—glucocorticoid (stress-adjusted), spironolactone (aldosterone antagonist), and estrogen replacement during expected puberty
- **21-Hydroxylase deficiency**—glucocorticoid and mineralocorticoid replacement
- **11-Hydroxylase deficiency**—glucocorticoid replacement and spironolactone (androgen and mineralocorticoid antagonist). Avoid bilateral adrenalectomy

Androgen Insensitivity Syndrome

Buzz Words: Normal-appearing female + primary amenorrhea + no sexual hair + absent cervix on pelvic exam + cryptorchid testes in labia majora or inguinal canal

Clinical Presentation: Adolescent female presents with primary amenorrhea.

MoD: XY genotype secretes Mullerian Inhibitory Factor → Degeneration of internal female sex organs → X-linked recessive defect of androgen receptor → Increased LH and testosterone due to negative feedback → Increased estrogen due to aromatase action on testosterone

Dx: Elevated testosterone, LH, and estrogen levels

Tx/Mgmt:
1. Gonadectomy to prevent malignancy
2. Estrogen replacement during expected puberty

GUNNER PRACTICE

1. A 55-year-old woman is brought to the emergency department by her husband after persistent nausea and vomiting in the setting of acute-onset abdominal pain for the past few hours. The husband states that the woman has been acting unusual since the onset of symptoms, and is now minimally conscious. The woman has a past medical history including type 1 diabetes mellitus. The husband recollects his wife complaining of chronic diarrhea. She takes a long-acting insulin at baseline and a short-acting insulin before each meal. Her pulse is 100/min, respirations are 20/min, and blood pressure is 95/65. Examination shows poor skin turgor, sunken eyes, dry oral mucous membranes, and a blistering erythematous rash around the mouth. Which of the following is the most appropriate next study to order?
   A. Serum glucagon level
   B. Insulin and C-peptide level
   C. Insulin, C-peptide, and sulfonylurea level
   D. Triphasic CT
   E. Serum somatostatin level

2. A 32-year-old man comes to your office with a chief complaint of diaphoretic episodes every few days, with associated heart palpitations and headaches. He has a history of treatment for anxiety disorder and asthma. The man tells you he is "at least lucky enough not to have cancer in the neck like my mother." His pulse in the office is 90/min, respirations are 14/min, and blood pressure is 175/110. A basic metabolic panel shows a calcium of 11.3 mg/dL and a phosphate of 1.8 mg/dL. Which of the following is the most appropriate next step after the work-up is complete?
   A. Observation
   B. DNA screening
   C. Total thyroidectomy
   D. Unilateral thyroid lobectomy
   E. Unilateral adrenalectomy
   F. Bilateral adrenalectomy

3. A 28-year-old woman presents to her pediatrician with an inability to breast feed her child 6 days post-vaginal delivery. She has no past medical history other than some hemophilia that runs in the family. Her pulse is 60/min, respirations are 16/min, and blood pressure is 130/84 while sitting and 98/68 when she stands. If she does not address this acute issue, which of the following symptoms may arise?
   A. Hemarthrosis
   B. Hypertension
   C. Constipation
   D. Hyperpigmentation
   E. Primary hypogonadism

ANSWERS: What Would Gunner Jess/Jim Do?

1. WWGJD? A 55-year-old woman is brought to the emergency department by her husband after **persistent nausea and vomiting** in the setting of **acute-onset abdominal pain for the past few hours.** The husband states that the woman has been acting unusual since the onset of symptoms, **and is now minimally conscious.** The woman has a past medical history including **type 1 diabetes mellitus.** The husband recollects his wife complaining of **chronic diarrhea.** She takes a long-acting insulin at baseline and a short-acting insulin before each meal. Her pulse is 100/min, **respirations are 20/min, and blood pressure is 95/65.** Examination shows poor skin turgor, sunken eyes, dry oral mucous membranes, and **a blistering erythematous rash around the mouth. Which of the following is the most appropriate next study to order?**

Answer: A, Serum glucagon level

Explanation: Pt has DKA (nausea, vomiting, acute abdominal pain, Kussmaul respiration, altered mental status) likely 2/2 glucagonoma, as indicated by symptoms of chronic diarrhea and necrolytic migratory erythema.

B. Insulin and C-peptide level → Incorrect. These laboratory studies distinguish insulinoma vs surreptitious insulin use in the setting of hypoglycemic symptoms (e.g., diaphoresis, syncope, seizures), which are not present in this patient.

C. Insulin, C-peptide, and sulfonylurea level → Incorrect. These laboratory studies distinguish insulinoma versus surreptitious insulin or sulfonylurea use in the setting of hypoglycemic symptoms (e.g., diaphoresis, syncope, seizures), which are not present in this patient.

D. Triphasic CT → Incorrect. Triphasic CT is used to localize glucagonoma after diagnosis is confirmed by laboratory studies.

E. Serum somatostatin level → Incorrect. This laboratory study evaluates for a somatostatinoma, which is capable of inducing a hyperglycemic state with steatorrhea, but would also present with gallstones rather than necrolytic migratory erythema.

2. WWGJD? A 32-year-old man comes to your office with a chief complaint of **diaphoretic episodes** every few days, with **associated heart palpitations and headaches.** He has a history of treatment for anxiety disorder

and asthma. The man tells you he is "at least lucky enough not to have cancer in the neck like my mother." His pulse in the office is 90/min, respirations are 14/min, and blood pressure is 175/110. A basic metabolic panel shows a calcium of 11.3 mg/dL and a phosphate of 1.8 mg/dL. Which of the following is the most appropriate next step after the work-up is complete?

Answer: E, Unilateral adrenalectomy

Explanation: Pt has symptoms of pheochromocytoma, laboratory studies consistent with hyperparathyroidism, and a first-degree relative with possible thyroid cancer. This clinical picture is diagnostic of MEN IIA syndrome. The next step is to address the pheochromocytoma first via unilateral adrenalectomy, so that it may not complicate medical or surgical management of the other neoplasias.

A. Observation → Incorrect. Observation is not appropriate in setting of pheochromocytoma, germline *RET* mutation, or hyperparathyroidism with serum calcium concentration of 1.0 mg/dL above ULN.

B. DNA screening → Incorrect. 1+ clinical symptom of MEN IIA syndrome in addition to first-degree familial history is diagnostic.

C. Total thyroidectomy → Incorrect. Must first address pheochromocytoma before prophylactic thyroidectomy.

D. Unilateral thyroid lobectomy → Incorrect. Must first address pheochromocytoma before prophylactic thyroidectomy. Unilateral lobectomy is not appropriate in setting of medullary thyroid carcinoma.

F. Bilateral adrenalectomy → Incorrect. Inappropriate in the setting of unilateral pheochromocytoma and could lead to Nelson syndrome.

3. WWGJD? A 28-year-old woman presents to her pediatrician with an inability to breast feed her child 6 days post-vaginal delivery. She has no past medical history other than some hemophilia that runs in the family. Her pulse is 60/min, respirations are 16/min, and blood pressure is 130/84 while sitting and 98/68 when she stands. If she does not address this acute issue, which of the following symptoms may arise?

Answer: C, Constipation

Explanation: Pt has agalactorrhea and orthostatic hypotension following a vaginal delivery complicated by hemophilia, hinting at a high likelihood of postpartum hemorrhage. This clinical picture is indicative of panhypopituitarism 2/2 Sheehan syndrome. Since hypothyroidism is one aspect of panhypopituitarism, we may expect the patient to develop the constellation of hypothyroid symptoms (hyporeflexia, bradycardia, constipation, weight gain, fatigue, percussion myoedema, myxedema, brittle hair, and cold intolerance).

A. Hemarthrosis → Incorrect. Hemarthrosis is a complication of hemophilia rather than Sheehan syndrome.

B. Hypertension → Incorrect. Hypopituitarism leads to a deficiency of ADH, cortisol, and thyroid hormones, which results in orthostatic hypotension due to an inability to regulate vasoconstriction.

D. Hyperpigmentation → Incorrect. Hypopituitarism leads to a decrease in ACTH synthesis from POMC, which results in decreased MSH, the byproduct that is typically attributed with the role of hyperpigmentation in primary adrenal insufficiency.

E. Primary hypogonadism → Incorrect. Hypopituitarism is classified as a hypogonadotropic hypogonadism.

Gunner Jim's Guide to Exam Day Success

Leo Wang and Hao-Hua Wu

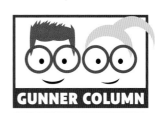

Do these three things to perform well on any shelf:

1. Master one review book.
2. Answer as many quality questions as you can.
3. Review questions on Excel (or other charting software).

"Master one review book."

The Surgery shelf is notorious for being one of the most difficult shelf exams you will take and requires a lot of knowledge to succeed. It can be particularly frustrating because anecdotally, most students who take this shelf claim that it is just another iteration of the Medicine shelf with a few more surgery-specific topics. Thus, this shelf can be the broadest of all of them.

The most important thing you can do prior to the start of your rotation is to identify the resource that best covers the material of your Surgery shelf and stick with it. You will NOT have time go through resource after resource to find the best one. Our augmented reality component provides the depth needed to explore the eclectic multimedia sources that you can use to prep for the exam.

Most of your learning takes place as you complete questions, so don't be discouraged if you cannot memorize every word of your review book as you did for step 1—this is not possible, even for the most accomplished physician. Instead, use your review book as a point of reference and annotate the margins.

If you see one topic come up in multiple chapters (or maybe even multiple shelf exams), make sure to write down the page numbers where it appears and flip to those pages every time you review. The more connections you make, the more you will master.

In addition, highlight themes that keep coming up. Anytime patients in the question stem have recently changed their medication regimen, suspect the medication change as the cause of their symptoms until proven otherwise. Another example is bleeding after surgical procedures, from neurosurgeries to joint replacements. Such bleeding should lead you to suspect coagulopathy.

"Answer as many quality questions as you can."

The key to success is practicing in an environment that simulates the pressure of test day, and nothing simulates that pressure better than taking practice questions under stringent time constraints.

After you identify your review book, select as many authoritative question banks as you can. We recommend *Gunner Practice, UWorld*, and *NBME Clinical Science* practice exams. Do at least 10 questions a day under timed conditions (1.5 minutes per question), starting on the first day of your rotation.

Remember, you can complete the same question multiple times in the course of study! In fact, it is recommended that you retry the questions you got wrong the first time around, so that you know you would get them right on the test.

It is also important that the questions you complete are of high quality. This means that the length and content of the question stems reflect what you would actually see on test day. Many question-bank resources make things too easy (giving you a false sense of confidence) or ask about material that would not show up on the exam (wasting your time).

Once you have selected your question bank resources, count the total number of questions and divide that by the number of days you have available for study. Then make sure you set a study plan where you can make at least two passes through your questions. The first pass is completion of all available questions. The second pass is completion of all the questions you got wrong or made a lucky guess on during your first pass. Seeing how many of the second-pass questions you can get right should serve as a nice confidence booster leading into exam day.

"Review Questions on Excel."

Your Way of Taking Notes on the Questions You Complete Is Vital to Your Success

The most effective strategy is to pick one take-home point for every question you complete and record it on an Excel sheet specific to your clinical rotation.

For instance, if you got a question about the treatment of sickle cell disease wrong, write "Tx of sickle cell" in column A of your Excel sheet and then "hydroxyurea" in column B. This will allow you to create an immediate flash card of a sort. When you review this material the following week, you can put your cursor over column A, say the answer out loud, and check your answer by shifting your cursor to column B. This will save you a lot of time and jump directly to the most important takeaway for each question. You can also make your own flash cards on the Gunner Goggles iOS app.

If you understand everything in the question-and-answer choices, don't record it in the Excel sheet.

If there are many things you don't understand in the question-and-answer choices, record the most important takeaway point and move on. For test day, it is better to be confident in what you know well than to undermine your confidence by fixating on what you are weak at.

By test day, you should have one Excel sheet that contains one important take-home point from every question about which you were unsure. The tabs on the bottom should be organized by question-bank resource. Such a sheet would ideally take only 3 or 4 hours to review, and that is something you could do on the day before the exam.

Last but not least, trust the process. Philadelphia 76ers fans endured years of painful basketball losses while Sam Hinkie rebuilt the team, but they were instructed to "trust the process."

Students often enter test day feeling anxious and overwhelmed, which can cause them to second-guess their answer choices. Trust the process—trust that you will have covered everything in leading up to the Surgery shelf exam and have some faith in your answer selections. After all, you were on this rotation for at least 8 weeks. For these reasons, don't second guess yourself. Your first instinct will usually be right.

In summary, Read, Apply, Review, and Trust the Process.

Index

Note: Pages followed by "*b*", "*t*", and "*f*" refer to boxes, tables, and figures respectively.

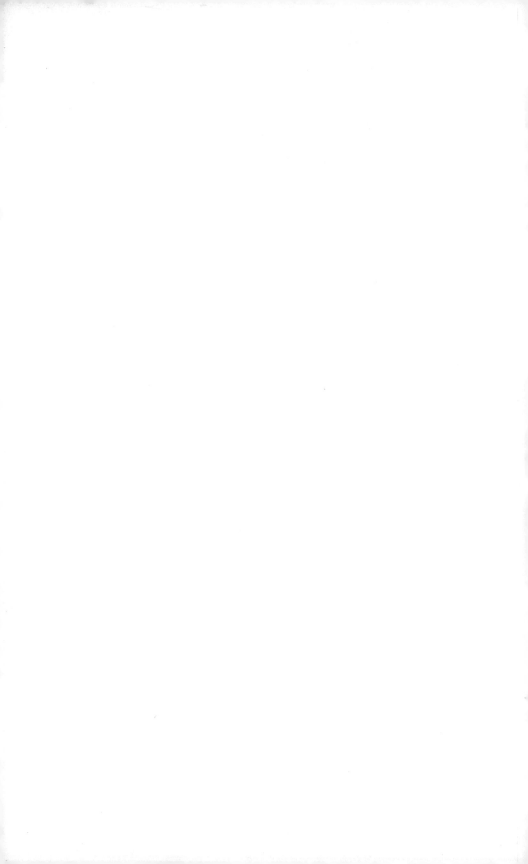